Clinical Guide to Positional Release Therapy

Clinical Guide to Positional Release Therapy

Timothy E. Speicher, PhD, ATC, LAT, CSCS

Positional Release Therapy Institute

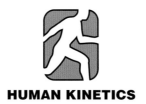

HUMAN KINETICS

Library of Congress Cataloging-in-Publication Data

Names: Speicher, Timothy E., 1969- , author.
Title: Clinical guide to positional release therapy with web resource /
  Timothy E. Speicher.
Description: Champaign, IL : Human Kinetics, [2016] | Includes
  bibliographical references and index.
Identifiers: LCCN 2015025912 | ISBN 9781450496247
Subjects: | MESH: Musculoskeletal Manipulations--methods--Handbooks.
Classification: LCC R733 | NLM WB 39 | DDC 615.53--dc23 LC record available at http://lccn.loc.gov/2015025912

ISBN: 978-1-4504-9624-7 (print)

The web addresses cited in this text were current as of November 2015, unless otherwise noted.

Acquisitions Editor: Joshua J. Stone; **Developmental Editor:** Judy Park; **Senior Managing Editor:** Carly S. O'Connor; **Copyeditor:** Patsy Fortney; **Indexer:** Nancy Ball; **Permissions Manager:** Dalene Reeder; **Senior Graphic Designer:** Nancy Rasmus; **Cover Designer:** Keith Blomberg; **Photograph (cover):** Neil Bernstein; © Human Kinetics; **Photographs (interior):** Neil Bernstein, unless otherwise noted; photos on pages 5, 50-55, 59, 64, 73, 75-77, 85, 87, 97, 99, 101, 102-103, 105, 107, 109-111, 113-116, 127, 129, 133-136, 139-141, 144, 146, 148, 161, 167, 169-172, 175, 177, 183, 185, 187-189, 202-205, 207, 209-211, 215, 217-218, 220-224, 241, 244-245, 247, 249, 251, 253, 255, 257, 266, 268-269, 271-274, 287-293, and 295-301 by Bradley W. Carroll; photos on pages 35 and 37 courtesy of Teara Galbrath; all photos © Human Kinetics; **Photo Asset Manager:** Laura Fitch; **Visual Production Assistant:** Joyce Brumfield; **Photo Production Manager:** Jason Allen; **Senior Art Manager:** Kelly Hendren; **Associate Art Manager:** Alan L. Wilborn; **Illustrations:** © Human Kinetics, unless otherwise noted; **Printer:** Versa Press

The video contents of this product are licensed for private home use and traditional, face-to-face classroom instruction only. For public performance licensing, please contact a sales representative at **www.HumanKinetics.com/SalesRepresentatives**.

Printed in the United States of America

10 9 8 7 6 5 4 3 2 1

The paper in this book is certified under a sustainable forestry program.

Human Kinetics
Website: www.HumanKinetics.com

United States: Human Kinetics
P.O. Box 5076
Champaign, IL 61825-5076
800-747-4457
e-mail: info@hkusa.com

Canada: Human Kinetics
475 Devonshire Road Unit 100
Windsor, ON N8Y 2L5
800-465-7301 (in Canada only)
e-mail: info@hkcanada.com

Europe: Human Kinetics
107 Bradford Road
Stanningley
Leeds LS28 6AT, United Kingdom
+44 (0) 113 255 5665
e-mail: hk@hkeurope.com

Australia: Human Kinetics
57A Price Avenue
Lower Mitcham, South Australia 5062
08 8372 0999
e-mail: info@hkaustralia.com

New Zealand: Human Kinetics
P.O. Box 80
Mitcham Shopping Centre, South Australia
5062
0800 222 062
e-mail: info@hknewzealand.com

E6296

This book is dedicated foremost to my life partner, Stephanie. I would not have had the capacity to write and complete this text without her unyielding support and perseverance; she endures much as I chase my dreams. I would also like to dedicate this book to my two daughters, Morgan and Marley, because they unknowingly provided me the energy and perspective to complete the book. And finally, to my mother; without her, nothing in my life would be possible.

I would also like to dedicate this book to my mentors and friends who believed in me when no one else did, who challenged me, and, most important, who revealed to me when I needed to change.

CONTENTS

TREATMENT FINDER

Anatomical Areas

Common Conditions

This book provides medical practitioners, educators, and students of preprofessional therapy and medical programs with evidence-based information on the clinical application of positional release therapy (PRT). It engenders an appreciation of the current evidence and theory supporting the clinical application of PRT for various patient populations and, more important, provides a simple way to assess and treat myofascial dysfunction with PRT. A gentle and passive technique, PRT has been advocated for the treatment of acute, subacute, and chronic somatic dysfunction in people of all ages (Speicher and Draper 2006).

Positional release therapy, which is also known by its parent term strain counterstrain (SCS), uses a position of comfort to resolve tissue dysfunction (e.g., pain, tightness, and spasm). Dr. Lawrence Jones, an osteopathic physician who first developed PRT in the 1950s, first called it positional release technique and later coined the term strain counterstrain (Jones 1964). Jones hypothesized that tissue dysfunction is the result of a strain–counterstrain mechanism. He proposed that when tissues are forced to adapt quickly to a sudden strain, the antagonist of the strained tissue counterstrains to stabilize the joint, muscle, or other structure insulted; the antagonist then becomes the root of the dysfunction requiring treatment. When he charted his patients' painful conditions, he found discrete tender points (myofascial restrictions) often manifested in specific locations, which he also believed were associated with nerve root innervations. As the technique has developed, multiple practitioners and researchers have advanced Jones' original theory and technique.

This text shares these advancements and the evidence they rest on to provide aspiring and seasoned PRT practitioners a straightforward approach to learning and implementing this therapy to improve the therapeutic outcomes of their patients. I came upon PRT by accident early in my career as a university professor of therapeutic modalities. A previous professor left me a syllabus that listed D'Ambrogio and Roth's PRT text (D'Ambrogio and Roth 1997). The authors claimed that PRT would result in a 75 to 100% pain reduction on the first treatment. I thought the claim must be too good to be true, but my neuroscience background suggested that it seemed plausible, if inflated. I thought that if a patient's pain could be reduced to this degree, I may have found the holy grail of therapy! Therefore, I attempted it on my track and field patients as well as my students. Unfortunately, I did not experience the profound pain reduction claimed. However, because I did have some marginal success, I stuck with it, although I struggled for many years with the method of treatment and charting of tender points outlined by D'Ambrogio and Roth.

I discovered from texts and trainings at conferences and workshops that there was not a systematic and straightforward way to learn and apply the technique or therapy, particularly to an athletic population. I was motivated to find a better way not only to apply PRT to my patients, but also to teach it to my students so that they could experience success on their initial attempts. I wanted them and their patients to have the holy grail experience that took me a decade to obtain. From my clinical practice, research, and teaching of PRT, I propose in this text a new paradigm for understanding, learning, and applying this therapy. Whether you are new to PRT or are a seasoned PRT practitioner, this book will help you build your therapy toolbox to improve your patient outcomes.

How This Book Is Organized

The book is organized by body region much like other PRT texts, but it deviates from Jones' original work in several major ways. In addition, the methods and techniques have been revised and built on. When available, evidence is provided for how PRT works and how it should be applied. This text does not use Jones' original tender point locations or associated segmental spinal level. Instead, tender points and methods for treating them are based on traditional anatomical structures that can be palpated. Many assessment and treatment methods and techniques as well as the documentation of tender points are also novel.

Each body region covered in the book contains an overview of common injury conditions and their myofascial triggers, differential diagnoses for consideration, and descriptions of how to treat specific anatomical structures (e.g., the plantar fascia), as well as treatment algorithms for specific injury conditions such as plantar fasciitis. The terms *near* and *far* are used to direct the clinician to the hand to use for application of the PRT treatments. The near hand is the hand closest to the treatment site or tissue, and the far hand is the farthest away from the treatment site or tissue. Each chapter also contains patient self-treatment techniques, where appropriate, and instructions for palpating specific anatomical structures. The content of the book has been organized and presented to match the structure of the preprofessional training of most health care practitioners. There are no complicated charting methods, hard-to-remember abbreviations, or difficult therapy applications. Scanning and mapping documentation forms are provided in the appendix to assist in the identification of key structures for assessment and documentation as well as to identify myofascial lesion patterns to help in the development of an individualized treatment road map. For each structure, I recommend recording pain during palpation using the numerical pain rating scale pre- and posttreatment, noting the approximate location of the pain.

Special Features of This Book

Several aspects of this PRT text, including palpation instructions, PRT techniques for special populations, and adjunctive treatments, are not found elsewhere.. Palpation is a core skill that enables successful diagnosis and the application of many orthopedic assessments and therapeutic techniques. Without proficient palpation skills and an anatomical and kinesiological knowledge

of the structures being treated, clinicians' success in the assessment and application of PRT will be diminished. Palpation of specific anatomical structures is thoroughly explained and demonstrated through visual media. Both the text and the visual media outline how to apply PRT and, where applicable, how to apply it to special populations such as children, the elderly, pregnant women, and athletes.

A web resource is included which showcases 60 detailed demonstrations of palpation and PRT techniques. The most common conditions and the techniques used to treat them are detailed, along with advice about adapting the techniques to other conditions and muscle groups. ▶ Video icons will direct you to the clip number on the web resource; if you are using an enhanced e-book your video will load directly below the technique's text and photo description. The web resource also includes all scanning and mapping forms, presented by anatomical region in the appendix, in reproducible form. ✋ To download printable PDF files and view videos, please read the pass code instructions found on the Accessing the Web Resource page and then visit **www.HumanKinetics.com/ClinicalGuide ToPositionalReleaseTherapy.**

Although PRT can be used as a stand-alone therapy, adjunctive therapies often help to create an optimal healing environment. Therefore, adjunctive therapies that complement PRT are outlined, such as ultrasound, electric stimulation, massage, taping, joint mobilization, and therapeutic exercise.

I am fortunate and honored to have had the opportunity to apply and advance the practice of PRT, and I hope that those who experience holy grail moments in their clinical practice, teaching, and research continue to move this transformative therapy forward. It is my vision that, as a result of this text, practitioners will no longer have to put the majority of their patients in pain to heal them and that PRT research, professional instruction, and clinical practice will serve as catalysts for the realization of this vision.

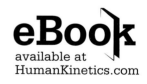

available at
HumanKinetics.com

ACKNOWLEDGMENTS

Clinical Guide to Positional Release Therapy would not have been possible without the work of the scholars, researchers, and clinicians who laid the foundation for its development and inception. However, all I have come into contact with directly or indirectly are a part of this text: the thousands of students I have had the opportunity to learn from, the unknowing author who contributed a key understanding, and the PRT course participants who challenged me and the teaching faculty at the Positional Release Therapy Institute to be better. Thanks to the teaching faculty at the institute who have provided unwavering support and dedication beyond what I ever expected. Also, thanks to my previous teaching assistants Kyle Torgerson and Andi Pigeon for being models and Brad Carroll and Teara Galbraith for their photography assistance.

Additionally, the support, patience, and expertise of the professionals at Human Kinetics were tremendous; without them, this book would not have been possible. They pushed me to open my mind to new ways of presenting material, challenged me to exceed my own limits, and were instrumental in keeping the spurs and reins on me when I needed them most.

Throughout *Clinical Guide to Positional Release Therapy* you will notice a reference to a web resource. This online content is available to you for free with the purchase of a new print book or an e-book. All you need to do is register with the Human Kinetics website to access the online content.

The web resource offers printable scanning and mapping evaluation forms along with video clips demonstrating techniques presented in the chapters. We are certain you will enjoy this unique online learning experience.

Follow these steps to access the web resource:

1. Visit www.HumanKinetics.com/Clinical GuideToPositionalReleaseTherapy.

2. Click the first edition link next to the corresponding first edition book cover.

3. Click the Sign In link on the left or top of the page. If you do not have an account with Human Kinetics, you will be prompted to create one.

4. After you register, if the online product does not appear in the Ancillary Items box on the left of the page, click the Enter Pass Code option in that box. Enter the following pass code exactly as it is printed here, including capitalization and all hyphens: **SPEICHER-7SN8-WR**

5. Click the Submit button to unlock your online product.

6. After you have entered your pass code the first time, you will never have to enter it again to access this online product. Once unlocked, a link to your product will permanently appear in the menu on the left. All you need to do to access your online content on subsequent visits is to sign in to www.HumanKinetics.com/ClinicalGuide ToPositionalReleaseTherapy and follow the link.

Click the Need Help? button on the book's website if you need assistance along the way.

Foundational Applications and Procedures

Part I provides an overview of the history and development of positional release therapy (PRT), foundational clinical applications and procedures, and theoretical and research findings to substantiate its use for treating somatic dysfunction and other ailments. PRT is an offshoot of its parent technique, strain counterstrain (SCS), and although most children look similar to their parents, differences exist and develop over time. Part I elucidates these differences and explains how clinicians can use PRT in a simplified and structured manner to treat a host of injury and disease conditions. Several established and emerging theories are presented along with evidence that explains how PRT may work to alleviate and eliminate somatic dysfunction.

CHAPTER 1

Introduction to Positional Release Therapy

CHAPTER OBJECTIVES

After reading this chapter, you should be able to do the following:

❶ Recall the historical development of positional release therapy (PRT).

❷ Understand how PRT works to treat painful tissues.

❸ Understand the difference between the application of strain counterstrain (SCS) and the application of PRT.

❹ Discuss the common assessment and documentation methods for tender and trigger points.

❺ Demonstrate how to apply PRT to relieve somatic dysfunction.

Positional release therapy, also known by its parent term strain counterstrain, is a therapeutic technique that uses a position of comfort of the body, its appendages, and its tissues to resolve somatic dysfunction. Somatic dysfunction is defined as a disturbance in the sensory or proprioceptive system that results in spinal segmental tissue facilitation and inhibition (Korr 1975). Jones (1973) proposed that as a result of somatic dysfunction, tissues often become kinked or knotted resulting in pain, spasm, and a loss of range of motion. Simply, PRT unkinks tissues much as one would a knotted necklace, by gently twisting and pushing the tissues together to take tension off the knot. When one link in the chain is unkinked, others nearby untangle, producing profound pain relief (Speicher and Draper 2006a).

Essentially, PRT is the opposite of stretching. For example, if a patient has a tight, tender area on the calf, the clinician would traditionally dorsiflex the foot to stretch the calf to reduce the tightness and pain. Unfortunately, this might lead to muscle guarding and increased pain. Using the same example, a clinician who employs PRT would place the tender point in the position of greatest comfort (plantar flexion), shortening the muscle or tissue in order to relax them. A gentle and passive technique, PRT has been advocated for the treatment of acute, subacute, and chronic somatic dysfunction in people of all ages (Speicher and Draper 2006b). Dr. Lawrence Jones, an osteopathic physician, is credited with the discovery of the therapy in the early 1950s; he initially called it positional release technique and later coined the term strain counterstrain (Jones 1964).

Jones described his clinical discovery as "a lucky accident and nothing more" (Jones, Kusunose, and Goering 1995, 2). After Jones failed to help a patient with severe back pain, the patient said that his greatest challenge was sleeping at night and that if he could find a comfortable position, he might get relief. Jones assisted the patient into various positions and discovered that a fetal position provided the greatest pain reduction. He left him in this position while he examined another patient. Upon his return, the patient arose without pain for the first time in four months. Jones didn't understand how placing a patient in a position of comfort for a short period of time could provide complete cessation of unrelenting pain after so many traditional therapies had failed. He then experimented with patient positioning with moderate success. Three years later he accidentally discovered that treatment of anterior pelvic tender points often relieved posterior pelvic pain. Based on this observation, Jones believed that tender points (TPs) were the result of a counterstrain mechanism: If a tissue is abruptly strained, the opposing tissue (antagonist) is counterstrained in its attempt to stabilize against the straining force, resulting in the production of antagonist TPs that prevent the agonist strained tissue from fully healing (Jones 1995).

Tender points, in contrast to myofascial trigger points (MTrPs), are not associated with hyperirritable bands of tissue, but are discrete areas of tissue tenderness that can occur anywhere in the body (Speicher and Draper 2006a). Myofascial trigger points are hyperirritable nodules of knotted muscular tissue that often entrap nerves and local vessels and cause pain, inflammation, and loss of function (Simons and Travell 1981). Myofascial trigger points, whether active or latent, are found in taut bands of muscular tissue. An active MTrP produces either local or referred pain or other sensory perception alterations with or without manual stimulation, whereas a latent trigger point requires manual stimulation to activate a potential pain or sensory response (Dommerholt, Bron, and Franssen 2006). Tender points can also be active or latent, but they are not commonly found within knotted muscle. Jones mapped TP locations based on segmental spinal levels, but TP locations have also been closely associated with the myofascial trigger point locations first described by Travell in 1949. Myofascial trigger points and possibly TPs may also be associated with ahi shi acupuncture points used for the treatment of pain (Hong 2000) as well as lymphatic reflex points (D'Ambrogio and Roth 1997). Melzack, Stillwell, and Fox (1977) asserted that not much difference existed between the locations of MTrPs and acupuncture points based on their finding of a 71% correlation. However, an investigation by Birch in 2003 of the correlation between trigger and acupuncture points reported in Melzack and colleagues' study found a correlation of only 18 to 19%. Birch (2003) and Hong (2000) contended that not all acupuncture points correlate with MTrPs, but they believe that ahi shi acupuncture points used for pain control do. Jones (1964) was the first to correlate the use of specific body positioning to reduce tender and trigger point associated tenderness and spasm (see figure 1.1). In the calf area alone there are different trigger, tender, acupuncture and reflex points related to pain in the soleus muscle, many of which

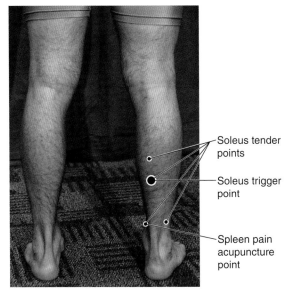

Soleus tender points

Soleus trigger point

Spleen pain acupuncture point

Figure 1.1 A comparison of trigger, tender, and acupuncture points.

overlap one another. Melzack et al. (1977) outlines these in greater detail.

This text not only presents and honors the foundational work of Jones, but also provides a user-friendly guide for the clinical application of PRT. Since Jones' seminal work, research and clinical case reports have continued to emerge to support its use and efficacy for the treatment of a variety of painful ailments linked to somatic dysfunction (Wong 2012), including restless leg syndrome (Peters, MacDonald, and Leach 2012). Positional release practitioners have also advocated for its use as a comprehensive therapy.

Strain Counterstrain

Even though more than 60 years have elapsed since the discovery of PRT by Jones, it is still not well known in the medical community or by the public. This may be because high-quality clinical trials have only recently begun to emerge (Wong 2012), and because the technique as originally presented has been cumbersome for health care students and practitioners to grasp and learn (Woolbright 1991).

On the surface, PRT appears to be simple; however, its ability to produce dramatic and profound clinical outcomes has perplexed clinicians, patients, and researchers for over half a century. When the therapy is examined through a neuroscience lens,

Text Abbreviations and Terms

ACh	Acetylcholine	MTSS	Medial tibial stress syndrome
AChE	Acetylcholinesterase	NPRS	Numerical pain rating scale
AChR	Acetylcholine receptor	OA	Osteoarthritis
ACL	Anterior cruciate ligament	OMT	Osteopathic manipulative therapy
ADP	Adenosine diphosphate	PAG	Periaqueductal gray matter
ATF	Anterior talofibular ligament	Pi	Inorganic phosphate
ATP	Adenosine triphosphate	PNF	Proprioceptive neuromuscular facilitation
CGRP	Calcitonin gene–related peptide		
CSS	Central sensitization syndrome	PRT	Positional release therapy
DPN	Diabetic peripheral neuropathy	SCS	Strain counterstrain
FHP	Forward head posture	SI	Sacroiliac
FRM	Fasciculatory response method	SR	Sarcoplasmic reticulum
GTO	Golgi tendon organ	T2D	Type 2 diabetes
ISTM	Instrumented soft tissue mobilization	TMD	Temporomandibular dysfunction
LBP	Low back pain	TMJ	Temporomandibular joint
LCL	Lateral collateral ligament	TnC	Troponin C
LE	Lower extremity	TPs	Tender points
LTR	Local twitch response	UE	Upper extremity
MCL	Medial collateral ligament	VAS	Visual analog scale
MCT	Mechanical coupling theory	VMO	Vastus medialis oblique
MTrPs	Myofascial trigger points		

an understanding of how it produces such remarkable pain relief becomes more difficult to grasp. Capturing neurological activity and resultant tissue responses has been challenging, but as a result of improved technology, along with ways to capture these outcomes, Jones' propositions are now being actively pursued and tested. Until recently, many dismissed PRT because ways to ascertain the mechanisms of how it worked were limited.

Howell and colleagues (2006) were the first to test changes in the stretch reflex after SCS treatments. They found that those with Achilles tendinitis had significantly reduced stretch reflexes after SCS treatment, lending support to Korr's (1975) theory of somatic dysfunction resulting from an increased gain or hypersensitivity of the stretch reflex. Korr proposed that the heightened stretch reflex was the result of muscle spindle dysfunction. His theory was based on the premise that the muscle spindle's sensitivity to stretch was heightened and sustained by increased gamma gain (intrafusal fiber neural activation), which enhances the sensitivity of the spindle and thereby elevates and maintains the stretch reflex (see figure 1.2).

In a follow-up examination of the effect of SCS on plantar fasciitis patients over a six-day treatment cycle, researchers found a significant reduction in the stretch reflex during the first two days, but not over time compared to controls (Wynne et al. 2006). The authors attributed the lack of congruence with Howell's initial findings to where the stretch reflex was measured. The triceps surae muscles were measured, not the intrinsic foot musculature where the treatment was administered.

Even in light of these results, the initial findings of Howell and colleagues (2006) have provided a framework for both understanding how PRT may work to reduce somatic dysfunction and a sound methodology for its future investigation. However, to date, the paucity of examination of the science behind the therapy as well as its conventional procedures of application has made teaching novice practitioners difficult (Woolbright 1991).

Tissue Assessment and Documentation

The traditional approach of SCS is problematic because its application procedures are frequently foreign to the novice's mental framework of how to locate, treat, and document tissue pain. Novices learn best when they can match a learning experience with something familiar (Speicher and Kehrhahn 2009). Moreover, beginners find it difficult to palpate while positioning a patient and to determine how hard to push while palpating. They also often elicit more pain and reflexive spasm from the patient as a result of overpressure during the assessment and reassessment portions of the treatment procedure advocated by Jones and others.

Even though the initial application procedures outlined by Jones (1973) have yet to be tested, they are still often advocated. Jones proposed that to find the position of comfort to resolve a TP, the practitioner should move the body segment and its tissues through their range of motion while

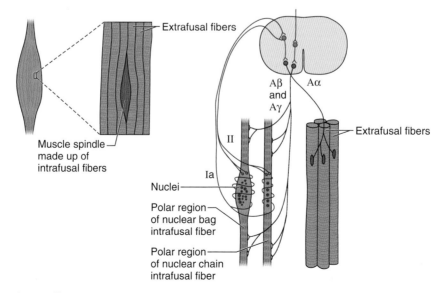

Figure 1.2 Muscle spindle.

palpating the TP with submaximal pressure. Once the position of comfort is found, tenderness to palpation would no longer be present. Brandt and Jones (1976) proposed that beginners should repeatedly probe the tender area while positioning to ascertain from the patient what position results in no tenderness, and that the experienced clinician would be able to experience the immediate relaxation of the TP to optimal positioning upon a slow return to neutral. "A period of only ninety seconds in a position of comfort will have a lasting beneficial effect every time, if we only return from it slowly" (Jones, Kusunose, and Goering 1995, 1). However, when attempting to both learn and teach these procedures, I did not achieve a lasting beneficial effect every time, no matter how slowly the positioning was returned. Even after years of practicing, learning, and teaching the proposed application procedures, mastery of the therapy proved elusive and frustrating.

The documentation schematic for determining tender point location and assessment proposed by Jones, Kusunose, and Goering (1995) and further developed by D'Ambrogio and Roth (1997) has been difficult to use clinically. D'Ambrogio and Roth's (1997) tender point palpation scale (TPPS) uses filled-in circles to indicate the location and intensity of pain that align with Jones' tender point locations (see figure 1.3). For example, if the left anterior scalene is tender, the reference points for treatment and documentation associated with this muscle may be either AC4 (anterior fourth cervical), AC5 (anterior fifth cervical), or AC6 (anterior sixth cervical), which are located on the anterior surface of the tips of the traverse processes of the cervical spine. Finding and remembering these locations is difficult for the novice practitioner and time-consuming in a busy clinical environment. Moreover, the method of documenting TP tenderness proposed by D'Ambrogio and Roth does not align well with traditional therapeutic education and training because the abbreviations are unfamiliar and too numerous and the method requires coloring circles to indicate levels of tenderness. Students would often ask why they couldn't just document that they were treating the anterior scalene and that its tenderness was 8 out of 10, rather than marking an extremely sensitive left AC6. As an instructor and positional release practitioner, finding traditional TP locations, using overpressure during assessment and positioning, and documenting tenderness using existing charting techniques were as much of a challenge for

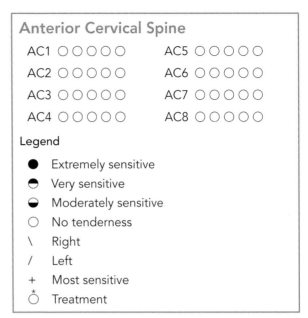

Figure 1.3 TPPS chart sample. This illustrates the legend and anterior cervical spine notations used in the tender point palpation scale. A full chart would cover all body areas and include patient and assessment date details. The open circles correspond to five potential treatment dates.

Adapted from D'Amrogio and Roth 1997.

me as for my students. Additionally, Wong and Schauer-Alvarez (2004) found very low reliability (K = .228–.327) and validity (r = .321–.451) of hip and adductor TPs using the TPPS.

The new method proposed in this text streamlines the assessment and documentation of tender tissues and aligns better with the traditional therapeutic training and experience of students and clinicians. Instead of Jones' tender point locations, I advocate the use of traditional musculoskeletal terminology (e.g., anterior scalene, muscle belly, origin, insertion, lateral epicondyle). Both novice students and seasoned practitioners recall and apply familiar and basic medical terminology more easily. Moreover, I advocate using the numerical pain rating scale (NPRS) for documenting the level of tenderness to palpation rather than D'Ambrogio and Roth's TPPS or the visual analog scale (VAS).

The prevailing methods used for assessing and documenting tender and trigger points in the clinical setting are the visual analog scale, tissue algometry, and the numerical pain rating scale.

Visual Analog Scale

The visual analog scale (VAS) has been advocated for charting tender and trigger point pain to palpation (Wong and Schauer-Alvarez 2004), but Williamson and Hoggart (2005) asserted that the numerical pain rating scale (NPRS) is more clinically relevant than the VAS because clinicians and patients find it easier to use and understand. Researchers (Delaney and McKee 1993; Jensen et al. 1986; Takala 1990) have also advocated the use of tissue algometry to assess the pressure sensitivity of trigger and tender points because of its ability to measure the degree of pressure applied by the clinician and its ability to provide quantitative data on initial and maximal patient sensitivity to pressure.

Tissue Algometry

Although tissue algometry for the purpose of measuring pressure patient sensitivity of trapezius trigger points has been found to show high interrater (ICC = .82–.92) and intrarater (ICC = .80–.91) reliability (Delaney and McKee 1993), Loveless and Speicher (2012) did not find a significant correlation of digital algometry assessment of upper trapezius active myofascial trigger points with either the VAS ($r = .14$) or NPRS ($r = .30$), but they did find a significant correlation between the VAS and NPRS ($r = .91$). Tissue algometry involves the application of a pressure meter with a hard tip to a tender tissue to assess the amount of force needed to illicit a pain response. Although tissue algometry may be a more objective measure for capturing trigger point tenderness in a research setting, clinically, it is difficult to use because the tip of the algometer can slide off the trigger point during assessment and is often painful over bony areas.

Dr. Chris Castel proposed that the application of algometry to trigger points may also produce an antinociceptive, or pain reducing, effect if it produces intense pain and ischemic compression, which could confound a determination of the effectiveness of the therapeutic intervention (personal communication, June 3, 2011). Gemmell, Miller, and Nordstrom (2008) and Aguilera and colleagues (2009) found that ischemic pressure on trapezius trigger points produced significant pain relief, which the authors attributed to a potential antinociceptive effect. Over the last 15 years, I have also observed novices and seasoned clinicians applying ischemic finger pressure to TPs during the assessment and treatment portions of PRT even after repeated instruction not to do so. This, coupled with the potential production of an antinociceptive effect, is why I do not advocate the use of tissue algometry for assessing tender and trigger points or the use of palpation during treatment positioning.

Numerical Pain Rating Scale

The NPRS is recommended in place of coloring in circles, as utilized in the TPPS, or marking a numberless line, as used in the VAS to indicate level of tenderness. The NPRS rates subjective pain on a scale of 0 to 10 (0 represents no pain and 10 represents the worst pain imaginable). Although the NPRS helped to capture point tenderness of tender and trigger points, it did not address how to avoid applying too much palpation pressure during the positioning of the patient. However, much like the accidental clinical discoveries Jones experienced, the revelation of how to accomplish this objective came from an accidental clinical discovery of my own while treating a patient.

While treating a patient with anterior scalene pain, I noted a local twitch response, or fasciculation, at the point of maximal tissue relaxation. However, it disappeared when I attempted to use Jones' palpation technique for determining optimal treatment positioning. What I discovered was that as the anterior scalene became relaxed, there was a resultant tissue fasciculation, or small oscillating tissue twitch or spasm. When I moved away from the position of comfort, the fasciculation would subside, but upon return, the fasciculation would strengthen in both amplitude and frequency. Not only did the fasciculation direct me to the most optimal treatment positioning, but it also told me how long to hold the position, which varied greatly from the 90-second rule established by Jones. If I released the position of comfort prior to the cessation of the fasciculation, even though 90 seconds had elapsed, TP relief was often muted. However, when I maintained the treatment position until the fasciculation subsided significantly or expired altogether, the patient most often reported full cessation of tenderness to palpation. As a result of these observations, I began to use the fasciculatory response of the tissue along with light pressure (~1 kg, or 2.2 lb) over either MTrPs or TPs at their most painful point while moving through a full range of motion to determine the most optimal treatment position and treatment time. As early as 1949, Hoover asserted that tissue restrictions would release when the tissue was placed in its most relaxed position within its range of motion, which he called functional technic, but it did not involve the use of the tissue's fasciculatory response.

Fasciculatory Response Method

After several years of investigation and using the fasciculatory, or twitch, response to treat tender tissues, I decided that it was the best method for guiding both PRT treatment positioning and duration. I called it the fasciculatory response method (FRM), which I proposed for the first time in 2006 (Speicher and Draper 2006). During the palpation portion of the assessment, the practitioner may feel a fasciculatory response with light palpation, but if not, the tender tissue will elicit a rise in amplitude and intensity of the fasciculation when the optimal treatment position is attained. Once this response is determined, the position is held until the fasciculation abates. After this time, the tissue is returned to a neutral resting state and reassessed.

Fasciculations have been shown to

- be occluded with too much finger pressure;
- often appear after a short time (30 to 60 seconds) while holding the tissue in the most relaxed position, when it was initially absent;
- be elicited or elevated with deep breathing regardless of its location;
- be enhanced when compression, distraction, or translation is applied to a joint or the tissue's respective fascia, along with the tissue's optimal treatment position;
- reappear upon return of the tissue or body segment to a neutral position, which requires additional treatment where it occurs in the range of motion;
- often result from another myofascial trigger (e.g., neurological impingement) or the influence of other TPs or MTrPs in another area—if the tissue does not stop fasciculating after five minutes; and
- have an increased cessation and release time that correlates to the amount of time the patient has had a painful condition.

The discovery and use of the FRM solved several challenges with teaching and applying PRT clinically. The FRM assists the practitioner in determining the optimal treatment position without having to induce patient discomfort, which may either cause more tissue restriction or facilitate an antinociceptive effect, clouding the treatment outcome. Not causing the patient discomfort may

also build patient trust in the therapy. The FRM also provides a definitive time for the application of positioning, which not only often reduces the time needed to hold a position, but more important, informs the clinician about when the tender point or myofascial trigger point release has been achieved, enhancing the therapeutic response to the therapy. However, fasciculations are present not only in TPs, but also in trigger points.

Local twitch responses (LTR), or fasciculations, have been found to be present in myofascial trigger points (Dommerholt, Bron, and Franssen 2006). When a trigger point is manually strummed or dry needled, a visible twitch contraction is often produced, which can be measured with electromyographic (EMG) monitoring. Gerwin and Dommerholt (2002), however, contended that an LTR in a MTrP can be identified with palpation alone and does not need a confirmation response from the patient. Clinical outcomes for the treatment of MTrPs with dry needling have been shown to improve when the LTR was produced with treatment and when the location of the treatment was on the trigger point (Hong 1994). Hong, Torigoe, and Yu (1995) found that needling trigger point locations in rabbits just half a centimeter (just under a quarter of an inch) from the MTrP resulted in less of a reduction of the LTR, versus when it was treated directly over the trigger point. Therefore, the criticality of the treatment location of an MTrP may explain Chaitow's (2002) assertion that light digital pressure is required during PRT treatment for a positive therapeutic effect to occur. If a TP is a variant of a MTrP, then it is also plausible that when submaximal pressure is applied over them, it will also elicit an LTR or a fasciculation to assist the release of the myofascial restriction as well as to inform the practitioner about when the release has occurred. The identification of LTRs in myofascial trigger points and their response to therapeutic needling sets the stage for further investigation of the fasciculatory response method advocated for use in PRT.

Strain Counterstrain Versus Positional Release Therapy

I am often asked how SCS and PRT differ (table 1.1). D'Ambrogio and Roth (1997) were the first to coin the term positional release therapy and also to advocate for its use as a total body therapy for the treatment of musculoskeletal dysfunction. They proposed that the entire body should be scanned or palpated for tender and trigger points to establish a map to guide treatment. I have adopted this global approach as well and the term PRT over SCS because SCS tends to suggest that TP restrictions are a result of this mechanism, which is not always the case. Also, when applied correctly, the technique originally laid out by Jones and further developed by other researchers and practitioners such as D'Ambrogio and Roth, Deig (2001), Chaitow (2002), Myers and colleagues (2006), and Speicher and Draper (2006a, 2006b) can be used as a stand-alone therapy and also integrated with other therapies. Although the development of trigger and TPs can be the result of an SCS mechanism, a multitude of triggers such as stress, pathological biomechanical abnormalities, disease states, and cumulative trauma may also produce trigger and TPs (Simons and Travell 1981).

Positional Release Therapy Guidelines

Taking into account that multiple triggers can cause somatic dysfunction, clinicians must conduct a thorough physical and biomechanical evaluation of the patient prior to treatment to determine the root of the pain. Given the differences in the evaluation and treatment of somatic dysfunction between SCS and PRT, I recommend the following PRT guidelines:

- The patient should feel no pain or discomfort during treatment.
- Use the FRM to guide treatment positioning and duration.

- Treat the most tender trigger or tender point first.
- If there is a concentration of equally tender points, apply treatment at the center point of the concentration.
- If there is a row of TPs, treat the one in the row that is most tender. If all are equally tender, apply treatment to the center of the row, which often releases the entire row.
- Anterior tissues are typically treated with flexion; posterior, with extension; and lateral, with side bending or rotation. However, treatment in all positions should include tissue manipulation in multiple planes; when possible, joint and or tissue distraction, compression, and translation should be used to enhance the magnitude of the release.
- If significant pain relief is not achieved (approximately 75 to 100%) after treatment, then repeat the procedure, return the tissue more slowly, and consider another cause of the pain (e.g., nerve impingement) or another area for treatment (e.g., opposing TPs).
- Inform patients that they may experience deep soreness up to 48 hours after the application of PRT, that they should not engage in vigorous physical activity for at least 24 hours to prevent reengaging the tissue restriction, and that the greatest pain relief may occur 48 hours after treatment.

▶ See video 1.1 for myofascial mapping procedures.

▶ See video 1.2 for general palpation procedures.

Table 1.1   Differences Between SCS and PRT

Domain	Strain counterstrain (SCS)	Positional release therapy (PRT)
Evaluation approach	Segmental	Whole body
Assessment of TPs and MTrPs	With palpation during positioning	With the FRM and feel of tissue relaxation during positioning
Treatment duration	Hold position for 90 seconds	Hold position until fasciculation subsides
Application of finger pressure	May or may not involve application of submaximal finger pressure	Submaximal finger pressure is applied
Application of joint manipulation	May or may not involve application of joint manipulation	Joint manipulation is attempted
Application of fascial manipulation	May or may not involve application of fascial manipulation	Fascial manipulation is attempted

General PRT Evaluation and Assessment Procedures

1. Conduct a thorough history and physical examination.
2. If the history and physical examination warrant, conduct a biomechanical evaluation to examine for pathological tissue-loading patterns.
3. Map the entire body through palpation to determine the presence of associated TP and MTrPs, if time permits. If time does not permit a full mapping, then identify additional tissue restrictions during subsequent sessions.
4. Record tenderness to palpation pre- and posttreatment using the NPRS.
5. Apply an amount of palpatory force that will determine tissue fasciculation, texture, and level of tonicity. Typically, light palpation of approximately one kilogram (2.2 lb, or enough to cause a slight dimpling of the skin) is all that is needed for superficial tissues.
6. Palpate the entire length or area of the tissue as well as its origin and insertion to determine the dominant tender or trigger point location or where they are most numerous.
7. Once the dominant TP or MTrP is located, lighten palpation to submaximal pressure to prevent occluding the fasciculatory response.
8. Once the treatment has been completed, reassess the dominant and surrounding TPs.

General Procedures for Assessing Tissue Relaxation and Fasciculation

1. Maintain submaximal finger pressure (slight dimpling of the skin) over the tender or trigger point throughout the treatment to assess tissue relaxation and fasciculation. Heavy pressure will occlude the fasciculation.
2. For tendinous structures such as the Achilles tendon and sternocleidomastoid, palpatory assessment should include the application of pincing. Pincing involves the application of light pressure of the tendon with the forefinger and thumb at the tendon's posterior borders while simultaneously rolling the pincing fingers upward against the tendon. Pincing a tendon or tissue does not involve pinching the tissue statically, but applying light pressure while allowing the tendon to roll under the pincing or pincer fingers.
3. Use the fasciculatory response method (FRM) coupled with the feel of tissue relaxation to determine the optimal treatment position and duration of treatment.
4. Engage the patient in deep breathing maneuvers when the fasciculation lessens to accentuate the relaxation response (Busch et al. 2012). The fasciculation commonly rises and falls during deep breathing.
5. If a fasciculation is not elicited during positioning, find the tissue's most relaxed position, engage the patient in deep breathing, and wait until it appears, which can take up to 60 seconds. In the rare case in which a fasciculation does not appear, hold the treatment position for at least three minutes. Because the ability to feel the fasciculatory response is learned, to gain early proficiency, start with an assessment of upper trapezius trigger points, which typically fasciculate strongly.
6. If possible, apply compression, distraction, and translation to the corresponding joint or tissue (or both) to facilitate additional tissue relaxation.
7. Hold the treatment position until the fasciculatory response has subsided considerably or has expired.
8. While maintaining the position of the palpation fingers over the treatment area, slowly return the tissue to a neutral position for reassessment.
9. If a fasciculation reappears during repositioning, treat the tissue again in the range in which the fasciculation manifests.

Most somatic conditions resolve after six to eight consecutive PRT sessions, but treatment time, duration, and methods to extend the pain relief often vary. When acute conditions are treated quickly after onset, often only one or two treatments are needed. The therapy is typically applied a minimum of once per week to assess the patient's response and to allow for adequate time for other therapeutic interventions. I have found over the last decade of clinical practice that patients respond best when the therapy is applied once or twice per week, but not prior to vigorous physical activity or an intensive rehabilitation session, particularly early in the treatment process. Moreover, I have observed that PRT applied after therapeutic exercise helps prevent the reengagement of tissue restriction. When it is used prior to joint manipulation or traction, better clinical outcomes are produced because the joint is no longer restricted by tissue or neural mechanisms.

Ultimately, the duration of the therapy session and when PRT is used in the treatment cycle depends on the clinician's goals. A comprehensive PRT session typically lasts one to two hours, but in acute situations, a single release may take only 5 to 10 seconds. Once a release has been achieved, there are several methods to extend it until the patient is seen again. Patients can perform self-treatments as many times as they feel is beneficial. Using ice, heat, or other complementary pain-relieving modalities after treatment is permissible and advocated to facilitate the healing process; however, they may confound the assessment of whether the PRT is producing the therapeutic effect. Therefore, patients with long-standing conditions, surgical interventions, or comorbidities may need additional complementary therapeutic interventions. If there is no change in the patient's pain or condition after three treatment sessions, the clinician should consider reevaluation, direct manipulative therapy options, or referral to determine another trigger or cause.

The osteopathic treatment philosophy states that the body has the ability to self-correct and heal itself if the right conditions exist, and the application of direct and indirect manipulative

Global PRT Indications and Contraindications

Indications

- Acute, subacute, and chronic pain
- Neuropathic pain
- Somatic referred pain
- Muscle spasm
- Tissue hypertonicity
- Range of motion deficit
- Joint hypomobility
- Fibromyalgia
- Central sensitization syndrome
- Peripheral sensitization
- Postconcussive syndrome
- Headache
- Myofascial pain syndrome
- Cumulative trauma
- Lymphatic compromise
- Hypoperfusion
- Muscular weakness
- Visceral dysfunction

Contraindications

Absolute:

- Open wounds
- Acute nerve root compression
- Infection
- Deep vein thrombosis
- Pain or neurologic symptomology during treatment
- Healing fracture
- Aneurysm
- Acute rheumatory conditions
- Hematoma
- Acute concussion

Relative:

- Herniated disc
- Vertebral stenosis
- Sutures
- History of motor neuron disease

Precaution:

Monitor the patient during marked cervical extension for vertebral artery compression signs.

therapy techniques may assist in this process (Still 1902). PRT is considered an indirect therapy because it does not attempt to reduce tissue restriction by means of applying force through the tissue barrier such as a thrust joint manipulation. However, in a study of 955 osteopathic physicians, 96% preferred direct techniques over indirect techniques (Johnson and Kurtz 2003). The authors did not explore the reasons for the preference, but attributed it to possibly time and reimbursement restraints and the organizational acceptance of direct manipulative therapy. They did contend, though, that effective osteopathic manipulative therapy often requires the practitioner to integrate multiple direct and indirect therapies for complex patient cases.

Summary

Positional release therapy is an exceptional therapeutic intervention for patients experiencing pain, spasm, and loss of range of motion as a result of somatic dysfunction. However, as powerful as PRT is for relieving somatic dysfunction, it may not be a stand-alone therapy for everyone. It is, however, an extremely effective tool for unlocking the healing process through its ability to decrease pain and restore normal tissue length. Through the use of the fasciculatory response method and the simplistic charting and treatment methods and procedures outlined in this text, PRT should produce powerful and lasting releases for patients. However, tissues may need to not only be released, but also restored or rehabilitated and their normalized state retained over time, which I have referred to as the three Rs of manual therapy. This book focuses on the first of the three, release, which I believe is the key to unlocking the healing process so that restoration and tissue maintenance can occur. Dr. Jones provided the first key; we need only learn how to turn it properly to open the door of healing for patients.

CHAPTER 2

Positional Release Therapy Research and Theory

CHAPTER OBJECTIVES

After reading this chapter, you should be able to do the following:

❶ Understand how sensory stimuli travel in the somatic nervous system and their influence on the development and maintenance of somatic dysfunction.

❷ Describe basic muscle spindle and Golgi tendon organ functions and understand how their manipulation may release tissue lesions.

❸ Articulate how the gamma motor neuron system affects spindle sensitivity and pain.

❹ Discuss the prevailing and emerging theories of somatic dysfunction.

❺ Understand the neurophysiological basis for how positional release therapy (PRT) assists in the resolution of somatic dysfunction and how it can be applied to clinical practice.

An understanding of how PRT promotes tissue healing through the manipulation of the somatic nervous system has only recently begun to emerge. The somatic nervous system provides the ability to experience and respond to pleasurable and painful stimuli. Stimuli perceived and transmitted by the somatic system are touch, temperature, pain, and body position or proprioception (Bear, Connors, and Paradiso 2007). This chapter explores how these four senses affect the somatic system based on foundational neurophysiological processes and prevailing and emerging theories of somatic dysfunction. This examination explains why somatic dysfunction may result in the development and persistence of osteopathic lesions. The clinical implications of the theory and research presented are also discussed.

Neurophysiological Foundations

A general overview of how stimuli travel in the nervous system is in order prior to discussing how they produce and sustain somatic dysfunction. Neurons located outside the spinal column are called first order neurons, those in the spinal cord are second order, and those in the cortex are third order (see figure 2.1). Sensory information from the periphery (first order) is transmitted toward the spinal cord (second order) segment's dorsal, or posterior, horn. Pleasurable and painful sensory information flows into the dorsal horn and loops into the ventral, or anterior, horn of the spinal segment via interneuron connectors. A sensory stimulus of sufficient magnitude will both activate and inhibit alpha motor neurons located in the ventral, or anterior, aspect of the segment. Additionally, alpha motor neuron activation can elicit a motor response from both the somatic and visceral tissue associated with its segmental innervation.

It is well known that when tissues are activated, inhibition also occurs (Byrne 1997). Therapy practitioners often use this principle during proprioceptive neuromuscular facilitation (PNF) stretching by manipulating the proprioceptors through a series of contractions interspersed with static stretching in diagonal patterns to gain greater tissue relaxation (Herbert and Gabriel 2002). Therefore, if tissues in a particular spinal segment are hyperactive, other tissues that the segment innervates may also be inhibited. The sensory to motor neuron pathway that directly controls the facilitation and inhibition of tissues forms a reflex arc known as the stretch, or myotatic, reflex (see figure 2.2). We have all had this reflex activated by having our deep tendon reflexes tested during a physical (e.g., the patellar tendon reflex). Simply, tissues subjected to an abrupt stretch produce an involuntary muscle contraction; however, pain can also activate this reflex. Although the myotatic reflex is localized to the first and second neuron levels, sensory information, whether from a painful or nonpainful origin, travels along two other primary neuronal pathways onward to the cortex.

Touch travels via the dorsal column–medial lemniscal pathway, whereas pain and temperature primarily travel along the lateral spinothalamic tract (see figure 2.1). Special consideration is paid to how pain travels through the spinal segment because when a painful stimulus is sent to the spinal cord, it may not only activate an efferent

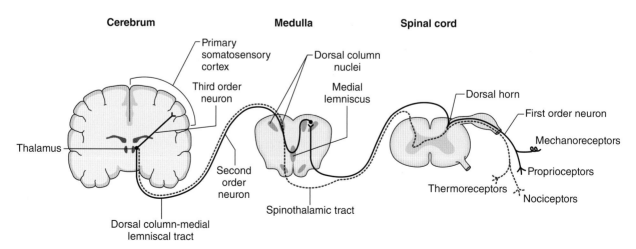

Figure 2.1 Somatic system neuron level organization.

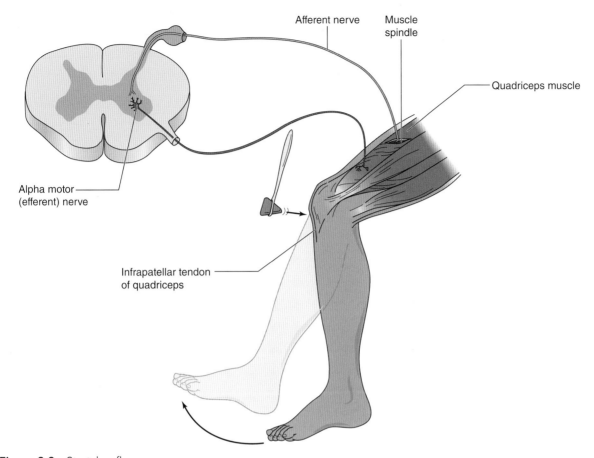

Figure 2.2 Stretch reflex.

motor response on the same side of the body where the stimulus occurred, but also produce a motor and inhibition response on the opposite side of the body (Kandel, Schwartz, and Jessell 2000). For example, during the withdrawal reflex (touching a hot stove), the activation and inhibition of anterior and posterior muscles on both sides of the body allow the person to both pull away and step back from the harmful stimulus. The reflexive cocontraction on the opposite side of the body is facilitated by the cross-spinal reflex at the spinal segment (Kandel et al. 2000). This may help to explain why tender and trigger points develop in both agonist and antagonist tissues as a result of an unanticipated abrupt movement, or what Jones (1973) termed a strain counterstrain (SCS) mechanism.

The segmental crossing of the pain pathway may also activate contralateral alpha motor neurons, which explains why people often develop lesions (trigger and tender points) on the side of the body opposite the involved side, in mirrorlike fashion. Moreover, ascending and descending intersegmental neurons transmit nociceptive information above and below a facilitated segment (Bailey and Dick 1992), which may also explain why one facilitated segment may spark the facilitation and inhibition of tissues at multiple spinal levels.

When pain ascends from the facilitated segment to higher-order neurons, such as the reticular formation in the brain stem and the somatosensory cortex, those at the brain stem play a major role in processing the pain response versus the perception of the pain at the somatosensory cortex. The medullary neurons of the periaqueductal gray matter (PAG) and raphe nuclei in the brain stem project to the dorsal horns to suppress activity of the nociceptor fibers (A delta and C fibers) at the dorsal horn where they terminate (Hocking 2013). These higher-order neurons have also been proposed to regulate gamma motor neuron activity (Capra, Hisley, and Masri 2007), which regulates the sensitivity of the muscle spindle to stretch and velocity change (Kandel et al. 2000).

Gamma motor neurons are located in the ventral, or anterior, horn of the spinal segment along with alpha motor neurons. Unlike alpha motor neurons, however, gamma motor neurons do not contract the extrafusal (striated muscle) fibers to produce joint movement. Gamma motor neurons contract the intrafusal fibers of the muscle spindle to regulate its sensitivity to stretch; however, activation of each type of fiber regulates the spindle differently (see figure 2.3).

Muscle Spindle

The muscle spindle is analogous to both how a bungee cord is constructed and how it responds to stretch. If a bungee cord is stretched, its sheath is elongated, but so are the internal strands, which produces the recoil. Each internal strand of the muscle spindle serves a specific function. The bag fibers respond primarily to the velocity of stretch and chain fibers, resting length, and joint position sense (Bear et al. 2007). The intrafusal and extrafusal fibers run parallel to one another. Because the intrafusal fibers are an internal component of an extrafusal fiber, changes in the length of the extrafusal fibers produce a response from the muscle spindle, and vice versa.

The ability of the muscle spindle to produce a recoil, or to spring back from a stretch, is based on its afferent sensory fiber orientation. The wire coil seen on the end of a bungee cord is similar to the way the primary (Ia) afferent nerve fiber is arranged around the intrafusal fibers of the muscle spindle (see figure 1.2). The annulospiral endings of the Ia afferent fiber wraps around all of the intrafusal fibers (dynamic, static, and chain) and

transmits spindle changes the fastest to the second order. Type II afferent fibers, on the other hand, are slower to respond because they are connected not to the dynamic nuclear bag fibers, but to the static nuclear bag and chain fibers of the spindle. The type II afferent fiber and its respective intrafusal spindle fibers predominantly transmit information to the second order about body position and resting tissue length. It has been proposed that hyperactivity of the spindle afferents causes a sustained stretch reflex to occur, driven by increased gamma gain at the higher-order neurons (Korr 1975). Howell and colleagues (2006) observed a significant reduction in the human triceps surae stretch reflex when SCS was applied to the triceps surae musculature and surrounding tissue.

Golgi Tendon Organ

Another proprioceptor that works in concert with the muscle spindle to control muscle contraction is the Golgi tendon organ (GTO). The GTO is located at the musculotendinous junction, but unlike the spindle, it is responsive only to changes in tension within the musculotendinous tissues (see figure 2.3). The GTO acts much like a brake on the spindle's fusimotor drive by communicating the level of tension of the overall complex to the second order on type Ib afferent fibers. The Ib afferent neural activity produced by GTO tension inhibits alpha motor neurons, thereby preventing the stretch reflex from damaging tissues when activated

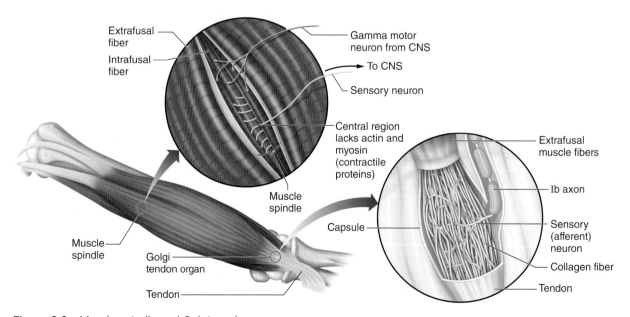

Figure 2.3 Muscle spindle and Golgi tendon organ.

(Moore 2007). The greater the amount of tension applied to the complex is, the more alpha motor neuron inhibition is produced (Moore 2007). The spindle and GTO provide highly efficient proprioceptive feedback and regulation to changes in tissue elongation and tension, but not without the gamma motor neuron system's influence.

Gamma Motor Neuron System

The gamma motor neuron system's activity is influenced by visual, sensory, and motor activity (Bear et al. 2007). It is responsible primarily for regulating the sensitivity of the muscle spindle to changes in dynamic stretch as well as static length, but does not directly regulate the GTO. Gamma motor activity is heightened when a person anticipates a taxing motor activity, such as lifting a heavy object or jumping, priming the muscle spindles for the demand (Kandel et al. 2000). Pain also modulates the activity of gamma motor neurons.

Inducing pain in the spinally innervated muscles of animals has been shown to both increase and decrease gamma activity of the spindles' intrafusal fibers at rest (Appelberg et al. 1983; Thunberg et al. 2002). These observations led Johansson and Sojka (1991) to propose a pathophysiological nociceptive model. Their hypothesis is that increased fusimotor activity is the result of an accumulation of inflammatory metabolites from voluntary static muscular contraction, which stimulates A delta and C fibers, thereby elevating the neural discharge of the spindle afferents, which alters the spindles' sensitivity to stretch during activity, but not at rest. However, validation of the influence of inflammatory metabolites on the stimulation of pain afferents and gamma motor neurons is lacking. Capra and colleagues (2007) did find that the algesic nociceptive chemical stimulation of jaw afferents in the rat both increased and decreased gamma motor neuron activity, but only at rest and not with jaw opening and closing. In the intervention group, a rise in the activity of static gamma–fusimotor activity was observed, but no effect was seen in dynamic gamma motor neuron activity levels during voluntary muscle activity. These findings both confound and lend support to Johansson and Sojka's (1991) nociceptive model of fusimotor metabolite stimulation.

Chemosensitive nociceptive afferents (pain fibers) have been shown to either inhibit or facilitate the static gamma–fusimotor activity of spinally innervated muscles at rest (Appelberg et al. 1983; Thunberg et al. 2002), but not during voluntary jaw muscular contraction (Capra et al. 2007). The presence of inflammatory metabolites produced from a painful mechanism may continue to affect spindle function and sensitivity via static gamma–fusimotor activity modulation at rest long after the initial insult has been removed.

However, in the absence of pain, dynamic and static gamma activity increase with muscle contraction (Byrne 1997). Consider what occurs when a bungee cord is slack. Because the cord fibers are no longer stretched, there is no need for recoil. When no stretch stimulus is placed on the muscle spindle, the neural rate coding, or activity of the spindle afferent fibers, becomes silent, but gamma motor neuron activity increases to contract the spindle (reset its resting length) to prime it for another stretch stimulus (Bear et al. 2007; Byrne 1997). The interplay between spindle silencing and gamma activation is known as alpha-gamma coactivation, which maintains muscle tone (Kandel et al. 2000), or spindle readiness.

The way the spindle and gamma system responds to slack may in part explain how PRT eliminates somatic dysfunction. When tissues are shortened, or placed in a position of comfort, the spindle's afferent discharge becomes silent, interrupting the myotatic reflex and the stimulation of the alpha motor neurons to contract the extrafusal fibers. When spindles are silenced, gamma activity at the spindle increases to restore the resting length of the spindle (Matthews 1981) and possibly the sensitivity level of the spindle. It has been proposed that when gamma drive or volume is high, an increased sensitivity of the spindle to stretch results, which in turn hypersensitizes the monosynaptic stretch reflex (Korr 1975). Decreased sensitivity of the spindle's stretch reflex has been observed with SCS in patients with plantar fasciitis (Howell et al. 2006), but the influence of this indirect therapy on the gamma system has not yet been evaluated in humans. Korr's proprioceptive theory (1975) states that when gamma volume is high, proprioceptor (muscle spindle) dysfunction results during rest and an osteopathic lesion (tender or trigger point) may result. Korr's theory is now bolstered by observations of altered static gamma–fusimotor activity to pain in the rat at rest (Capra et al. 2007) and a reduction of reflex arc activity when plantar foot spindles are shortened with an indirect positional release technique (Howell et al. 2006).

Somatic Dysfunction and the Osteopathic Lesion

Historically, the basis of somatic dysfunction was founded on the concept of the osteopathic lesion. Korr (1947) proposed that a lack of somatic system homeostasis manifests from joint derangement, also termed an osteopathic lesion. Korr described the osteopathic lesion as having five distinct attributes (1947, 191):

1. Hyperesthesia of the muscles and vertebrae
2. Hyperirritability, reflected in altered muscular activity and altered states of muscular contraction
3. Changes in the tissue texture of muscle, connective tissue [fascia], and skin
4. Changes in local circulation and in the exchange between blood and tissues
5. Altered visceral and other autonomic functions

The lesion has been proposed to be associated with a hyperirritable spinal segment (Hocking 2013; Korr 1947) and shown to possess a low stimulus threshold (Hubbard and Berkoff 1993). Even when the body is at rest, the lesion's associated motor neurons are easily activated to produce muscle contraction (Hong and Yu 1998; Hubbard and Berkoff 1993; Kostopoulos et al. 2008). Korr proposed that the main culprit in sensitizing the anterior horn cells, which regulate the efferent motor stimulation of extrafusal muscle tissue, was the postural, mechanical, and articular derangements resulting in alterations in the length–tension relationship between muscle and connective tissue—and that the change in length directly affects the proprioceptors (e.g., muscle spindle, mechanoreceptors, and nociceptors). Korr proposed not only that the spinal segment receiving afferent (sensory) impulses from the proprioceptors becomes hyperstimulated when an osteopathic lesion is present, but also that the segments above and below and all tissues receiving efferent innervation from the hyperstimulated segments also become facilitated. There has been considerable speculation and debate to date as to why and how lesions develop, as well as why they often persist, producing a multitude of theories and promising research to answer these questions.

Integrated Hypothesis Theory

Positional release therapy's ability to reduce somatic dysfunction has been thought to result primarily from the reduction of aberrant neural activity and the mediation of inflammation and circulation through manipulation of the somatic nervous system. Some of the earliest theories of somatic dysfunction, such as Korr's proprioceptive theory (1975), focused on the muscle spindle as a primary culprit. Later theories moved toward a more integrated perspective, starting with the integrated hypothesis (Simons, Travell, and Simons 1999), which proposes that proprioceptors, the central nervous system (CNS), and biomechanical factors work together to produce and maintain somatic dysfunction, particularly the formation of trigger points. The crux of the integrated hypothesis theory is that electrical activity at the motor end plate (the neuromuscular junction where the alpha motor neuron interfaces with the muscle) becomes dysfunctional as a result of excessive acetylcholine (ACh) release into the synaptic cleft at the junction.

Hocking (2013) contended that trigger point activation and maintenance is modulated at the alpha motor neurons within the dorsal horn, not at the motor end plate. Hocking's central modulation hypothesis affirms that excessive ACh neuromuscular junction release causes increased motor end plate noise, or neural activity, but that the increased ACh release at the neuromuscular junction is elicited as a result of prolonged central sensitization at the alpha motor neurons, not at the motor end plate. Over time this causes a decrease in alpha motor neuron plateau depolarization levels, propagating the spontaneous release of ACh at the motor terminal. Hocking asserted that the decreased alpha motor neuron plateau depolarization "is the cause, not the result of the local energy crisis that perpetuates the TrP [trigger point]" (2013, 4).

Impaired regulation of ACh release and uptake coupled with a hypoxic, or low, O_2 tissue environment has been proposed to cause a depletion of adenosine triphosphate (ATP), causing an ATP energy crisis (McPartland 2004; Simons, Travell, and Simons 1999). ACh release activates nicotinic ACh receptors (nAChRs) on the postsynaptic membrane, sparking an action potential to cause extrafusal fiber muscle contraction (Matthews 1981). McPartland (2004) explained that excessive release of ACh either as a result of injury, genetic predisposition, or another insulting mechanism may produce sustained muscle contraction that compresses local sensory nerves within the muscular tissue. The increased release of ACh and resultant sustained muscular contraction compresses local vessels much like pinching off the flow of water from a garden hose, resulting in reduced tissue oxygenation and ATP levels.

ATP serves a critical role in regulating muscle contraction. ATP is the fuel for the calcium pump, enabling the reuptake of calcium back into the sarcoplasmic reticulum, and powers muscle contraction by assisting the actin and myosin filaments to couple (attach) and uncouple (detach) from one another (Bear et al. 2007). Additionally, ATP inhibits the release of ACh (Dommerholt, Bron, and Franssen 2006). The increased demand for muscular contraction in the absence of a lack of fuel (ATP and O_2) to power muscle contraction produces an energy demand that cannot be met, causing a release of proinflammatory metabolites (e.g., prostaglandin, leukotrienes, substance P) locally in the tissues to further sensitize nociceptors (McPartland 2004). The release of proinflammatory metabolites may also cause vascular endothelial dysfunction resulting in hypoperfusion of tissues (Larsson et al. 1999; Maekawa, Clark, and Kuboki 2002), producing mitochondrial damage, oxidative cellular distress, and tissue edema (Rosas-Ballina et al. 2011), which has been attributed to the formation of trigger points (McPartland and Simons 2006).

Simons and colleagues (1999) hypothesized that once a trigger point forms, it generates nociceptive input to the CNS, producing central sensitization of the spinal segment. Central sensitization results from a constant barrage of nociception at the dorsal horn of the spinal cord, producing ectopic nociceptive impulses (McPartland 2004) from the second-order neurons. The abnormal pain impulses generated at the spinal cord can occur even when the insulting force has been removed and tissues are no longer acutely injured. Phantom limb pain, in which an amputee experiences pain in a limb that is no longer there, is a classic example of this phenomenon. Gerwin, Dommerholt, and Shah (2004) expanded on the integrated hypothesis of trigger point formation through a presentation of recent data of the well-known factors that cause the formation of trigger points, but provided additional propositions as to why trigger points persist.

Expanded Integrated Hypothesis

The expanded model (figure 2.4) presented by Gerwin and colleagues (2004) adds substantial evidence to support the basic tenets of Simons and colleagues' (1999) integrated hypothesis, and builds on the model put forth by Shaw (2003). Their further discussion on the role of unaccustomed muscle contraction, tissue acidity, calcitonin gene–related peptide (CGRP), and hypoperfusion may help to clarify why somatic dysfunction sometimes persists beyond the acute stage of healing. (For a full review, see Gerwin et al. 2004.)

A precipitating event that Gerwin and colleagues (2004) attributed to the onset of somatic dysfunction is unaccustomed or unexpected maximal muscle exertion of either an eccentric or concentric nature. Repeated eccentric contractions have been shown to damage sarcomeres and the vascular network within the muscular tissue environment (Stauber et al. 1990). Damage of the muscle's fibrils and vascular supply produces a release of proinflammatory mediators that not only disturbs the excitation–contraction coupling system of the sarcomere (Proske and Morgan 2001), but also limits the supply of oxygen to the tissues, which produces capillary restriction (McPartland and Simons 2007). The capillary restriction and damage may impair cellular and tissue perfusion, resulting in greater acidity, or lower tissue pH (Sluka, Kalra, and Moore 2001; Sluka et al. 2003), thereby activating nociceptors, which sparks the release of calcitonin gene–related peptide (CGRP) from the motor terminal (Gerwin et al. 2004; Shah et al. 2003).

CGRP is as an amino acid peptide that is well known for its ability to exert powerful peripheral vasodilation, but it has also been implicated in the mediation of the neural inflammatory response along with substance P (O'Halloran and Bloom 1991). CGRP exists side by side with ACh at the motor nerve synapse. When CGRP is elevated, ACh at the motor terminal increases because CGRP increases acetylcholine receptor (AChR) phosphorylation and prolongs the time ACh has to dock with its receptor channels at the postsynaptic membrane (Gerwin et al. 2004; Shah et al. 2003). Typically, acetylcholinesterase (AChE) breaks down ACh at the postsynaptic terminal (McPartland and Simons 2006), but AChE is pH dependent, and when pH is low, AChE production is decreased (Gerwin et

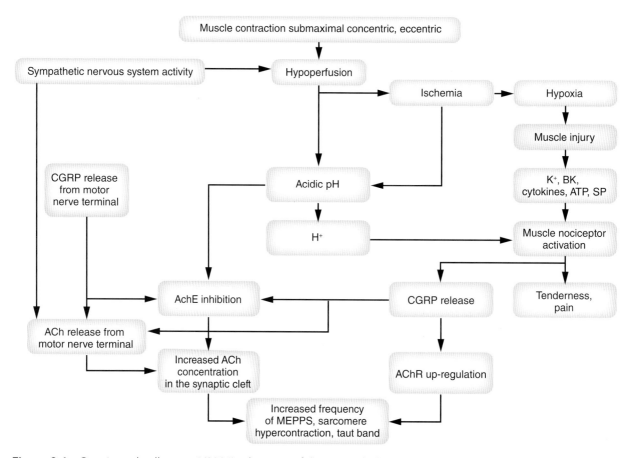

Figure 2.4 Gerwin and colleagues' (2004) schematic of the expanded integrated hypothesis of trigger point formation. Ach: acetylcholine; AChE: acetylcholinesterase; AChR: acetylcholine receptors; ATP: adenosine triphosphate; BK: bradykinin; CGRP: calcitonin gene-related peptide; H+: protons; K+: potassium; MEPP: miniature endplate potentials; SP: substance P.

Springer and *Current Pain and Headache Reports*, volume 8(6), 2004 of publication, 468-475, "An expansion of Simons' integrated hypothesis of trigger point formation," R.D. Gerwin, figure 1, ©2004. With kind permission from Springer Science and Business Media.

al. 2004; Kovyazina et al. 2003). Therefore, ACh continues to rise at the neuromuscular junction because it cannot be removed effectively from its postsynaptic receptors by the limited amount of AChE. Also, its release is inhibited as a result of low levels of ATP and oxygen. To compound the rise in ACh at the synaptic cleft, CGRP also downregulates AChE to limit ACh, but CGRP release increases when pH is lowered, further limiting the breakdown and inhibition of ACh.

In sum, Gerwin and colleagues (2004) contended that, in part, an elevated level of CGRP drives trigger point chronicity by producing and enhancing the presence of ACh. This results in a flood of nociceptor signals at the dorsal horn, which over time leads to neuroplastic changes that continually activate nociceptor fields within the spinal segment, but also above and below the facilitated segment. This is due to the cortical tract arrangement of the spinal segments.

Preceding theories have highlighted muscle contraction, hypoperfusion, neuroactive peptides, pain, and proprioceptive dysfunction as some of the primary causes of the production and maintenance of somatic dysfunction at multiple spinal segmental levels. Speicher and Draper, however, posited in 2006 that metabolic, neurochemical, and proprioceptive influences propagate structural dysfunction at the actin–myosin filaments, augmenting the development and maintenance of somatic dysfunction.

Mechanical Coupling Theory

The mechanical coupling theory (MCT) proposed by Speicher in 2006 posits that somatic dysfunction is produced and maintained through metabolic, neurochemical, and proprioceptive influences that produce a structural dysfunction of the fusimotor complex (figure 2.5). The MCT adds to previous models of somatic dysfunction through its attention on the influence of the ATP energy crisis on ATP hydrolysis and filament coupling. Under homeostatic conditions, thick myosin protein filaments mechanically couple and uncouple with thin actin protein filaments to produce muscular contraction (Matthews 1981). As described by Vandenboom (2004), the regulation of the mechanical coupling process is driven by the conversion of chemical energy to mechanical energy from the following process:

> During the excitation/contraction coupling (ECC) process, calcium (Ca2+) ions released from the sarcoplasmic reticulum (SR) bind to troponin C (TnC) to activate the thin filament and allow myosin to interact with actin. Formation of this myofibrillar complex allows myosin to transduce the free energy liberated by the hydrolysis of adenosine triphosphate (ATP) into mechanical work against the thin filament. (p. 331)

A further understanding of how a disturbance in the mechanical coupling process may result in and sustain somatic dysfunction can be gleaned from Vandenboom's (2004) foundational work on myofibrillar fatigue.

Whereas increased calcium ion (Ca^{2+}) concentrations at the sarcoplasmic reticulum (SR) increase myofibril contractility (McPartland and Simons 2007; Proske and Morgan 2001), Ca^{2+} concentration is reduced in the presence of fatigue (Vandenboom 2004), which has been linked to a reduction in muscular function and force production (Proske and Morgan 2001). Regardless of an increase or decrease of Ca^{2+} at the SR, an increased or decreased amount can produce SR dysfunction and, in turn, impair myofibrillar protein function (Proske and Morgan 2001). Thick myosin proteins hydrolyze (break apart) ATP to liberate its free energy to power the myosin–actin crossbridge power stroke to produce muscle contraction (Vandenboom 2004). The myosin heads contain nucleotide sites that regulate the binding ability of the actin filaments (Matthews 1981). Coursing along the thin actin filaments is a chain of regulatory proteins ensconced in the tropomyosin protein that forms the tropomyosin–troponin complex (figure 2.6) The complex contains the subunit protein TnC, which regulates the nucleotide-binding

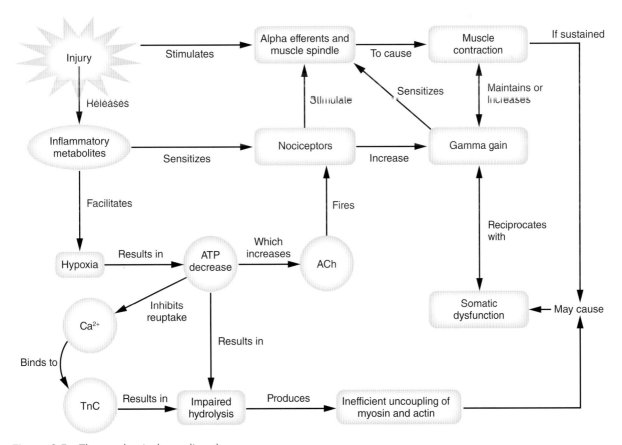

Figure 2.5 The mechanical coupling theory.
© Timothy E. Speicher

Sarcomere

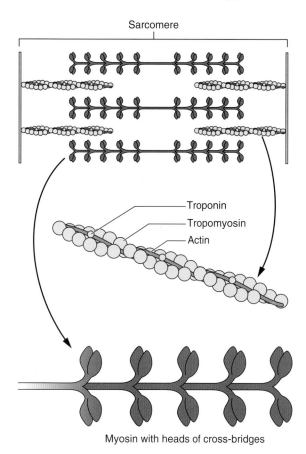

Troponin
Tropomyosin
Actin

Myosin with heads of cross-bridges

Figure 2.6 The tropomyosin–troponin complex.

sites for the actin protein on the myosin filament, covering and uncovering them through a cascade of neurochemical reactions (Matthews 1981). The interaction of calcium and TnC plays an integral role in the exposure of these binding sites and hence in the regulation of muscular contraction.

As previously discussed, when Ca2+ levels at the SR are high and ATP levels are low, an energy crisis, or what Vandenboom (2004) termed a chemical crisis, ensues. McKillop and Geeves (1993) proposed a model that elucidates how the binding of Ca2+ with TnC influences both myosin and actin filament interactions. When calcium levels are low, actin filament binding to the myosin head is blocked, impairing the ability of the actin–myosin proteins to produce a strong crossbridge connection. However, "a strongly bound cross-bridge [in the presence of high Ca2+ levels] has a high affinity for actin and can generate force and perform work against the thin filament" (Vandenboom 2004, 333).

Houdusse and colleagues (1997) highlighted that when TnC is in the presence of calcium, it serves as a switch to power ATP hydrolysis. When

ATP is hydrolyzed during the crossbridge power stroke, Pi (inorganic phosphate) and ADP (adenosine diphosphate) are released as by-products to work in concert with ATP to regulate the coupling and uncoupling of myosin and actin filaments (Vandenboom 2004). However, Vandenboom pointed out that if ADP release is inhibited, which occurs in the presence of lowered pH, then ATP will fail to uncouple the filaments, creating a "rigor cross-bridge . . . not capable of generating further force" (p. 335). The inefficiency of the coupling and uncoupling process produces a structural dysfunction and deformation of the filament complex, assisting in the maintenance of its coupled position, which may result in the recalcitrant taut band or knot observed with osteopathic lesions. ATP helps to prime the myosin–actin complex for recoupling or attachment, much like how gamma motor neurons help to prime, or ready, the muscle spindle for stimulation.

The inefficiency of the uncoupling of the myosin–actin filaments as a result of low ATP and TnC and calcium binding may explain why increased strength has been observed when hip trigger and tender points have been released with SCS (Wong and Schauer-Alvarez 2004). Not only are the actin–myosin filaments in a structural position to produce work because they have been uncoupled, but the ATP, Pi, and ADP balance has also been restored to assist in the coupling process. However, if calcium and ACh levels remain high in the presence of TnC, myofibrillar binding may be sustained, resulting in myofibrillar fatigue that produces an inefficient coupling of the actin–myosin filaments (Vandenboom 2004).

The mechanical coupling theory builds on existing models of somatic dysfunction by affirming the cascade of neurometabolic events that occurs when tissue is damaged. The discovery of the impairment to ATP hydrolysis and its impact on the coupling of actin—myosin crossbridges may further research into this mechanism and others that produce and sustain somatic dysfunction. Even though the theoretical foundation for somatic dysfunction and its associated trigger and tender points is solidifying, further research is needed to test the propositions and explore how they may translate to the clinical application of PRT for the treatment of somatic dysfunction.

Based on my clinical experience with PRT as well as its instruction, I have chosen not to include in this text the traditional tender point locations originally outlined by Jones, in order to encourage practitioners to explore the entire tissue during palpation. Even though common tender and trigger point locations have been identified across patient conditions and populations, most practitioners are often surprised to find undocumented points during examination. In the absence of a thorough palpation examination and exploration, critical dominant tender and trigger points may be missed. In part, this is why this text has moved away from the traditional point-by-point approach and toward a more exploratory approach when investigating somatic lesions and, hence, why the palpation of specific tissue structures is emphasized. Although not all tissues that can be treated with PRT have been presented in this chapter or text, those readily palpable and frequently affected by somatic lesions are presented. However, the clinical training and experience of the practitioner should be paramount when ascertaining the origin and cause of the patient's somatic dysfunction.

Clinical Implications

Although it may be tempting to treat PRT as a panacea for somatic dysfunction, it is just one tool for facilitating the resolution of somatic dysfunction, albeit a versatile and powerful one. During the acute inflammatory process, PRT can be used to limit muscle spasm, improve blood flow, and limit the neurochemical cascade that results in the formation of osteopathic lesions. Controlling the formation of these lesions early may reduce the propensity for central sensitization, ischemia, and tissue atrophy. One of the major concerns during the acute stage of healing is protecting the tissue from further damage by controlling the inflammatory response (Knight and Draper 2012). By mitigating the unbridled release of proinflammatory mediators and ACh and limiting capillary restriction, practitioners can avoid a dive into the abyss of chronic inflammation, thereby facilitating an optimal environment in which the patient can move into the repair phase of the healing process.

To heal adequately in the repair phase, tissues need adequate blood flow to receive nourishment. Most important, pain must be controlled to permit the range of motion needed for encouraging phagocytosis and fibroplasia (Knight and Draper 2012). However, when lesions do develop, range of motion is often restricted (Jones 1973), resulting in irregular scar formation and potentially weakening the tissue and making it more susceptible to further injury when stressed. If pain is not controlled, then the patient will likely regress into the inflammatory phase, delaying healing and producing unwanted scar tissue. Also, uncontrolled or intentionally delivered pain from direct therapeutic interventions may entrench and spread somatic dysfunction to other areas of the body, affecting strength, range of motion, and functional movement patterns. If PRT is applied to tissue lesions during this phase of healing, perfusion should improve to deliver critical blood flow to facilitate fibroplasia and tissue nourishment. Moreover, if blood flow is adequate, the primary culprit of somatic dysfunction, ACh, will be marginalized.

For patients who do not progress through the repair phase and fall into a state of chronic inflammation, PRT can assist in freeing them from its grip. It does so by decreasing the gamma gain that may be driving a sustained myotatic reflex, interrupting the myotatic reflex by silencing the muscle spindles' aberrant neural discharge and increasing perfusion to blood-thirsty tissues, resetting the neural firing patterns of type II spindle afferents, decreasing GTO inhibition from a reduction in musculotendinous tension produced by a lesion, and potentially recalibrating nociceptive fields and alpha motor neurons at the dorsal horn to eradicate central sensitization.

Summary

With an understanding of the foundational neurophysiological underpinnings of how sensation and pain affect the somatic system, the theories that may explain the development and persistence of somatic dysfunction, as well as their implications for the clinical practice of PRT, aspiring positional release therapists will be poised to understand, learn, and apply PRT to a multitude of conditions arising from somatic dysfunction. The age-old concept of no pain, no gain is not easily set aside in the current therapeutic culture and training environment. Although there is a place for direct painful therapies, the option of accomplishing the same or a more optimal therapeutic outcome with an indirect technique such as PRT may be more appealing once we understand how pain travels throughout the somatic system. Pain does not reside only where it is caused or felt, but permeates the entire somatic system, crossing the spinal column and facilitating multiple segmental levels and the tissues they innervate, both somatic and visceral. Additionally, pain, either felt or caused, also activates other spinal reflexes such as the cross-spinal reflex that could produce tender and trigger points in antagonist musculature or in unintended areas of the body. Although acute pain or that induced by a therapist may be a trigger for the development of osteopathic lesions, multiple metabolic, neurochemical, and proprioceptive influences may work together to produce and sustain somatic dysfunction and a resultant structural dysfunction of the fusimotor complex.

Korr's proprioceptive theory (1975) laid the foundation for other theories of somatic dysfunction to follow. Simons and colleagues' (1999) integrated hypothesis of trigger point formation encapsulated Korr's idea that the muscle spindle was dysfunctional. However, Simons et al. (1999) postulated that the primary culprit in spindle dysfunction is motor end plate dysfunction and central sensitization, which has been supported since the theory's introduction. The theory has been bolstered and expanded on further. Gerwin and his colleagues (2004) provided additional evidence to support the integrated hypothesis through their expanded model and proposed additional mechanisms that may lead to the development and maintenance of trigger points such as unaccustomed muscle contraction, tissue acidity, calcitonin gene–related peptide (CGRP), and hypoperfusion. Speicher affirmed and incorporated these somatic dysfunction theories into his mechanical coupling theory (2006). This theory places a spotlight on how metabolic, neurochemical, and proprioceptive influences may work together to develop and sustain a dysfunctional fusimotor complex, leading to the inefficient coupling and uncoupling of myosin–actin filaments. Although not all theories of somatic dysfunction have been presented in this text, the ones that have provide a guide for how to integrate PRT into the overall treatment plan for both acute and chronic maladies.

Regardless of where it is used in the healing process, PRT is a nonpainful therapeutic intervention that limits pain and spasm and restores range of motion. Compelling evidence is mounting that supports the use of this therapy for the treatment and prevention of somatic dysfunction in all populations and clinical settings (see table 2.1). As evidence builds to support the efficacy of this therapy, I suspect that we will look back and wonder what took so long for PRT to become a cornerstone of our therapeutic foundation and treatment philosophy.

Table 2.1 Primary Somatic Dysfunction Neurometabolic Events

Neurometabolic event	Increased ↑	Decreased ↓	Supporting literature	Potential PRT impact
Inflammatory metabolites	X		McPartland 2004; Proske and Morgan 2001; Reinöhl et al. 2003	Decrease
Tissue pH		X	Gerwin et al. 2004; Sluka et al. 2001; Sluka et al. 2003	Increase
Stretch reflex arc activity	X		Howell et al. 2006; Wynne et al. 2006	Decrease
Gamma activity	X		Appelberg et al. 1983; Capra et al. 2007; Thunberg et al. 2002	Decrease
ACh	X		Dolezal et al. 1992; Dommerholt et al. 2006; Maekawa et al. 2002; Simons et al. 1999; Wessler 1996	Decrease
AChR	X		Dolezal et al. 1992; Gerwin et al. 2004; McPartland and Simons 2006	Decrease
AChE		X	Gerwin et al. 2004; Kovyazina et al. 2003; McPartland and Simons 2006	Increase
ATP		X	Dommerholt et al. 2006; McPartland and Simons 2007; Reinöhl et al. 2003; Wessler 1996	Increase
Calcium release	X		McPartland and Simons 2007; Proske and Morgan 2001; Vandenboom 2004	Decrease
TnC calcium binding	X		Houdusse et al. 1997; McKillop and Greeves 1993; Vandenboom 2004	Decrease
Nociception	X		McPartland 2004; Reinöhl et al. 2003	Decrease
Motor end plate activity	X		Hong and Yu 1998; Hubbard and Berkoff 1993; Kostopoulos et al. 2008	Decrease
Tissue perfusion		X	Gerwin et al. 2004; Larsson et al. 1999; Maekawa et al. 2002; Rosas-Ballina et al. 2011	Increase
CGRP release	X		Domhnall and Bloom 1991; Gerwin et al. 2004; Shah et al. 2003	Decrease

CHAPTER 3

Special Populations

CHAPTER OBJECTIVES

After reading this chapter, you should be able to do the following:

❶ Understand important considerations when working with special populations.

❷ Articulate special considerations and therapeutic interventions to be taken when working with youth and elderly patients.

❸ Treat unique injury conditions such as mastectomy pain based on somatic lesion patterns.

❹ Apply special therapeutic considerations and precautions when treating competitive athletes and pregnant clients with positional release therapy (PRT).

❺ Clinically approach the evaluation and treatment process for patients with diseases and disabilities such as obesity, diabetes, and fibromyalgia through the lens of PRT.

The use of PRT for the treatment of somatic dysfunction provides both opportunities and challenges when working with diverse patient populations. Although every patient is unique, I have found over the course of my clinical experience that some groups require special considerations during the evaluation and treatment process. These include youth and elderly patients, patients recovering from mastectomies, competitive athletes, pregnant women, and clients with disease and disability.

This book provides the nuts and bolts of how to apply PRT to a variety of tissues and injury conditions, although the life, work, and sport demands of clients often dictate how they are evaluated, how PRT is applied, and how they are managed throughout the recovery process. For example, women who are carrying a child at some point are not able to lie prone, and an elderly patient who has progressive knee osteoarthritis is unable to tolerate joint compression or rotation. Situations such as these require the therapist to alter the evaluation and treatment approach to ensure the safety of the patient and the effectiveness of the therapeutic interventions.

Youth and Elderly Patients

Besides the obvious characteristics of young and elderly patients, both groups are unique in their receptiveness to PRT. I have noted that clients in both groups who are treated with PRT appear to heal at a faster rate than middle-aged patients do. Considering the metabolism of the young, it is not surprising that they bounce back quickly when treated with PRT, but this does not explain the return to pain-free activity experienced by the elderly. Two plausible explanations are age-related differences in cellular signaling and lower levels of physical and psychological stress.

Altered Cellular Senescence Signaling

It is well documented that human tissue declines in efficiency with age. Campisi and colleagues (2011) laid out a convincing hypothesis for the reason our tissues and their respective cellular responses to stress decline with age; they attribute it primarily to alterations in cellular senescence signaling. "Cellular senescence generally refers to the essentially irreversible loss of proliferative ability that

occurs when cells experience potentially oncogenic stimuli" (Campisi et al. 2011, 3). Essentially, when proliferative cells are damaged or stressed, they are at risk of mutating and initiating tumorigenesis, or tumor growth. According to Campisi and colleagues (2011, 3), stressed or damaged cells can cause an "increase in mRNA levels and secretion of numerous cytokines, chemokines, growth factors and proteases," which they termed senescence-associated secretory phenotype (SASP). Cytokines and chemokines (e.g., IL-1β) and growth factors such as transforming growth factor (TGF-β), vascular endothelial growth factor (VEGF), and IL-8, among other inflammatory mediators, enable the healing process to progress (Gouin and Kiecolt-Glaser 2011). However, the continued presence of these inflammatory mediators may or may not be advantageous to healing. For example, in cataract patients younger than 40 years of age, Dawes, Duncan, and Wormstone (2013) found higher levels of TGF-β than in older patients as well as reduced cellular signaling activity in aged patients despite high levels of ligand availability. The authors postulated that the decrease in growth factors and higher senescence levels found in their older patients may be the result of their shortened telomeres and impaired healing ability.

Telomeres are DNA sequences that cap the ends of chromosomes, enabling cells to divide; however, as the cells divide, the telomeres become shorter resulting in cell aging. The enzyme telomerase is more abundant in young people than in older people, which keeps the cells from breaking down to a great degree (Blackburn 1991). The breakdown of cells, however, may release SASP to repair the stressed or damaged cells, which may activate senescent cells to limit fibrosis during repair (Campisi et al. 2011). Senescent cells are eliminated by the immune system, but they are found in greater number in aged tissues, which may be from a decline in functionality of the immune system and increased oxidative stress as a result of the inefficiency of the mitochondria (Campisi et al. 2011).

Decreased Physical and Psychological Stress

Research suggests that cellular signaling is more robust early in life, enabling the healing process to advance with little complication. As we age, however, our cellular signaling systems, intended to rid our bodies of damaged cells, become less efficient, leading to delayed healing and an array of diseases and illnesses such as cancer (Campisi et al. 2011). Therefore, an increase in cellular signaling along with the preservation of telomeres may explain, in part, why young people treated with PRT heal more quickly than older people do. However, the more expedient return to homeostasis in older people is likely due to the lower levels of physical and psychological stress at this stage of life, which may limit cellular stress. We can also assume, then, that recovery from somatic dysfunction during midlife may be hampered by increased psychological and physiological stress from work and life demands.

In their examination of the impact of stress on wound healing, Gouin and Kiecolt-Glaser (2011) presented compelling research that affirms the negative impact of psychological and physiological stress on healing. The authors pointed out that psychological stress activates the hypothalamic-pituitary-adrenal and sympathetic-adrenal-medullary axes, resulting in the increased production of glucocorticoids and catecholamines, which have been shown to retard wound healing in both humans and animals. The researchers also reported on studies that demonstrated improved healing in people who perceived greater support from their partners and were surrounded by a supportive social network. Conversely, women who discussed marital strife demonstrated lower levels of proinflammatory cytokines (IL-1β, IL-6, TNF-α).

McPartland and Simons (2006) also pointed out that psychological and physical stress can impair the ability of acetylcholinesterase (AChE) to deactivate acetylcholine (ACh). "Intrasynaptic ACh must be deactivated; otherwise, it will continue to activate nicotinic ACh receptors (nACRs) in the muscle cell membrane" (McPartland and Simon 2006, 6). Excess ACh has been strongly linked to the development and persistence of myofascial trigger points (Gerwin, Dommerholt, and Shah 2004). Although the young and old have plenty to be stressed out about, I propose that a diminished level of psychological and physical stress coupled with less exposure to repetitive movements and postures at work result in less of a demand on the somatic system in these populations, enabling them to capitalize on the application of PRT unlike other age groups. Even though the young and elderly populations may attune better to PRT, special precautions should be exercised when applying PRT to the elderly.

Treating Elderly Patients With Low Bone Mass and Osteoarthritis

The elderly may be particularly prone to the development of somatic dysfunction as a result of aging telomeres, decreased cellular signaling efficiency, and the presence of osteoporosis and osteoarthritis. Based on data from the 2005-2008 National Health and Nutrition Examination Survey, 49% of all adults over the age of 50 have low bone mass—a precursor to osteoporosis, which 9% of the sample possessed (Looker et al. 2012). Values were assessed at either the femoral neck or lumbar spine, which are common areas of osteoarthritis in the aged population (Murphy and Helmich 2012). The prevalence of low bone mass was found to be 39% at the femoral neck and 27% at the lumbar spine. However, the prevalence for osteoporosis at these sites was flipped: 4% at the lumbar spine and 3% at the neck of the femur. Therefore, nearly 50% of people over the age of 50 have low bone mass, and roughly 10% are osteoporotic. Bearing these statistics in mind, PRT is an excellent modality to use with this population because of its gentle, nonforceful nature. However, the amount of force used during joint compression, rotation, and distraction should be based on patient comfort and joint feel. If low bone mass is suspected, a bone mineral density test will help to ascertain the integrity of the bone, particularly when working with the hip, pelvis, and spine.

The potential presence of osteoarthritis (OA) also calls for special considerations in the application of PRT. Based on available epidemiological data, Murphy and Helmich (2012) estimated that approximately 27 million U.S. adults have clinical OA, which accounts for more than 10% of the U.S. population. Although OA can emerge in the young and throughout life, the incidence rises with age (Murphy and Helmich 2012). Nguyen and colleagues (2011) reported that OA is the most common cause of knee pain in people over the age of 50 and the primary reason for knee replacement. Although aging may increase the risk for knee OA (Murphy and Helmich 2012), obesity is also a strong risk factor (Nguyen et al. 2011).

Guillemin and colleagues (2011) found similar results in a population-based survey of a multiregional sample in France. The authors found that the incidence of OA increased with age, and that OA was more prevalent among those with obesity. An additional modifiable risk factor for OA is excessive mechanical stress on the job, such as that experienced in agriculture, construction, cleaning, and retail occupations. Zidron and colleagues (2005) found a high prevalence of somatic dysfunction among 103 Kenyan elders, which was associated with caregiving intensity, being female, and being engaged in manual labor such as farming.

Although there are no studies yet linking somatic dysfunction to OA in a U.S. population, somatic dysfunction is often present among patients with OA. Osteoarthritis typically is caused by microtrauma to the joint over time, which results in inflammation and pain. The inflammation and pain can cause thickening of the joint capsule and the formation of osteophytes, which can disturb the normal function of the joint and produce dysfunctional movement patterns. Murphy and Helmick (2013) reported that the three most commonly found activities with functional limitations among arthritic patients were bending, stooping, and walking.

Although young patients can develop OA, advanced OA is more typical in the aged population and results in more deeply rooted joint structure and function alternations, somatic dysfunction, and functional movement impairment (Cooper et. al 2013). When applying PRT to older people with osteoporosis, osteoarthritis, or both, therapists must be cognizant of how patient positioning and the application of force during positioning may affect them (see figure 3.1). Therapists should take

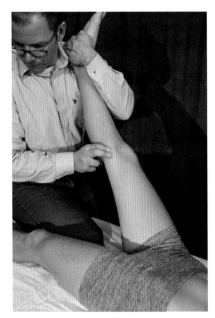

Figure 3.1 PRT pes anserine treatment for an OA patient.

the following into consideration when using PRT with OA patients, particularly the elderly:

CLINICIAN THERAPEUTIC INTERVENTIONS
Osteoarthritis

- To avoid evoking pain and irritation, exercise caution when moving the joint through the range of motion and when applying joint compression and rotation. Osteoarthritic joints often present with diminished osteo- and arthrokinematic movement, and pain is often elicited when attempting to move beyond the available range of motion.
- Consider requesting a radiograph to ascertain the severity of the OA.
- Address modifiable risk factors with the patient such as weight loss and occupational and ADL (activities of daily living) modifications.
- Ascertain whether an underlying condition exists that may be causing increased joint loading such as a significant leg length discrepancy or a prolonged pronation phase during gait.
- Educate the patient on the use of nonimpact exercises that will help to stabilize and nourish the joints.
- Provide the patient with educational and stress management resources. A popular resource is the Arthritis Program of the U.S. Centers for Disease Control and Prevention.

Treating Young Patients With Osteopathic Lesions

The therapist must be attentive when applying force during PRT to the young to avoid disturbing epiphyseal growth. However, the most important thing to remember when working with children is to address osteopathic lesions immediately before they cause central sensitization and functional movement impairments that may manifest late into life and during sport participation. As early as 1958, Bates and Grunwaldt reported that myofascial pain with trigger areas was a "common clinical entity in childhood" (p. 208). The authors reported on myofascial pain and "trigger areas" in children as young as three years of age and presented a variety of chronic myofascial pain conditions, such as headache, that were treated successfully with ethyl chloride spray and procaine hydrochloride injection.

In a recent pilot study, researchers investigated the impact of trigger point–specific physiotherapy on tension-type headaches in nine female children ages 5 to 15 (von Stülpnagel et al. 2009). The physiotherapy was applied to the shoulders, neck, and head twice a week over the course of a month and consisted of active and passive stretches, deep-stroking massage, trigger point pressure release, and heat and electrical stimulation. The authors determined improvement through participant self-reported journaling of headache intensity and frequency throughout the treatment phase of the study as well as changes in pain based on the visual analog scale (VAS). Self-reported symptoms reduced by 67.7%; and symptoms reported using the VAS, by 74.3%. The authors attributed the reduction in headache symptoms to interrupting the nociceptive input to the caudal trigeminal nucleus, thereby mitigating the central sensitization caused from myofascial trigger points (MTrPs).

Little is known to date about the prevalence of MTrPs and tender points in children, what treatments are most effective for this population, and how the pathophysiology and treatment of MTrPs may differ between children and adults. Additionally, investigations into the long-term consequences of osteopathic lesions in children are lacking. However, based on the clinical implications of chronic active and latent trigger points on the persistence of somatic tissue disorders and function in adults, the early treatment of osteopathic lesions in children warrants significant attention by researchers and clinicians. Therapists should take the following into consideration when using PRT with young patients with osteopathic lesions:

CLINICIAN THERAPEUTIC INTERVENTIONS
Osteopathic Lesions in the Young

- Examine children who complain of persistent pain for the presence of osteopathic lesions.
- To avoid central sensitization development in children that may persist late into adulthood, treat osteopathic lesions quickly.
- Reduce the use of compressive or traction forces at the joints, and use these forces cautiously to avoid disturbing epiphyseal growth.

- Consider ordering a radiograph to ascertain the presence of epiphyseal growth disturbance in the presence of an associated injury mechanism.
- Ensure that a parent or legal guardian is present during treatment, particularly when working in sensitive areas.
- When young patients do not respond readily (within two or three sessions) to PRT, investigate other causative or underlying factors that may account for the persistence of their somatic dysfunction.
- Educate young patients and their caregivers about other therapeutic measures to optimize their treatment and healing.

Mastectomy Patients

Cancer is the leading cause of death in developed countries and ranks second in developing countries (Mathers, Fat, and Boerma 2008). Approximately 12.7 million cases of cancer occur each year globally, of which 7.6 million result in death. In 2008 the most frequently diagnosed cancer in women was breast cancer (1.38 million cases worldwide); it accounted for 14% (458,400) of cancer deaths (Jemal et al. 2011). In 2000 Andrews, Cofield, and O'Driscoll reported that 1 in 10 American women were affected by breast cancer in their lifetimes. In 2014 the American Cancer Society estimated that one in eight American women (12.4%) are afflicted with invasive breast cancer, equating to 232,670 new cases annually. Of these cases, 62,570 will be new cases of carcinoma situ, an early form of breast cancer; however, 40,000 of the cases overall will result in death. Breast cancer rates are two to five times higher in developed countries such as the United States and the United Kingdom, which has been attributed primarily to early detection and the reduction in the use of combined postmenopausal hormone therapy (Jemal et al. 2011). Fortunately, improvements in the medical management of the disease have resulted in a five-year survival rate of 89% (Ebaugh, Spinelli, and Schmitz 2011).

According to Jemal and colleagues (2011), risk factors for developing breast cancer in women are a long menstrual history (1.2–1.3 RR), nulliparity (1.3–1.4 RR), the recent use of postmenopausal hormone therapy (1.3–2.0 RR), late age at first birth (1.1–1.4 RR), alcohol consumption (1.2–1.4 RR), and obesity (1.3–1.6 RR). However, the greatest relative risk (5–30 RR) factor for breast cancer has been observed in women who possess a genetic germ-line mutation on chromosome 17q, known as BRCA1, which confers a 39 to 62% lifetime risk (Easton, Ford, and Bishop 1995). The strongest preventive breast cancer recommendation from the National Comprehensive Cancer Network (NCCN) is for women to maintain an acceptable body mass index (BMI) and to remain active throughout life. When preventive measures fail, surgical and radiation interventions are often pursued to address the disease.

The classical treatment for breast cancer based on 2014 NCCN guidelines includes two options: breast conservation therapy consisting of a lumpectomy followed by radiation therapy, or a more aggressive approach such as mastectomy with or without radiation. Regardless of the option chosen, complications often result (Andrews et al. 2000) and can persist for several years or more if left unchecked (Ebaugh et al. 2011). Complications that often result from classical treatment are shoulder and chest wall pain, subcutaneous fibrosis, decreased shoulder range of motion, lymphedema, impaired scapulothoracic function, axillary web syndrome, shoulder girdle weakness and altered alignment (Fourie and Robb 2009), and shoulder girdle somatic dysfunction (Ebaugh et al. 2011). One reason a mastectomy patient may complain of shoulder pain and dysfunction is that the somatic dysfunction that ensues from surgery may cause rotator cuff disease (Ebaugh et al. 2011). Shoulder girdle somatic dysfunction, whether driven by active or latent osteopathic lesions, impairs range of motion, strength, and scapulothoracic rhythm (Lucas et al. 2004), which may inhibit the rotator cuff's ability to stabilize the humeral head in the glenoid fossa. This can result in the impingement of the supraspinatus tendon at the subacromial arch (Ebaugh et al. 2011).

Although early detection and survival rates have improved over time, no therapeutic interventions have been found to be superior in addressing the associated surgical complications of mastectomy (Ebaugh et al. 2011; Todd et al. 2008). In our clinical practice, we have found PRT to be an extremely effective tool to address postmastectomy pain, shoulder girdle weakness and range of motion deficits, and resultant shoulder and chest wall somatic dysfunction. Most patients report pain-free ADLs within six weeks.

The application of PRT to this population opens the door for effective rehabilitation to occur because it frees hypertonic tissues, thereby taking pressure off lymphatic and vascular tissues. This may improve perfusion-engendering tissue homeostasis, increase strength, and restore shoulder girdle function and range of motion. Most important, PRT dramatically reduces pain at rest and with ADLs, allowing postmastectomy patients to resume normal life and sport activities without physical impairment. Therapists should take the following into consideration when using PRT with mastectomy patients:

CLINICIAN THERAPEUTIC INTERVENTIONS
Postmastectomy

- Perform an evaluation to determine the magnitude of shoulder girdle dysfunction.
- Examine the affected tissues for the presence of axillary web syndrome, which may need additional therapeutic and surgical interventions to resolve.
- Perform PRT first; then treat recalcitrant tissues with therapeutic ultrasound or another deep heating modality to facilitate collagen reorganization under range of motion restoration procedures.
- Use myofascial release and massage post-PRT treatment to increase blood flow, relax tissues, and further fascial unwinding.
- Educate the patient about chronic pain control methods such as meditation, visual imagery, ADLs, and palliative modalities.
- Initiate a progressive therapeutic program to address deficits found in the initial evaluation.
- Teach the patient how to self-release affected tissues.

Patient Self-Treatment Interventions

- Perform self-release daily.
- Perform a daily self-massage for five to eight minutes on affected tissues.
- Stretch affected tissues daily or after physical activity.
- Apply palliative modalities to control pain and spasm.
- Meditate or perform relaxation pain control techniques daily to reduce chronic pain.

Treatment Points and Sequencing

1. Sternum
2. Xiphoid

3. Pectoralis minor

4. Pectoralis major

5. Serratus anterior

6. Intercostals

7. Trapezius (upper)

8. Subclavius

9. Infraspinatus

10. Teres minor

11. Rhomboids

12. Levator scapulae at the shoulder

Competitive Athletes

Critical to treating competitive athletes is addressing injuries and resultant osteopathic lesions as quickly as possible. If the clinician can treat the injury or painful tissue lesion(s), be it a myofascial trigger point (MTrP) or tender point (TP), the potential for these osteopathic lesions and their root injuries to cause alterations in nervous system function may be mitigated. Mense (2003) proposed that if muscle pain is not treated in a timely manner, the prolonged stimulation of inhibitory interneurons may cause dorsal horn neuroplastic changes that can lead to functional reorganization of the spinal dorsal horn. This can cause nociceptive neurons to become dysfunctional and hyperactive, leading to the development of chronic pain. Mense noted that clinicians should "abolish the muscle pain as early and effectively as possible to prevent the central nervous system alterations. If a patient already has developed alterations in the nociceptive system, treatment will be difficult and long-lasting because alterations need time to disappear" (2003, 423). Therefore, evaluating acute and subacute patients for MTrPs and TPs at the time of injury and throughout the recovery process is critical to prevent central sensitization (see figure 3.2). As pointed out previously, an evaluation may reveal both painful active and nonpainful latent trigger points. Both should be treated, because nonpainful latent trigger points have been shown to negatively affect muscle activation and the movement of the shoulder girdle as well as the distal musculature in the arm; conversely, treating them has been shown to normalize muscle activation patterns (Lucas, Polus, and Rich 2004).

Unfortunately, regardless of whether an injury is acute or chronic, most competitive athletes have both active and latent osteopathic lesions because

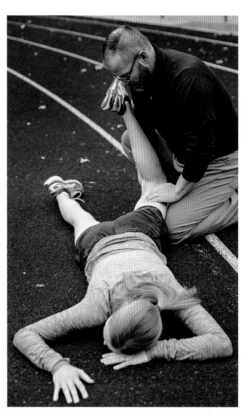

Figure 3.2 On-field PRT hamstring procedure performed on a track and field athlete.

of the nature of athletic activity, which requires a significant amount of repetitive eccentric work, muscular action over sustained periods leading to fatigue, and the need to react to unforeseen forces (e.g., getting stiff-armed in American football). Repetitive eccentric muscular contractions have been shown to disrupt the cytoskeleton of the muscle fiber, disturb its cellular processes, increase its size because of the contracture, and produce shortening leading to the production of painful taut bands of tissue (Fridén and Lieber 1998). Itoh, Okada, and Kawakita (2004) found active MTrPs in the forearm among 15 healthy subjects after a bout of eccentric exercise of the extensor digitorum. The hyperirritable taut bands that developed in the elbow of subjects demonstrated increased tenderness, altered electrical activity assessed through EMG analysis, and referred pain into the distal extremity.

The demand of eccentric work experienced during training and competition coupled with a lack of sleep from a hectic schedule, academic and competitive stress (Gouin and Kiecolt-Glaser 2011; Salinis and Webbe 2012), an underlying nutritional deficiency such as in the female athlete triad

(Gerwin 2005; De Souza et al. 2014), or previous injury (Sytema et al. 2010) may play a role in the development and persistence of osteopathic lesions in the competitive athlete. Moreover, Simons (2004) suggested that complaints of regional pain or pain of sudden onset as a result of sustained or sudden muscle overload or repetitive activity may help determine the presence of clinically relevant myofascial trigger points. Therefore, when working with competitive athletes, the following considerations should be taken into account:

CLINICIAN THERAPEUTIC INTERVENTIONS
Injured Athletes

- Use PRT to treat acute injury immediately or as soon as possible.
- Consider additional triggers that may propagate the development and persistence of osteopathic lesions (e.g., nutritional deficiency, hormonal disturbance, lack of sleep, stress, muscular fatigue, previous injury).
- Consider prescreening athletes for active and latent MTrPs and TPs prior to the start of the season or at its completion to develop a preventive PRT and therapeutic treatment regimen.
- Keep in mind that because PRT may produce marked soreness, particularly among chronic pain patients, treatment prior to a game or practice could negatively affect performance. For patients with chronic pain, apply PRT on an off day or after practice to ascertain their post-PRT soreness response. If there is no soreness response, then using PRT prior to or during competitive periods should not be problematic.

Pregnant Patients

Most women experience low back and pelvic pain at some time during pregnancy and postpartum. Pennick and Liddle (2013) reported that more than two thirds of pregnant women experience back pain, and one fifth experience pelvic pain. The severity of lumbopelvic pain has been reported to increase throughout pregnancy, limiting activities of daily living, sleep, and work (Lillios and Young 2012; Pennick and Liddle 2013). There is no clear consensus about why women develop low back and pelvic girdle pain during pregnancy, but it is believed to be due to anatomical and physiolog-

ical changes that occur during pregnancy such as increased ligamentous laxity, weight gain, and altered pelvic biomechanics (Ritchie 2003).

Ritchie (2003) proposed that as a woman progresses through term, the gravid uterus promotes the pelvis to rotate forward, which increases lumbar lordosis, thereby placing an increased mechanical strain on the low back. The shift of the pelvis forward places a call on the sacroiliac ligament to resist its forward rotation. However, as the ligaments become more lax as the hormone relaxin is released, they lose their ability to resist the forward shift, resulting in more low back strain (Ritchie 2003). The hormone relaxin also causes widening of the pubic symphysis at approximately the 10 to 12th week of pregnancy, which may produce inflammation and tenderness (Ritchie 2003). As a result of increased fluid production and retention during pregnancy, women may also experience transient carpal tunnel syndrome and de Quervain syndrome (Khorsan et al. 2009). However, when the clinician is faced with a pregnant woman who complains of hip pain, other differential diagnoses should be considered such as a rupture of the pubic symphysis, osteitis pubis, osteonecrosis and transient osteoporosis of the hip, and lumbar disc pathology (Ritchie 2003). Although low back and pelvic girdle pain are prevalent during pregnancy, no therapeutic intervention to date has demonstrated a superior effect on pregnancy-related low back and pelvic pain and disability (Pennick and Liddle 2013).

The authors of several systematic studies (Boissonnault, Klestinski, and Pearcy 2012; Ee et al. 2008; Lillios and Young 2012; Pennick and Liddle 2013) have examined the efficacy of therapeutic interventions for the treatment of pregnancy-related low back and pelvic girdle pain. The primary interventions examined have been traditional physical therapy, aquatic exercise, osteopathic manipulative therapy (OMT), acupuncture, and physical and manual therapy combined. Although no therapeutic intervention was found to be more effective than any other for relieving pregnancy-related low back and pelvic pain, evidence suggests that when exercise and acupuncture are tailored to the stage of pregnancy, lumbopelvic pain is reduced (Ee et al. 2008; Pennick and Liddle 2013). However, a low level of evidence exists for using exercise alone to reduce low back and pelvic pain during pregnancy or postpartum (Lillios and Young 2012; Nilsson-Wikmar et al. 2005; Pennick and Liddle 2013). Lillios and Young (2012) and

Pennick and Liddle (2013) noted a greater reduction in pregnancy-related low back and pelvic pain when aquatic exercise or acupuncture was used over traditional physical therapy; however, Ee and colleagues (2008) reported only a limited level of evidence for the use of acupuncture. Likewise, the use of spinal manipulative therapy (SMT) or OMT for the treatment of pregnancy-related low back and pelvic pain has also yielded only limited support (Khorsan et al. 2009; Licciardone et al. 2010; Pennick and Liddle 2013).

Based on the evidence to date, Clemente-Fuentes, Pickett, and Carney (2013) suggested that both physical therapy and aquatic therapy and acupuncture (including auricular acupuncture) will help to relieve low back pain and improve function and that OMT may improve disability slightly. Even though the use of acetaminophen and corticosteroid injections have been found to be safe for use during pregnancy for reducing lumbopelvic pain (Clemente-Fuentes et al. 2013), nonprescription pain-relieving alternatives are advocated and sought after by pregnant women (Ritchie 2003) because of the unknown consequences of pain medications on fetal development.

Remaining active during pregnancy may also mitigate pregnancy-related pain (Ritchie 2003). Women who have been exercising previously and are not expected to have a complicated pregnancy are encouraged to continue exercising. Competitive athletes engaging in strenuous exercise while pregnant should receive close medical attention (Pivarnik, Perkins, and Moyerbrailean 2003) because eccentric exercise may result in the development of somatic dysfunction (Fridén and Lieber 1998). Although there have not been any studies to date examining the use of PRT for the treatment of pregnancy-related back and pelvic pain, PRT is an excellent therapeutic alternative to mitigate a pregnant patient's low back and pelvic girdle pain (see figure 3.3) because of its exceptional ability to treat somatic dysfunction with a passive, gentle approach. When working with pregnant women, therapists should take the following considerations into account:

Pregnancy-Related Pain

- The patient should be positioned for treatment in the most comfortable position (e.g., side-lying).

- Because joints will be more lax as the patient progresses through pregnancy, the amount of joint compression and distraction applied during PRT should be decreased accordingly.
- With slight modification, almost all PRT treatment positions can be done safely in a side-lying position.
- The placement of a pillow or bolster between the thighs and knees during treatment often reduces strain to the lumbopelvic area.

Populations With Disabilities and Disease

Although PRT has not been widely reported in the literature to cure physical or emotional disability or disease, the therapy can dramatically improve quality of life by reducing pain and spasm, improving function and enhancing overall well-being, and reducing hospital length of stay. Schwartz (1986) advocated the use of counterstrain, or PRT, for hospital patients suffering from acute illness. Schwartz commented that the therapy is an excellent prescription for nearly all bedridden patients, particularly those suffering from pain and somatic dysfunction as a result of acute

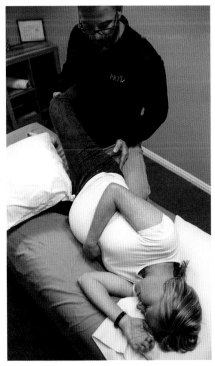

Figure 3.3 A piriformis PRT procedure performed on a pregnant woman.

fracture, postsurgical pain, and osseous metastatic disease, provided they can be moved without complication.

Radjieski, Lumley, and Cantieri (1998) reported a significant decrease in length of hospital stay by 3.5 days in pancreatitis patients treated with both OMT and traditional care versus patients treated with traditional care alone. In their randomized and blinded pilot study ($N = 14$), some patients were treated with primarily counterstrain and myofascial release and rib manipulation ($n = 6$), whereas those in the control group ($n = 8$) received standard care. The researchers hypothesized that the use of OMT for this population helped to improve intracellular function "through improved circulation and respiration, and by decreasing or intercepting prolonged sympathetic activity" (p. 265). As previously discussed, pain and the somatic dysfunction that ensues can heighten sympathetic activity, disturbing the homeostasis of the entire human organism. Although we must exercise caution when interpreting pilot study findings, further rigorous investigations of the use of PRT for the treatment of patients with disease or disability both in and outside a hospital setting are warranted based on the therapy's potential clinical implications for this population.

I am regularly surprised at how PRT helps those with disabilities and disease reestablish homeostasis. Patients often report treatment effects such as improvements in energy, mood, mental concentration, sleep, eating habits, and function with activities of daily living and recreation, as well as decreased depression. Although it is not within the scope of this text to discuss all of the diseases and disabilities that can be treated with PRT, the ones highlighted have shown promise and often require special considerations during the evaluation and treatment process.

Patients With Obesity and Diabetes

A person can be born with a disability, but disablement can also manifest over a lifetime from conditions such as obesity and diabetes. According to the World Health Organization (World Health Organization [WHO] 2014), obesity is a global burden both from a health care and a financial standpoint. The WHO reported in 2008 that 1.4 billion adults worldwide suffered from obesity, and women outpaced men. In 2013 the organization estimated that 42 million children worldwide were classified as either overweight or obese. Obesity is now identified as one of the top five reasons for death worldwide and often presents with associated comorbidities (Ellulu et al. 2014; Horne et al. 2014) such as diabetes, cardiovascular disease, metabolic syndrome, osteoarthritis, headache, and migraine.

Chai and colleagues (2014) found a 40 to 80% increased risk for migraine in those with progressive obesity, and the increase peaks during the childbearing years. However, the authors did not find a tenable connection between tension-type headache and obesity in adults. Oakley and colleagues (2014) reported that the current evidence suggests a possible connection between obesity and headache disorders in the pediatric population, including tension-type headaches.

In light of rising childhood overweight and obesity figures (Ellulu et al. 2014) and the reported negative impact on quality of life and risk for developing illness and musculoskeletal impairments such as osteoarthritis (Blagojevic et al. 2009), experts contend that the disease must be curbed. In addition, clinicians will likely be faced with treating obese patients of various ages, including the young, who possess not only one or more of the health problems associated with the disease, but also the pain they produce (Vincent et al. 2012). Obese patients often present with persistent musculoskeletal and joint pain (Ellulu et al. 2014; Vincent et al. 2012) and resultant somatic dysfunction caused by the abnormal and excessive loading of joints, particularly at the knee and hip (Blagojevic et al. 2009; Toivanen et al. 2010).

Based on a literature review, Finckh and Turesson (2014) proposed that obesity may be a risk factor for rheumatoid arthritis (RA), particularly in young women. The researchers suggested that adipocytes may be one of the causes because those found in adipose tissue release adipokines. Adipokines are cell-signaling proteins that have varied metabolic functions, but they are both pro-inflammatory and anti-inflammatory (Kwon and Pessin 2013). However, in both obese humans and rodents, pro-inflammatory adipokines are more prevalent than anti-inflammatory adipokines (Kwon and Pessin 2013), which may cause increased and sustained pain in the obese because of a heightened inflammatory response (Finckh and Turesson 2014). Moreover, obese patients also present with comorbidities the longer they are obese (Ellulu et al. 2014), especially type 2 diabetes (T2D), which is the most widely recognized (Toivanen et al. 2010). Therefore, clinicians should take the following into account when working with obese patients:

CLINICIAN THERAPEUTIC INTERVENTIONS
Obese Patients

- Obese patients should be placed on a lifestyle and behavioral modification program if they are not formally engaged in one.
- The somatic dysfunction and pain obese patients exhibit typically respond more slowly to treatment until a healthy weight or body composition is attained.
- Investigate whether obese patients have comorbidities and how they are currently managing them, as well as the association of those conditions with the patients' pain and somatic dysfunction.
- Older obese patients are more likely to have comorbidities such as T2D or OA. Therefore, consider decreasing the amount of compression, distraction, mobilization force, and palpatory pressure used during treatment.
- When assessing obese patients for osteopathic tissue lesions, place them on their side or in a position that uses gravity to move the adipose tissue away from underlying structures to be palpated.
- Use a high-low table, bolsters, and an exercise ball to alleviate the strain of performing PRT on obese and overweight patients.
- Perform a biomechanical and functional assessment for obese patients to ascertain whether an underlying biomechanical or functional impairment is causing or complicating their condition.

According to the American Diabetes Association (ADA), 29.1 million Americans, or 9.3% of the population, were afflicted with diabetes in 2014, resulting in direct medical and reduced productivity costs of $245 billion that year. Diabetes is also known to result in multiple complications and a myriad of comorbid conditions such as peripheral neuropathy (Martin et al. 2014), hypertension, and cardiovascular disease (ADA 2014). Diabetic patients may also present with joint pain (Schett et al. 2013) and somatic dysfunction, which typically moves upward from the feet. Symptoms tend to worsen as the disease progresses (Martin et al. 2014). Although type 1 diabetes is found in obese

patients and among 5% of the general U.S. population, type 2 diabetes (T2D) is more prevalent among the obese (ADA 2014). Obesity is known to be associated with underlying medical and psychological conditions that inhibit weight loss, although such conditions are less frequent causative factors than poor health style and behavioral choices (Toivanen et al. 2010).

Even though PRT may improve somatic dysfunction among patients with both obesity and diabetes, the foremost therapeutic intervention should be to help patients attain a healthy lifestyle that not only moves them out of obesity, but also helps them control and manage their diabetes. Both cardiorespiratory exercise and resistance training are advocated for the T2D obese patient regardless of the stage of the disease to help them regain a healthy weight and control of the disease (Schett et al. 2013). Regular physical activity may also help the type 2 obese diabetic patient avoid the development of knee and hip osteoarthritis.

Schett and colleagues (2013) examined 927 men and women between 40 and 80 years of age with T2D over a period of 20 years and found that T2D was an independent risk factor for the development of osteoarthritis (OA) based on the incidence of hip or knee arthroplasty, which was found to be independent of age and BMI. An increased probability for arthroplasty was observed among patients with a high BMI and also as patients aged. The findings of this study point to a metabolic influence on the development of OA among type 2 diabetics, bridging several of the disease and disability conditions discussed thus far. Diabetes, obesity, arthritis, and headache often appear in combination among chronic patient populations regardless of age or physical activity level. Therefore, clinicians should consider the therapeutic interventions discussed thus far in this chapter in addition to the following when treating the diabetic patient:

CLINICIAN THERAPEUTIC INTERVENTIONS
Diabetes

- Evaluate the lifestyle or physical activity behaviors of type 2 diabetic (T2D) patients for potential modification.
- Progressive T2D patients may present with cardiovascular disease, diabetic peripheral neuropathy (DPN), or autonomic cardiovascular neuropathy. Consult with the patient's

> continued

**Clinician Therapeutic
Interventions: Diabetes** > *continued*

attending physician prior to initiating a physical activity modification program (Colberg et al. 2010).

- Because patients with DPN have increased pain, altered sensation, and decreased perfusion in their extremities (Martin et al. 2014), exercise caution when attempting to locate and demarcate osteopathic tissue lesions. Currently, no studies have examined the impact of PRT on DPN patients or those with any diabetic condition; however, the diabetic patient often reports pain reduction, improved sensation, and increased tolerance to ambulatory pressure after the application of PRT.

- Post-PRT massage and the exercise of distal extremities are advocated to facilitate further tissue perfusion.

- The resolution of somatic dysfunction among T2D patients is often predicated on their ability to maintain a healthy weight.

Patients With Fibromyalgia

First described as rheumatic thickenings of tissue in 1816 by Balfour in Stockman (1920), widespread painful somatic lesions have been a topic of debate and speculation since (Smith, Harris, and Clauw 2011). The tissue thickenings observed by Stockman (1920) were painful to palpation, widely distributed throughout the body, and often in an irregular pattern. Because the lesions were initially thought to be associated with inflammation as the result of trauma, the term *fibrositis* was adopted to describe the condition (Gowers 1904). In 1945 Kelly commented that the condition was often thought to be "psychogenic" because of its mysterious nature and recalcitrant response to treatment. Kelly (1945), however, was convinced that fibrositis was not psychogenic, but a result of a reflex phenomenon that produced tender myalgic spots that referred pain to deeper tissues that could manifest anywhere in the body but appeared to have an affinity for musculotendinous junctions. In 1948 Korr also identified these myalgic spots, which he described as osteopathic lesions that resulted in widespread somatic dysfunction and pain.

Until the early 1990s, the term *fibrositis* was used by the rheumatic community to describe the presence of widespread painful tissue lesions. However, Smythe and Moldofsky (1977) and others who followed them determined that patients with fibrositis often demonstrated symptoms other than just painful tissue lesions, such as sleep disturbance, which could also be produced in healthy people when deprived of sleep. Moreover, the presence of widespread somatic lesions and their resultant pain was observed among those with other somatic disorders such as irritable bowel syndrome and headache, suggesting that fibrositis was associated with a much larger spectrum of disorders than first thought (Smith et al. 2011). When it became apparent that somatic tissue lesions resulted from factors and conditions other than inflammation, the term *fibrositis* was abandoned and *fibromyalgia* was adopted (Wolfe et al. 1990).

The American College of Rheumatology (ACR) in 1990 was the first to provide criteria for the classification of fibromyalgia, which provided the initial framework for a standard of diagnosis and research of this condition (Wolfe et al. 1990). In their attempt to provide a framework, Wolfe and colleagues (1990) examined 293 patients with fibromyalgia and 265 controls who were not deemed to have fibromyalgia, but who had other painful conditions such as lumbago. The researchers investigated primarily the presence of painful tender points in 30 anatomical sites throughout the body through dolorimetry and manual palpation and previously identified global indicators such as sleep disturbance, fatigue, morning stiffness, anxiety, and sensitivity to auditory stimuli. Among fibromyalgia subjects, the primary findings were axial and extremity tender points of moderate sensitivity at 18 of the 30 anatomical sites investigated and secondary complaints of generalized whole body pain, sleep disturbance, fatigue, and morning stiffness. These findings led investigators to classify fibromyalgia as a condition requiring a prolonged history of widespread pain and the presence of moderately sensitive tender points in multiple regions of the body, including the axial skeleton and extremities. (See Wolfe and colleagues [1990] for a full review of the ACR classification of fibromyalgia.)

The 1990 ACR classification of fibromyalgia has served as an excellent guide for numerous studies that have followed, but the identification of tender points in the clinical setting based on the ACR criteria, although useful for research purposes, has been deemed unrealistic and unnecessary for diagnosis (Smith et al. 2011). Instead, it is advocated that global complaints of pain, fatigue, and sleep disturbance be considered the primary criteria for diagnosis (Smith et al. 2011). Smith and colleagues provided an excellent in-depth review of the research supporting the rationale for the shift away from the use of tender points and toward the use of the revised criterion. They suggested various survey tools to assess them such as the fibromyalgia assessment status (FAS) index. The new evaluative criteria expand the definition of fibromyalgia beyond the symptoms of pain and its resultant somatic dysfunction. However, reports of pain and findings of tissue tenderness, although no longer considered central to a diagnosis, should not be abandoned (Smith et al. 2011). Although more clarity is developing on how to define or diagnose fibromyalgia, widespread pain, fatigue, and sleep disturbance remain central to its diagnosis. However, "the pathophysiology of fibromyalgia remains uncertain but is believed to be largely central in nature" (Smith et al. 2011, 217).

Fibromyalgia has been proposed to have both direct and indirect costs that are comparable to those of osteoarthritis (Smith et al. 2011). Thus, it is critical that we understand why the condition develops and explore how best to address its etiology. Smith and colleagues (2011) reported the primary symptoms of fibromyalgia as "multi-focal pain, fatigue, sleep disturbances, and cognitive or memory problems" with secondary symptoms of "psychological distress, impaired functioning, and sexual dysfunction" (p. 217). These symptoms are also often present in many other somatic conditions (Gerwin 2005; Smith et al. 2011; Wolfe et al. 1992), raising the question of whether fibromyalgia is a unique condition or simply a manifestation of multiple injury and disease mechanisms (Gerwin 2005). Wolfe and colleagues (1992) examined the presence of localized tenderness (tender points) and taut, painful muscle bands (myofascial trigger points) in patients diagnosed with both fibromyalgia and myofascial pain syndrome and also among healthy subjects. The researchers found that both disease groups possessed tender points, but those with myofascial pain syndrome possessed them in greater proportions. Even though the study had significant methodological limitations, its preliminary finding that myofascial pain syndrome patients possess more trigger points than tender points has continued to be the differentiating factor between the two conditions (Gerwin 2005), although both appear to be triggered by and persist for similar reasons.

Fibromyalgia and many somatic conditions are often precipitated by underlying conditions such as infection, psychological stress, a disease state, or trauma. However, "there is no objective tissue pathology or standard to which "[the] disease" can be anchored" (Smith et al. 2011, 274), which makes diagnosis and treatment challenging. Gerwin (2005) also suggested that fibromyalgia may ensue from a metabolic insufficiency caused by a deficiency in vitamin D, iron, and vitamin B_{12} and from hormonal imbalances caused by hypothyroidism.

Rather than being a single entity, fibromyalgia appears to be part of a larger continuum of somatic conditions such as irritable bowel syndrome, myofascial pain syndrome, tension-type headaches, and migraines, leading some researchers to group them because of their overlapping clinical symptoms. Yunus (2008) proposed a collective term for these somatic conditions, central sensitivity syndrome (CSS), because it is now believed that patients along the somatic spectrum have a "fundamental problem with pain or sensory amplification rather than a structural or inflammatory condition in the specific region where the pain is being experienced" (Smith et al. 2011, 219). Additional mechanisms that may also be at play are neurogenic inflammation, dysfunction of the autonomic nervous system, and hypothalamic pituitary dysfunction (Smith et al. 2011).

Smith and colleagues (2011) provided an in-depth review of the evidence supporting the pathophysiology of fibromyalgia, which is worth reviewing. They discussed evidence pointing to why there may be an amplification of pain and sensory-processing centers in CSS patients. They posited that an imbalance exists between the release and reuptake of neurotransmitters in the central nervous system, which is responsible for increasing the sensitivity, or "gain," of the pain and sensory-processing centers, thereby facilitating central sensitization to occur. The hyperactivity or increased volume of the pain and sensory-processing centers may in part explain why fibromyalgia patients experience widespread chronic pain and subsequently a poorer quality of life than those who do not have the condition.

Historically, the predominant therapy for treating fibromyalgia, or CSS, has been pharmacological. Pharmacological therapies showing promise include: tricyclic antidepressants, selective serotonin reuptake inhibitors, serotonin-norepinephrine reuptake inhibitors, and alpha-2-delta ligands such as gabapentin and pregabalin, gamma-hydroxybutyrate, and tizanidine (Smith et al.

2011). The central purpose of these pharmacological compounds is to regulate and reestablish the balance between neurotransmitter release and reuptake. However, many patients seek a nonpharmacological approach to treating CSS. PRT may be an excellent one because of its ability to decrease afferent sensory reflexes, pain, and sensory amplification by reducing gamma gain at the third-order neuronal level. How PRT affects neurotransmitter release and reuptake has not yet been established, and to date, no studies have examined its use as a primary therapy intervention for the treatment of fibromyalgia.

Salient PRT and Fibromyalgia Research Findings

- Imaging studies reveal that fibromyalgia patients are hypersensitive to all sensory stimuli, including sensory pressure and auditory, heat, cold, and electrical stimuli.
- Fibromyalgia patients demonstrate an increased sensitivity, or gain, to painful pressure.
- Those with fibromyalgia show elevated cerebrospinal fluid levels of pronociceptive neurotransmitters such as substance P, glutamate, nerve growth factor, and brain-derived neurotrophic factor and decreased levels of serotonin, norepinephrine, and dopamine.
- CSS patients show a strong genetic and familial predisposition.
- CSS patients do not experience significant pain relief with endogenous opioids.
- CSS patients may possess a metabolic or nutritional deficiency.
- A multifaceted approach to treatment should be pursued, consisting of pharmacological therapy, education, mild to moderate exercise, cognitive behavioral therapy, and PRT.

My clinical experience with fibromyalgia patients suggests that many of them fall somewhere on the somatic dysfunction spectrum with varying degrees of symptomology and impairment. Moreover, many CSS patients report an early trauma in life that caused what they believe is a spreading of pain throughout the body. However, some patients also report an underlying disease condition that they believe may have caused the condition, such as Lyme disease or irritable bowel syndrome. Typically, CSS patients fall into one of two prognostic categories: those whose somatic dysfunction resolves with treatment and those whose condition does not resolve but their quality of life does with treatment. The disease or somatic condition of people in the latter category often does not resolve because of an underlying trigger or disease condition that cannot be treated, such as an autoimmune dysfunction. Therefore, when working with CSS patients or those diagnosed as having fibromyalgia, clinicians should perform a thorough investigation into the factors that may have precipitated the condition as well as its maintenance.

CLINICIAN THERAPEUTIC INTERVENTIONS
Fibromyalgia

- Perform a thorough history and diagnostic workup to identify causative or perpetuating factors for the patient's condition.
- Consider requesting a blood chemical profile to identify any nutritional deficiencies.
- Assess and document the patient's quality of sleep and pain and fatigue levels throughout the assessment and treatment process.
- Use a multimodal treatment approach consisting of manual, behavioral, nutritional, and pharmacological therapy coupled with progressive therapeutic exercise and stress management interventions.
- Assess and treat the patient's somatic dysfunction according to the area of concentration and the level of intensity. However, also consider the 18 designated fibromyalgia tender point locations identified in the 1990 ACR criteria as key areas for treatment.
- Palliative modalities such as heat, cold, and light massage may be helpful for those who cannot tolerate deep manipulative stimuli. For patients who cannot tolerate these palliative modalities, focus on the application of PRT until pain and sensory amplification has diminished; then implement these complementary modalities for further pain control and healing.

Summary

Although PRT is a safe, nonpainful, and passive modality for the treatment of somatic dysfunction, each patient and special population requires modifications to the application of the therapy. More important, internal and external factors must be taken into account such as age, level of physical activity, surgical history, body composition, disability, and underlying disease or comorbidities because they may affect the assessment and treatment of the condition. Some underlying disease states may not be remedied through therapeutic, surgical, or pharmacological interventions, but many of the somatic conditions discussed in this chapter possess underlying triggers or mechanisms that, if addressed, will help to resolve the patient's condition. A prime example is obesity. It is accepted that being overweight or obese perpetuates a host of injury and disease conditions (Ellulu et al. 2014). For example, the obese are at greater risk for the development of knee osteoarthritis (Blagojevic et al. 2010), type 2 diabetes (Toivanen et al. 2010), headache (Chai et al. 2014), breast cancer (Jemal et al. 2011), rheumatoid arthritis (Finckh and Turesson 2014), and chronic pain (Vincent et al. 2012). If the therapist can help the patient address his obesity, then many of the associated conditions will also be addressed. However, by the time chronic pain patients seek treatment, they often possess widespread pain and a poor quality of life, typical of the ACR 1990 definition of fibromyalgia. These patients are often in too much pain to engage in exercise, even of light intensity, as a result of worn-out joints, pain, weakness, or fatigue. The balancing act the clinician must perform is to reduce the patient's somatic dysfunction with PRT and complementary therapies while addressing underlying disease(s) and trigger(s) without further aggravating the condition.

The list of special populations that may benefit from PRT presented in this chapter is not exhaustive. However, all typically show signs of pain and sensory amplification resulting from central sensitization that negatively affects their quality of life. What may first be a simple ankle sprain may over time develop into fibromyalgia, resulting in widespread pain, fatigue, and sleep disturbance. The clinical presentation of fibromyalgia may be one of many somatic dysfunctions on a spectrum of chronic pain disorders that share a similar pathogenesis among all populations and age groups irrespective of diagnosis. With this in mind, clinicians must address somatic dysfunction early and correct structural and mechanical abnormalities as well as precipitating factors such as nutritional, hormonal, and physical activity issues to prevent somatic dysfunction from becoming widespread.

PRT Techniques by Anatomical Area

Part II presents therapeutic techniques for the lower quarter, pelvis, spine, upper quarter, and cranium. The foot is divided into dorsal and plantar structures, and the pelvis is divided into anterior and posterior structures. The spine is organized according to orientation: cervical, thoracic, and lumbar. In the upper quarter, the shoulder, wrist, and hand are divided into anterior and posterior structures, and the elbow and forearm are divided into anterior, medial, lateral, and posterior structures. Cranial therapy is divided into osseous and muscular structures. Structures' origins, insertions, actions, and innervations, if applicable, are presented to help practitioners determine the origin of the lesion. Additionally, instructions for locating and palpating structures are provided coupled with clinician procedures for treatment with positional release therapy (PRT). The terms *near* and *far* are used to direct the clinician to the hand to use for application of the PRT treatments. The near hand is the hand closest to the treatment site or tissue, and the far hand is the farthest away from the treatment site or tissue. When possible, instructions for patient self-treatment are included. Common injury conditions are also presented for each body region to guide practitioners in treating them with PRT. The myofascial scanning and mapping documentation forms in the appendix can help practitioners capture and map evaluation and treatment outcomes as well as identify myofascial lesion patterns so that they can form individualized treatment road maps.

CHAPTER 4

Foot

CHAPTER OBJECTIVES

After reading this chapter, you should be able to do the following:

1. Identify the factors that may influence the development of somatic dysfunction at the foot.

2. Locate and palpate foot structures to be treated with positional release therapy (PRT).

3. Apply PRT techniques to treat the foot.

4. Appreciate how common injury conditions such as plantar fasciitis may be treated based on myofascial lesion patterns.

The incidence of lower-quarter injury in athletic and recreational populations is staggering, as is its potential economic cost. Shibuya and colleagues (2014) reported that 280,933 foot and ankle fractures and dislocations occurred in the United States between 2007 and 2011. Of those, 92.74% were non-work-related; 55.7% occurred at the ankle, and the greatest number occurred in the foot at the metatarsals (12.5%). Given the magnitude of fracture alone, it is not surprising that one in five middle-aged to older Americans suffers from foot pain (Thomas et al. 2011). Although extrinsic factors such as skill level, shoe type, and playing surface are important to take into account when evaluating a patient presenting with lower-quarter injury and somatic dysfunction, potentially modifiable intrinsic factors such as anatomical alignment, muscle tightness, range of motion, and strength and tissue imbalance may have the greatest potential to be influenced by PRT. The literature review by Murphy, Connolly, and Beynnon (2003) revealed little consensus among prospective studies on these factors; however, the literature suggests that these factors may play a role in the predisposition of lower-extremity (LE) injury and possibly the development of somatic dysfunction. It would stand to reason that if somatic dysfunction reduces strength, as seen in the Wong and Schauer-Alvarez hip study (2004), then it could also affect the stability and function of the lower-extremity articulations and tissues, specifically at the foot.

However, the hip articulation is not the only driver of kinematic movement in the lower extremity. The role of distal kinematics and foot type or posture for the predisposition of lower-quarter injuries such as Achilles tendinopathy, patellofemoral syndrome, medial tibial stress syndrome (MTSS), and iliotibial band friction syndrome has received considerable attention (Dowling et al. 2014; Neal et al. 2014). However, most foot studies are retrospective and involve the analysis of static foot posture, which may lack clinical relevance once the patient ambulates (Dowling et al. 2014).

A long-standing theoretical assumption has been that an increased navicular drop, or a "flat foot posture," increases the risk for MTSS, and that a high arch, or pes cavus foot, increases limb stiffness. Both foot postures are thought to increase the risk of lower-extremity injury (Neal et al. 2014; Tong and Kong 2013). However, foot posture assessment methods such as the navicular drop test and foot posture index have resulted in mixed causation findings (Neal et al. 2013). It is possible that these assessment methods are not sensitive enough to detect dynamic changes when the patient ambulates (Dowling et al. 2014).

To date, systematic reviews of foot posture, either static or dynamic, have yielded only limited evidence to support the association between altered foot posture and the risk for lower-quarter injury. However, Neal and colleagues (2014) reported strong evidence for an increased risk of MTSS among patients with a static pronated foot posture with very limited evidence of a propensity for patellofemoral pain. As well, Dowling and colleagues (2014) found very limited evidence that dynamic foot function is a risk factor for the development of lower-extremity injury. The authors did indicate that the clinical assessment of lower-quarter kinematics was a significant challenge because most clinicians lack access to sophisticated kinematic analysis technology as well as expertise in using it and interpreting the outcomes. Kinematic research findings thus may not be clinically relevant based on the multifactorial nature of lower-quarter injury and the difficulty of assessment in the clinical environment. However, age and body composition are easily assessed in the clinical environment.

As discussed in chapter 3, the older population may be more susceptible to injury as a result of the aging process. According to Hill and colleagues (2008), foot injury afflicts more than 30% of the aged population, which has been associated with falls (Spink et al. 2011). In a systematic review, losses in strength, range of motion, balance, and flexibility were assessed as potential risk factors that could be mitigated by the use of a foot and ankle (FA) exercise intervention program. Investigators, however, found only limited evidence to support the use of an FA exercise intervention program to reduce the risk of falling in this population. Significant improvements occurred only in balance and flexibility (Schwenk et al. 2013), which may improve foot function and reduce the risk of falling.

Obese patients may be more susceptible to osteoarthritis from increased joint loading. Abnormal foot function has also been observed in the obese population (Butterworth et al. 2014). The authors found among the obese strong associations among decreased balance, increased dynamic pronation, and increased plantar pressure during ambulation. However, because of methodological variations in the assessment of foot structure across studies, a direct relationship between body composition (fat

Common Anatomical Areas and Conditions for PRT

- Fibromyalgia
- Sprains and strains
- Osteoarthritis

- Tendinopathy
- Bursitis

Dorsal Structures

- Lisfranc sprain
- Morton's neuroma
- Osteoarthritis

- Dorsal compression syndrome
- Turf toe

Plantar Structures

- Plantar fasciitis
- Metatarsalgia
- Morton's neuroma

- Sesamoiditis
- Bone spur

mass) and foot structure was not possible. Butterworth and colleagues (2013) posited that foot pain experienced in the obese population may be the result not only of altered foot mechanics but also of "metabolic and inflammatory mediators produced by adipose tissue" (p. 7), which, if coupled, may create somatic dysfunction of the lower quarter in this population.

In my clinical observation of thousands of patients who have presented with lower-quarter somatic dysfunction, the majority of lesions are the result of compensatory biomechanical loading patterns such as prolonged stance pronation, weak hip abductors, leg length discrepancy, muscle imbalance, excessive weight, and prior injury. The somatic or myofascial lesion patterns often manifest from either a functional or structural abnormality, which overloads the tissues; the tissues respond by forming osteopathic lesions in defense.

However, it is imperative that therapists consider other triggers in the assessment process to identify and address any underlying disease process, visceral facilitation, or neurological derangement.

Unfortunately, at this time scant literature exists examining the effect of PRT on lower-extremity intrinsic and extrinsic factors in isolation or in combination. The body of PRT literature has tended to focus on facial, spinal, pelvic, and upper-quarter painful conditions (Wong 2012).

Positional release therapy research is starting to gain a footing on explaining how the therapy provides significant pain relief and correction of somatic dysfunction. However, until the gaps in the PRT literature are filled, clinical experience and feedback from patients about what they value from their clinical experience with PRT will inform the positional release therapist about how to approach lower-quarter somatic dysfunction.

Dorsal Interossei

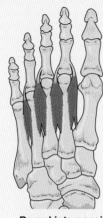

Dorsal interossei

The dorsal interossei are bipennate muscles, each with two heads. Their action occurs relative to the midline of the foot (second digit). Although the majority of the intrinsic lumbrical muscles lie on the plantar aspect of the foot, they may be indirectly palpated along with the dorsal interossei as a group between the metatarsal bones.

Origin:	Metatarsal bones (1-4)
Insertion:	First: Medial surface of the second proximal phalange and extensor digitorum tendons
	Second to fourth: Proximal phalanges and extensor digitorum tendons
Action:	Toe abduction and metatarsophalangeal (MP) joint extension
Innervation:	S2-S3 (lateral plantar nerve)

Palpation Procedure

- Place the foot in a relaxed position.
- Stabilize the plantar aspect of the forefoot with one hand.
- With the other hand, apply moderate pressure between the metatarsals with the fingers.
- Palpate the entire length of the dorsal interossei along the metatarsal shaft.
- Note the location of any tender points or fasciculatory response along the muscle.
- Once you have determined the most dominant tender point or fasciculation (or both), maintain light pressure with the pad(s) of the finger(s) at the location throughout the PRT treatment procedure until reassessment has occurred.

PRT Clinician Procedure

- The patient is prone with the knee flexed to 90° and the shin supported with either your thigh or a bolster.
- With the ulnar aspect of your far hand or forearm, apply downward compression over the forefoot, moving the ankle into dorsiflexion.
- Use the fingers of your near hand to assess and monitor the treatment position and fasciculatory response.
- Apply eversion and inversion of the forefoot with your far hand or forearm (a greater amount of inversion for the first through third metatarsals and eversion for the fourth and fifth metatarsals).
- Alternate: Grasp the lateral forefoot with your far hand for positioning and force application.
- Corollary tissues treated: Metatarsals

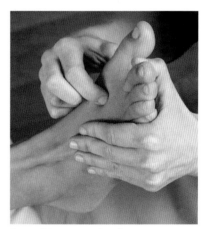

Dorsal interossei palpation procedure.

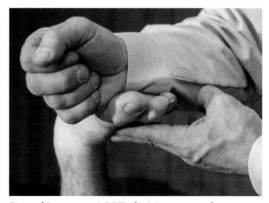

Dorsal interossei PRT clinician procedure.

 See video 4.1 for the dorsal interossei PRT procedure.

Cuneiforms

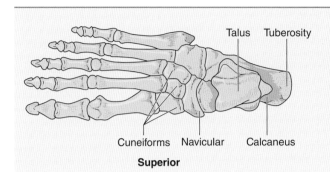

Superior

Three cuneiforms comprise the midfoot. Each lies behind its respective metatarsal (the first cuneiform behind the first metatarsal, and so on), and all communicate with the navicular bone. The first cuneiform serves as an attachment site for the tibialis anterior and tibialis posterior muscles. The cuneiforms are a common site of midfoot ligament sprains.

Palpation Procedure

- Place the foot in slight dorsiflexion to relax the extensor structures of the dorsal foot.
- Palpate the shaft of the first metatarsal up to its proximal base.
- Glide your fingers just over the joint space or valley between the first metatarsal proximal base and the first cuneiform.
- Moving medially onto the second, or middle, cuneiform, you will feel a distinct rise as you gain the ridge of the second cuneiform.
- Continue to slide your fingers laterally off the ridge of the middle cuneiform and into the next valley, where you will find the third, or lateral, cuneiform behind the third metatarsal.
- Note the location of any tender points or fasciculatory response between and over the cuneiforms.
- Once you have determined the most dominant tender point or fasciculation (or both), maintain light pressure with the pad(s) of the finger(s) at the location throughout the PRT treatment procedure until reassessment has occurred.

PRT Clinician Procedure

- The patient is prone with the knee flexed to 90° and the shin supported with either your thigh or a bolster.
- With your far hand or forearm, apply downward compression over the midfoot, moving the ankle into dorsiflexion.
- Apply eversion and inversion of the midfoot with your far hand or forearm (greater inversion for the first and second cuneiforms, less for the third) for fine-tuning.
- Alternate: Grasp the midfoot with your far hand for positioning.
- Corollary tissues treated: Cuneiform interosseous ligaments and talus

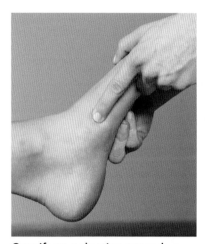

Cuneiform palpation procedure.

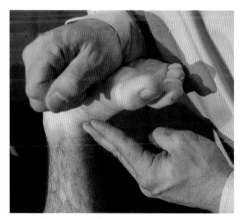

Cuneiform PRT clinician procedure.

Talus

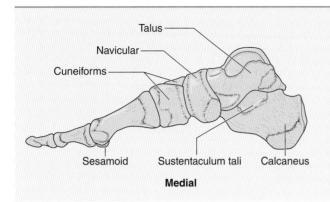

Talus
Navicular
Cuneiforms
Sesamoid
Sustentaculum tali
Calcaneus
Medial

The talus is a cube-shaped bone with a body, neck, and head configuration. The posterior portion of the talus is narrower than the front, and when the ankle is dorsiflexed, a wedge is formed within the talocrural joint. This moves the ankle into a closed-pack position, increasing the stability of the ankle and limiting inversion and eversion.

Palpation Procedure

- Place the ankle in a relaxed open-pack position (plantar flexion).
- Place your fingers at the center of the ankle joint at the level of the malleoli between the extensor tendons. This location is over the anterior dome of the talus.
- While palpating on the bony surface of the talus, move the ankle through dorsiflexion and plantar flexion to feel the roll of the anterior dome.
- The medial and lateral heads of the talus can be palpated by sliding the fingers in either direction from its anterior dome. To expose each head more fully, invert the foot to expose the lateral head and apply eversion to expose the medial head. Also, the medial head is located just proximal to the navicular tubercle.
- Note the location of any tender points or fasciculatory response over the talus.
- Once you have determined the most dominant tender point or fasciculation (or both), maintain light pressure with the pad(s) of the finger(s) at the location throughout the PRT treatment procedure until reassessment has occurred.

PRT Clinician Procedure

- The patient is prone with the knee flexed between 60 and 90° and the shin supported with either your thigh or a bolster.
- Grasp the calcaneus with your far hand and apply compression downward while moving the ankle into dorsiflexion.
- Apply inversion, eversion, and rotation with your far hand to fine-tune the treatment location.
- Corollary tissues treated: Extensor digitorum tendons

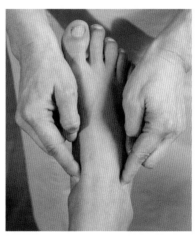

Talus palpation procedure.

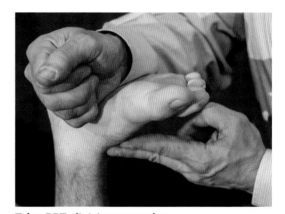

Talus PRT clinician procedure.

Extensor Digitorum Longus Tendons

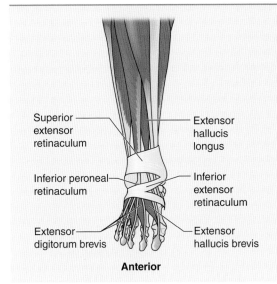

Superior extensor retinaculum

Extensor hallucis longus

Inferior peroneal retinaculum

Inferior extensor retinaculum

Extensor digitorum brevis

Extensor hallucis brevis

Anterior

The four extensor digitorum longus tendons are lateral to the extensor hallucis longus tendons on the dorsal foot and come together proximal to the ankle joint to form the common tendon of the extensor digitorum longus muscle. This muscle is sandwiched between the tibialis anterior and peroneal muscles.

Origin: Lateral tibial condyle, upper three quarters of the medial shaft of the fibula, interosseous membrane, deep crural fascia

Insertion: Second through fifth middle and distal phalanges

Action: Extension of toes 2 through 5, ankle dorsiflexion (accessory), foot eversion (accessory)

Innervation: L5-S1 (deep peroneal nerve)

Palpation Procedure

- Place the ankle and foot in a relaxed but slightly dorsiflexed position.
- Ask the patient to dorsiflex the ankle and extend the toes to visibly bring out the extensor tendons.
- Either pince or strum over the tendons.
- Note the location of any tender points or fasciculatory response between and over the tendons.
- Once you have determined the most dominant tender point or fasciculation (or both), maintain light pressure with the pad(s) of the finger(s) at the location throughout the PRT treatment procedure until reassessment has occurred.

PRT Clinician Procedure

- The patient is prone with the knee flexed to 90° and the shin supported with either your thigh or a bolster.
- Grasp the calcaneus with your far hand and place the forearm of the same hand on the plantar foot with an emphasis on the second through fifth metatarsals, or rays.
- Move the foot into dorsiflexion and apply toe extension with forearm pressure.
- Apply eversion and inversion to the foot with your far forearm for fine-tuning.
- Corollary tissues treated: Cuneiform interosseous ligaments, extensor hallucis longus

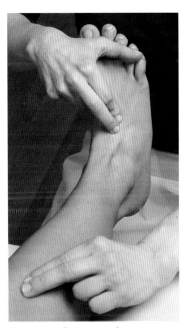

Extensor digitorum longus tendon palpation procedure.

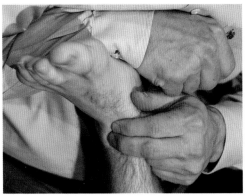

Extensor digitorum longus tendon PRT clinician procedure.

Extensor Digitorum Brevis

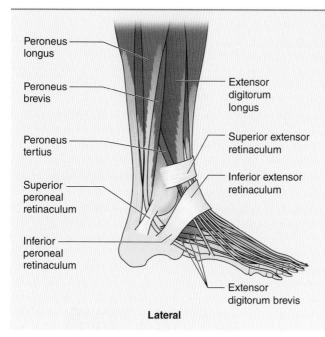

Peroneus longus

Peroneus brevis

Peroneus tertius

Superior peroneal retinaculum

Inferior peroneal retinaculum

Extensor digitorum longus

Superior extensor retinaculum

Inferior extensor retinaculum

Extensor digitorum brevis

Lateral

The extensor digitorum brevis muscle belly lies beneath the extensor digitorum longus tendons approximately 2 cm (about 3/4 in.) anterior to the lateral malleolus on the dorsolateral aspect of the foot. When the toes and ankle are extended, the small, round belly of this muscle becomes visible.

Origin: Dorsal surface of the calcaneus, lateral talocalcaneal ligament, inferior aspect of the extensor reti-naculum

Insertion: Second through fourth toes via the extensor tendon longus ten-dons. Some consider the extensor hallucis tendon a part of the extensor digitorum brevis.

Action: Second through fourth MP exten-sion, great toe MP extension

Innervation: L5-S1 (lateral branch of the deep peroneal nerve)

Palpation Procedure

- Place the ankle and foot in a relaxed but slightly dorsiflexed position.
- Move approximately 4 cm (1.5 in.) distal from the lateral malleolus toward the fifth toe while moving under the extensor tendons.
- Ask the patient to extend the toes and ankle along with eversion to bring the muscle belly of the extensor digitorum brevis out over the cuboid.
- Note the location of any tender points or fas-ciculatory response over the muscle.
- Once you have determined the most dominant tender point or fasciculation (or both), maintain light pressure with the pad(s) of the finger(s) at the location throughout the PRT treatment procedure until reassessment has occurred.

PRT Clinician Procedure

- The patient is prone with the knee flexed to 90° and the shin supported with either your thigh or a bolster.
- Grasp the heel with your far hand and place your wrist and forearm of the same hand on the plantar foot.
- Move the ankle into dorsiflexion and marked eversion with the far hand, wrist, and forearm.
- Rotate externally and apply a compressive force downward with the far hand, wrist, and forearm.

- Corollary tissues treated: Peroneal tendons

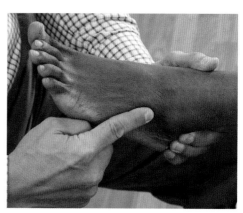

Extensor digitorum brevis palpation procedure.

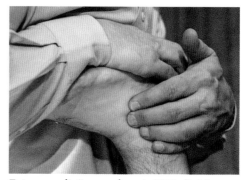

Extensor digitorum brevis PRT clinician procedure.

Plantar Aponeurosis

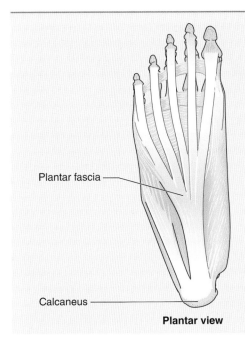

The plantar aponeurosis, also known as the plantar fascia, is a dense triangular avascular connective tissue that covers the majority of the foot's plantar muscles. The plantar fascia stabilizes the arch during ambulation.

Origin: Plantar aspect of the calcaneus. The central portion originates at the medial calcaneal tubercle, which is a common site for irritation.

Insertion: Proximal phalanx on each side of the toes

Action: Stabilizes the arch through the windlass mechanism; assists in stabilizing the calcaneus during push-off during the gait cycle

Innervation: S1-S2 (tibial nerve, medial and lateral branches)

Plantar fascia

Calcaneus

Plantar view

Palpation Procedure

- Place the patient in a prone position with the foot in a relaxed position.
- Ask the patient to pull the big toe toward the shin to accentuate the fibers of the plantar aponeurosis for palpation.
- Strum across the aponeurosis with firm pressure from its distal insertions to its proximal origin at the medial calcaneus.
- Note the location of any tender points or fasciculatory response of the tissue, particularly at its origin at the calcaneus.
- Once you have determined the most dominant tender point or fasciculation (or both), maintain light pressure with the pad(s) of the finger(s) at the location throughout the PRT treatment procedure until reassessment has occurred.

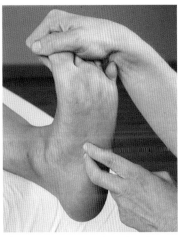

Plantar aponeurosis palpation procedure.

> continued

Plantar Aponeurosis > *continued*

PRT Clinician Procedure

- The patient is prone with knee flexed to ~60° and the shin supported with either your thigh or a bolster.
- Place the toes in the sulcus of your dominant shoulder to promote phalangeal flexion.
- Move the ankle into marked plantar flexion with your far hand.
- Apply calcaneal caudal traction with the far hand.
- Apply calcaneal eversion or inversion based on the location of the lesion with the far hand.
- Also with the far hand, apply calcaneal internal or external rotation based on the location of the lesion.
- Corollary tissues treated: Quadratus plantae, flexor digitorum brevis, flexor digitorum longus

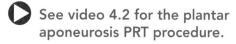 See video 4.2 for the plantar aponeurosis PRT procedure.

Patient Self-Treatment Procedure

- If there is adequate flexibility at the knee and hip, place the foot on the opposite thigh. If there is not enough flexibility to accomplish this positioning, place the foot on the opposite shin.
- Grasp the dorsal forefoot and toes, moving them into flexion and abduction with a cupping or cradling mechanism.
- Place the fingers of the other hand over the anterior aspect of the ankle and the thumb of the same hand at the back of the heel.
- While flexing and compressing the forefoot and toes inward, translate the calcaneus toward the toes to encourage relaxation of the plantar fascia. If a finger of either hand can reach the area of tenderness, place it over this area to ascertain the fasciculatory response of the tissue.

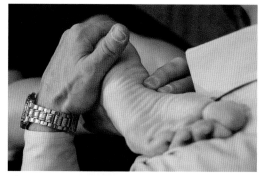

Plantar aponeurosis PRT clinician procedure.

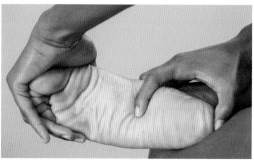

Plantar aponeurosis patient self-treatment procedure.

Flexor Hallucis Brevis

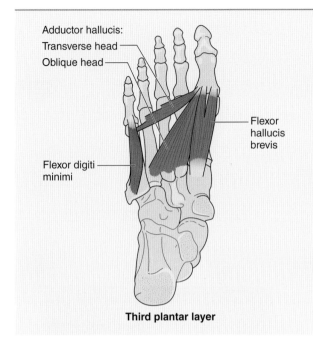

Adductor hallucis:
Transverse head
Oblique head

Flexor digiti minimi

Flexor hallucis brevis

Third plantar layer

The plantar muscles are arranged in four layers from superficial to deep based on the covering of them by the plantar fascia; the longer muscles are closer to the fascia. Even though the flexor hallucis brevis muscle is located within the deep third layer, its contraction can be palpated by having the patient flex the big toe against resistance.

Origin: Plantar cuboid and third cuneiform surfaces, posterior tibialis tendon, medial intermuscular septum

Insertion: Medial and lateral surfaces of the proximal phalanx of the first toe

Action: First toe MP flexion and abduction

Innervation: S1-S2 (medial plantar nerve)

Palpation Procedure

- The patient is prone with the foot in a relaxed position.
- Strum across the flexor hallucis brevis proximal to the first metatarsal head, moving toward the plantar navicular.
- Note the location of any tender points or fasciculatory response of the muscle.
- Once you have determined the most dominant tender point or fasciculation (or both), maintain light pressure with the pad(s) of the finger(s) at the location throughout the PRT treatment procedure until reassessment has occurred.

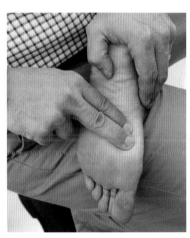

Flexor hallucis brevis palpation procedure.

> continued

Flexor Hallucis Brevis > *continued*

PRT Clinician Procedure

- Place the toes and forefoot in the sulcus of your hip to promote phalangeal flexion.
- Place the ankle in marked plantar flexion.
- Apply calcaneal caudal traction with your far hand while placing the forefinger of the same hand over the flexor hallucis brevis, if possible.
- Place the first metatarsal into plantar flexion with your near hand while applying inward rotation.
- Both hands can apply a valgus force using the fore- and hindfoot for fine-tuning.
- Corollary tissues treated: Plantar fascia, quadratus plantae, flexor digitorum brevis and longus, flexor hallucis longus, plantar interossei, lumbricals

 See video 4.3 for the flexor hallucis brevis PRT procedure.

Patient Self-Treatment Procedure

Use the plantar fascia self-treatment with the exception of emphasizing first metatarsal plantar flexion and rotation.

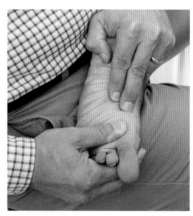

Flexor hallucis brevis PRT clinician procedure.

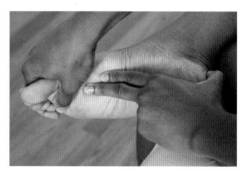

Flexor hallucis brevis patient self-treatment procedure.

Abductor Hallucis

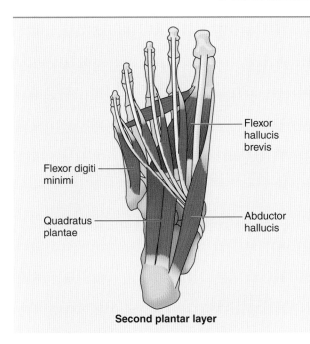

Flexor hallucis brevis

Flexor digiti minimi

Quadratus plantae

Abductor hallucis

Second plantar layer

The abductor hallucis muscle helps to form the medial arch of the foot and is one of the plantar muscles that is most easily palpable. Some people can abduct the great toe, which brings out the abductor hallucis' distinct muscle belly.

Origin: Medial calcaneal tuberosity, plantar aponeurosis, flexor retinaculum

Insertion: Base of the medial side of the first proximal phalanx, medial sesamoid, flexor hallucis brevis tendon

Action: Big toe MP abduction and flexion

Innervation: S1-S2 (medial plantar nerve)

Palpation Procedure

- Place the foot in relaxed plantar-flexed position off the end of the treatment table or on your thigh.
- Palpate the bulk of this muscle at the posterior aspect of the medial heel and trace it forward to the big toe.
- Plantar flexion of the big toe against resistance will bring out the muscle belly for palpation.
- Note the location of any tender points or fasciculatory response at the muscle and its attachments.
- Once you have determined the most dominant tender point or fasciculation (or both), maintain light pressure with the pad(s) of the finger(s) at the location throughout the PRT treatment procedure until reassessment has occurred.

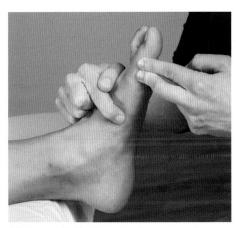

Abductor hallucis palpation procedure.

> continued

Abductor Hallucis > *continued*

PRT Clinician Procedure

- The patient is prone with the knee flexed to ~60° and the ankle on your thigh.
- Place the ankle in marked plantar flexion.
- Grasp the heel with your near hand and the forefoot with your far hand to apply a valgus force at the midfoot.
- Use a finger from either hand to monitor the tissue lesion.
- While applying the valgus force, invert the heel with your near hand.
- Apply compression of the calcaneus toward the toes with your near hand.
- Rotate the first ray into flexion and internal rotation with your far hand.
- Corollary tissues treated: Plantar navicular, plantar fascia, quadratus plantae, flexor digitorum brevis and longus, flexor hallucis longus, plantar interossei, lumbricals

Patient Self-Treatment Procedure

Use the self-treatment procedure for the plantar fascia, but focus on inverting the calcaneus while applying a valgus force at the forefoot while rotating the first ray into flexion and internal rotation.

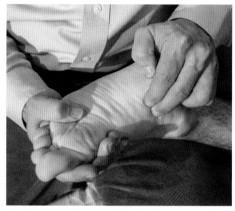

Abductor hallucis PRT clinician procedure.

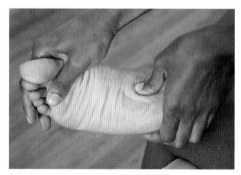

Abductor hallucis patient self-treatment procedure.

Abductor Digiti Minimi

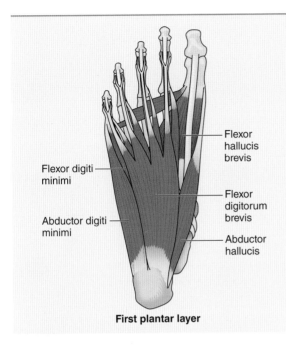

Flexor hallucis brevis

Flexor digiti minimi

Abductor digiti minimi

Flexor digitorum brevis

Abductor hallucis

First plantar layer

The abductor digiti minimi is a superficial muscle that lies along the lateral border of the foot. Its orientation along the fifth toe and metatarsal allows it to both flex and abduct the fifth toe.

Origin:	Lateral and medial calcaneal processes of the tuberosity, plantar aponeurosis, intermuscular septum
Insertion:	Lateral aspect at the base of the fifth proximal phalanx
Action:	Abducts the big toe, flexes the fifth MP
Innervation:	S1-S3 (lateral plantar nerve)

Palpation Procedure

- Place the foot in a relaxed plantar-flexed position off the end of the treatment table or on your thigh.
- Palpate this muscle between the lateral heel and lateral plantar surface of the fifth toe.
- Abduction and flexion of the fifth toe against resistance will accentuate the contraction of this muscle for palpation.
- Note the location of any tender points or fasciculatory response of the muscle and its attachments.
- Once you have determined the most dominant tender point or fasciculation (or both), maintain light pressure with the pad(s) of the finger(s) at the location throughout the PRT treatment procedure until reassessment has occurred.

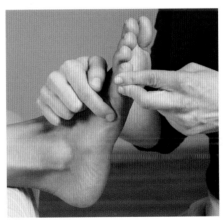

Abductor digiti minimi palpation procedure.

> continued

Abductor Digiti Minimi > *continued*

PRT Clinician Procedure

- Position the patient prone with the ankle flexed on your thigh.
- Place the ankle in slight plantar flexion.
- With your near hand at the forefoot, grasp the heel with your other hand and use a finger from either hand to monitor the lesion.
- Apply compression of the heel toward the toes with your far hand to promote phalangeal flexion.
- Using both hands, apply a varus force to the midfoot by adducting the forefoot and hindfoot (the fifth ray should approximate toward the calcaneus).
- Internally rotate the forefoot with the near hand for fine-tuning.
- Corollary tissues treated: Plantar cuboid, plantar fascia, quadratus plantae, flexor digitorum longus

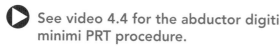 See video 4.4 for the abductor digiti minimi PRT procedure.

Patient Self-Treatment Procedure

Use the self-treatment procedure for the plantar fascia, but focus on compressing the heel toward the toes while flexing, adducting, and rotating the forefoot towards the heel.

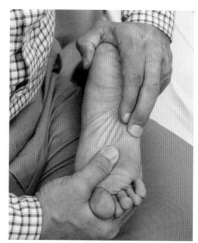

Abductor digiti minimi PRT clinician procedure.

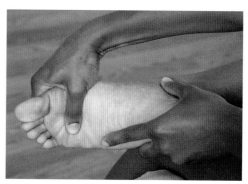

Abductor digiti minimi patient self-treatment procedure.

Plantar Interossei and Lumbricals

The plantar interossei and lumbricals are deep intrinsic muscles that lie on the plantar surface of the metatarsals rather than between them, as seen with the dorsal interossei. They have been grouped here because the PRT treatment of these muscles affects the release of both. Deep palpation over these structures elicits their tenderness, and their fasciculation will be felt during treatment.

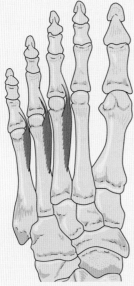

Plantar interossei

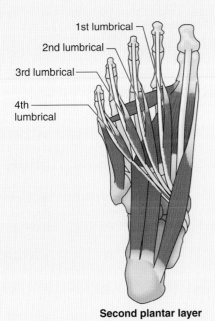

1st lumbrical
2nd lumbrical
3rd lumbrical
4th lumbrical

Second plantar layer

Origin: Plantar interossei: Plantar surface of the third through fifth metatarsals

Lumbricals: Flexor digitorum longus tendon

Insertion: Plantar interossei: Medial side of the proximal phalange of the same toe, dorsal digital expansion

Lumbricals: Proximal second through fifth phalanges, dorsal expansion of the extensor digitorum longus tendons

Action: Plantar interossei: Third through fifth toe adduction, MP flexion; assists interphalangeal (IP) extension

Lumbricals: Second through fifth metacarpal phalangeal (MP) flexion; assists proximal interphalangeal (PIP) and distal interphalangeal (DIP) extension

Innervation: Plantar interossei: S2-S3 (lateral plantar nerve)

First lumbrical: L5-S1 (medial plantar nerve)

Second through fourth lumbricals: S2-S3 (deep branch of the lateral plantar nerve)

> continued

Plantar Interossei and Lumbricals > *continued*

Palpation Procedure

- Place the foot in a relaxed plantar-flexed position off the end of the treatment table or on your thigh.
- Palpate the density or firmness of the muscle contraction for these tissues over the plantar surfaces of the metatarsals while the patient flexes the toes against resistance.
- Note the location of any tender points or fasciculatory response of the muscles and over the metatarsal shafts.
- Once you have determined the most dominant tender point or fasciculation (or both), maintain light pressure with the pad(s) of the finger(s) or the thumbs at the location throughout the PRT treatment procedure until reassessment has occurred.

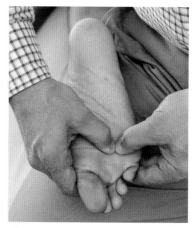

Plantar interossei and lumbricals palpation procedure.

PRT Clinician Procedure

- The patient is prone with the knee flexed to ~60° with the ankle on your thigh.
- Cup the forefoot with your far hand while resting the dorsum of the foot on your thigh in maximal plantar flexion while your near hand monitors the lesion.
- Compress the metatarsal shafts together with your far hand while applying toe flexion.
- Apply rotation for fine-tuning with the far hand.
- Corollary tissues treated: Flexor digitorum brevis and longus, flexor hallucis longus and brevis

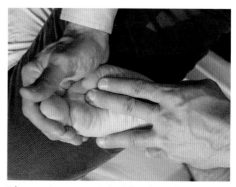

Plantar interossei and lumbricals PRT clinician procedure.

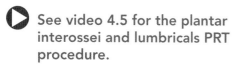 See video 4.5 for the plantar interossei and lumbricals PRT procedure.

Patient Self-Treatment Procedure

- Use the self-treatment procedure for the plantar fascia, but do not translate the heel toward the toes.
- The focus of the positioning should be on compressing the metatarsal shafts toward one another while applying toe flexion and rotation.

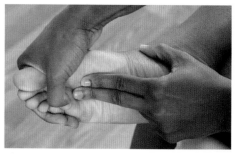

Plantar interossei and lumbricals patient self-treatment procedure.

Metatarsalgia

Metatarsalgia, or forefoot pain, is considered a symptom of another condition in the foot, such as Morton's neuroma (Bauer et al. 2014). The condition can be acute as a result of high-impact activities, but it typically results from an overload of the plantar foot structures over time from kinetic chain compensation. The clinician must first determine and address the causative factors for this condition to ensure that the releases are sustained. If the foot continues to be irritated, the tissue lesions will likely return.

Common Signs and Symptoms

- Pain at and between the metatarsal heads
- Point tenderness over and between the metatarsal heads
- Decreased ability to bear weight on the affected structures

Common Differential Diagnoses

- Morton's neuroma
- Sesamoid fracture
- Metatarsal stress fracture
- Hallucis rigidis

Clinician Therapeutic Interventions

- Determine the root of the patient's condition (e.g., faulty biomechanics, particularly at the first and second metatarsals, plantar warts, leg length discrepancy, training alteration, surface change, shoe alteration).
- Consider requesting a radiograph or MRI to rule out fracture and nerve impingement at the forefoot and midfoot areas.
- Scan and treat the structures in the order presented in the Treatment Points and Sequencing box. However, base your treatment sequencing off the most dominant (tender) points first.
- Follow PRT with thermal ultrasound or laser, joint and/or neural mobilization, and myofascial massage.

Treatment Points and Sequencing

1. Plantar interossei and lumbricals
2. Flexor hallucis brevis
3. Plantar aponeurosis
4. Abductor hallucis
5. Abductor digiti minimi
6. Dorsal interossei
7. Posterior tibialis
8. Medial gastrocnemius
9. Soleus
10. Popliteus

- Implement open- and closed-chain strengthening for the intrinsic foot, pretibial, hip, and core muscles.
- Implement PNF stretching of the triceps surae complex and plantar foot tissues.
- Consider using a metatarsal pad to spread and elevate the metatarsals, but base its use on patient response.
- Address any other insulting factors or conditions.
- Slowly progress the patient to dynamic physical activity.

Patient Self-Treatment Interventions

- Perform self-release on a daily basis or when irritated.
- PNF stretch the plantar foot structures and triceps surae complex after exercise on a daily basis. Do not stretch if it produces pain because doing so may result in additional tissue lesions.
- Perform self-massage for five to eight minutes daily after stretching.
- Ice-massage the affected area when irritated. If greater relief occurs with heat, apply heat (e.g., warm whirlpool or Jacuzzi). (*Note:* Consult with the clinician about where you are in the healing process, which will determine whether to apply heat or ice.)

Plantar Fasciitis

When the arch is irritated, the engagement of the windlass mechanism places strain on the plantar tissues (Bolgla and Malone 2004), which can activate the myotatic reflex and reinitiate the inflammatory process. Therefore, the clinician must work to determine how best to limit reengagement of the myotatic reflex to prevent the patient from entering a chronic cycle of inflammation every time he takes a step or bears weight. Converse to the traditional therapeutic approach of using an aggressive stretching protocol to treat this condition, the PRT approach is to release the tissue lesions prior to stretching and to avoid causing pain with any therapeutic intervention because doing so often reengages the myotatic reflex and tissue lesions.

Common Signs and Symptoms

- Pain at the medial heel or within the arch (or both), particularly upon waking ambulation
- Sharp, burning pain upon landing or push-off, a dull constant pain at rest, or both
- Pain that subsides with the cessation of weight bearing

Common Differential Diagnoses

- Heel spur
- Posterior tarsal tunnel syndrome
- Calcaneal fracture

Clinician Therapeutic Interventions

- Determine the root of the patient's condition (e.g., faulty biomechanics, movement faults, heel spur, leg length discrepancy, training, surface, shoe alteration).
- Consider performing a biomechanical analysis to evaluate faulty mechanics that may be overloading the plantar fascia.
- Consider requesting a radiograph to rule out a heel spur or calcaneal fracture if the pain is located at the heel and has been chronic.
- Scan and treat the structures in the order presented in the Treatment Points and Sequencing box. However, base your treatment sequencing off the most dominant (tender) points first.

Treatment Points and Sequencing

1. Plantar aponeurosis
2. Flexor hallucis brevis
3. Plantar interossei and lumbricals
4. Dorsal interossei
5. Posterior tibialis
6. Medial gastrocnemius
7. Soleus
8. Popliteus
9. Semitendinosus
10. Pes anserine
11. Iliotibial band
12. Adductor magnus
13. Gluteus medius
14. Piriformis
15. Psoas

- Follow PRT with thermal ultrasound, PNF stretching, and myofascial massage of the plantar fascia.
- Using KT Tape or arch taping in the initial stage of rehabilitation helps to reduce pain in some patients.
- Apply instrumented soft-tissue mobilization (ISTM) if recalcitrant tissue adhesions are present.
- Implement open- and closed-chain strengthening for the intrinsic foot, pretibial, hip, and core muscles with a focus on controlling eccentric internal rotation during ambulation.
- Have the patient use temporary or custom orthotics initially and, most important, upon waking ambulation and throughout the day to prevent reirritation.
- Slowly progress the patient to dynamic physical activity.

Patient Self-Treatment Interventions

- Perform self-release on a daily basis or when irritated. Some patients report significant relief with self-release upon waking.
- Use a supportive sandal or shoe upon waking to flatten the arch when stepping out of bed.
- PNF stretch the plantar fascia and gastrocnemius soleus complex after exercise on a

daily basis. Do not stretch if it produces pain because doing so may result in additional tissue lesions.

- Use a night splint or plantar fasciitis sock if it helps.
- Perform self-massage for five to eight minutes daily after stretching.

- Ice-massage the plantar fascia on a stretch when irritated. If greater relief occurs with heat, apply heat (e.g., warm whirlpool or Jacuzzi). (*Note:* Consult with the clinician about where you are in the healing process, which will determine whether to apply heat or ice.)

Summary

Often, injury conditions of the lower quarter are a result of intrinsic and extrinsic factors, such as biomechanical or structural abnormalities, changes in footwear or playing surface, or weak proximal hip structures. Emerging evidence points to altered foot structure, age, and obesity as additional risk factors for foot pain and somatic dysfunction. Therefore, it is essential to evaluate for the influence of these and other causative factors. Clinicians must also consider proximal neurological conditions such as disc pathology or disease conditions that may present as typical lower-quarter painful conditions. Regardless of the origin of the condition, it is essential to determine the root of the somatic dysfunction. However, conditions of the foot, such as plantar fasciitis, are commonly the result of abnormal compensatory gait mechanics, which overload the capacity of the tissues to adapt. A thorough scanning and mapping procedure often reveals a pattern that can be correlated with the findings of a gait analysis and standard orthopedic examination.

CHAPTER 5

Ankle and Lower Leg

CHAPTER OBJECTIVES

After reading this chapter, you should be able to do the following:

1 Recall the factors that may influence the development of somatic dysfunction at the ankle and lower leg.

2 Locate and palpate ankle and lower-leg structures to be treated with positional release therapy (PRT).

3 Apply PRT techniques to treat the ankle and lower leg.

4 Demonstrate the ability to treat common injury conditions such as Achilles tendinopathy based on myofascial lesion patterns.

Injuries to the ankle and lower leg are common, and both initial and recurrent injury can pose long-term consequences. Smith, Harris, and Clauw (2011) proposed that even a simple ankle sprain early in life may trigger the development of fibromyalgia. Of all lower-quarter injuries that do occur, ankle sprain is the most common (Doherty et al. 2015; Swenson et al. 2013). A total of 3,140,132 ankle sprains were reported in the United States in 2010, an incidence of 2.15 per 1,000 (Waterman et al. 2010). More ankle sprains occurred in people between the ages of 10 and 19, and males 15 to 24 years old had the highest rate (Waterman et al. 2010).

The majority of ankle sprains (49.3%) occur during athletic activity, and most (41.1%) occur in basketball players (Waterman et al. 2010). A systematic review of American high school athletes (football, soccer, volleyball, basketball, wrestling, baseball, softball) between 2005/2006 and 2010/2011 revealed that athletic trainers (ATs) reported 1,370,545 ankle sprains, which accounted for 16.7% of all the injuries reported (Swenson et al. 2013). In contrast to Waterman's findings that ankle sprains occur more frequently among young males, Swenson and colleagues (2013) found that in gender-comparable sports such as soccer, girls were more likely (RR = 1.46) to sustain sprains than boys were. The authors proposed that girls may be more susceptible than boys to ankle sprain as a result of a lack of motor development, weak hip abductors, or a hormonal influence. Doherty and colleagues (2015) also found an elevated incidence of ankle sprain among females over males (13.6 vs. 6.94 per 1,000 exposures). The highest rate was found among children, and it decreased throughout the life span. Unlike Swenson and colleagues (2013), Doherty and colleagues (2015) believe that the differences seen in ankle sprain incidence between the sexes cannot be explained by neuromuscular, hormonal, or anatomical differences, but may be related more to training behavior. However, the most significant factor found for ankle sprain regardless of gender was a previous history of sprain; Swenson and colleagues (2013) reported that 15.7% of ankle sprains were recurrent.

The type of ankle sprain most often seen is the lateral, or inversion, ankle sprain, which is attributed to the lack of bony block to inversion and weak lateral ligaments (Doherty et al. 2015). Disability from ankle sprain results in time lost not only from athletic competition, but also from school, work, and military duty (Doherty et al. 2015). Recurrent sprains may produce chronic ankle instability (Doherty et al. 2015) and ankle joint osteoarthritis (Valderrabano et al. 2006). With the potential for the development of long-term sequelae of early-onset osteoarthritis and fibromyalgia, there is a critical need to address ankle injury early and to use preventive measures.

Once a fracture has been ruled out, it may be prudent to apply PRT to an ankle sprain as soon as possible to avoid the onset of somatic dysfunction, either in the field or at the emergency department (ED). In a prospective randomized control trial by Eisenhart, Gaeta, and Yens (2003), adults (N = 55) with an acute ankle sprain without fracture received a single session of osteopathic manipulative treatment (OMT) from an osteopathic physician in the ED. The treatment consisted of PRT (also called strain counterstrain), muscle energy, and joint manipulation. The OMT intervention group (n = 28) demonstrated a significant reduction of pain and swelling and improved range of motion over the control group that received standard care (ice, anti-inflammatories, and bracing). Of those returning for follow-up examination (75%) one week later, OMT patients demonstrated a significantly better range of motion than controls did. The authors attributed their finding to improved arthrokinematics of the ankle as a result of edema and pain reduction, which may have restored patients' functional anatomy more quickly. Therefore, it may be plausible that more OMT or manual therapy over a longer period of time would produce improved outcomes over a one-time application.

Cleland and colleagues (2013) examined whether the application of low- and high-velocity joint manipulations to the talocrural and proximal and distal tibiofibular joints by a physical therapist twice per week for four weeks would produce better functional outcomes and pain reduction over a home exercise program alone. Although those who received manual therapy did show greater improvement in pain and function at four weeks and at a six-month follow-up, the difference between the groups was not robust enough to indicate a significant minimal clinically important difference (MCID). However, at a six-month follow-up, the patients who received only home exercises showed double the rate of recurrence compared to those in the manual therapy and exercise group, although the finding was not statistically significant. Joint mobilization combined with exercise may appear to be more helpful than exercise alone for ankle sprain recovery, but the authors attributed the differences to a lack of compliance with the home exercise program, the therapeutic touch of the clinician, and a possible placebo effect given that no sham intervention was used.

Beyond acute trauma to the ankle mortise, cumulative trauma to the ankle and lower leg may result in chronic inflammatory conditions such as Achilles tendinopathy and medial tibial stress syndrome (MTSS), which may predispose people to stress fractures. Franklyn-Miller and colleagues noted in 2012 that lower-extremity injury rates for military recruits was approximately 20 to 50%, and the most frequent injury was lower-limb stress fractures (Zadpoor and Nikooyan 2011), compared to 25 to 65% among the nonmilitary running population. Nielsen and colleagues (2012) proposed that the majority of running-related injuries (RRIs), including lower-limb fractures and overuse injuries, are related not only to previous injury, but also to training error (novice runners committed the most errors). Although their systematic review findings were inconclusive in regard to the impact of training error on RRIs, Newman and colleagues (2013) found MTSS to be significantly related to fewer years of running experience.

A multitude of factors may pose an increased risk for the onset of ankle and lower-limb injury. Early preventive measures such as the reduction of training errors and improved hip abductor strength and proprioception could help curb the incidence of injury. However, because lower-limb injury will occur, the question is whether an early PRT intervention would help to reduce the time lost and improve therapeutic outcomes. Based on the ability of PRT to reduce pain, restore range of motion, improve strength, and potentially improve the perfusion of tissues, this would seem to be the case. However, research is needed on how PRT affects lower-leg and ankle injuries directly as well as how PRT integrates with other therapies for this body region to answer this question.

TREATMENT
Common Anatomical Areas and Conditions for PRT

Anterior Structures
- Exertional compartment syndrome
- High ankle sprain
- Nonacute contusion

Posterior Structures
- Exertional compartment syndrome
- Achilles tendinitis
- Retrocalcaneal bursitis
- Os trigonum

Medial Structures
- Tarsal tunnel syndrome
- Medial tibial stress syndrome

Lateral Structures
- Fibular head displacement
- Peroneal tendinitis
- Peroneal nerve entrapment

Tibialis Anterior Muscle

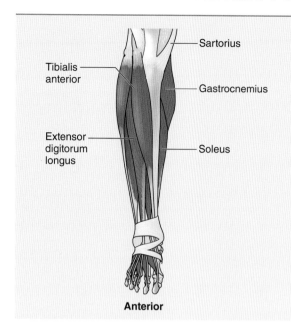

Sartorius
Tibialis anterior
Gastrocnemius
Extensor digitorum longus
Soleus

Anterior

The tibialis anterior muscle belly is located at the upper two thirds of the tibia and immediately lateral to its bony ridge. The tendon of this muscle, one of the most prominent of the foot, traverses medially across the ankle joint. The muscle and its tendinous orientation assists to slow foot and ankle pronation during the initial phases of gait.

Origin: Lateral tibial condyle and upper two thirds of the lateral tibial surface

Insertion: First (medial) cuneiform and the base of the first metatarsal

Action: Ankle dorsiflexion, foot inversion and adduction (supination) at the subtalar and midtarsal joints; supports the arch during ambulation

Innervation: L4-L5 and often S1 (deep peroneal nerve)

Palpation Procedure

- The patient can be placed supine or prone, but the tissue must be relaxed.
- Find the ridge, or tibial crest, of the tibia and move just laterally off of it at its upper two thirds to find the tibialis anterior muscle belly.
- Resistive ankle dorsiflexion with inversion will bring out the belly of the muscle under the fingers.
- Once found, strum across the muscle and then follow its course to its tendinous aspect.
- Note the location of any tender points or fasciculatory response at the muscle or tendon and their attachments.
- Once you have determined the most dominant tender point or fasciculation (or both), maintain light pressure with the pad(s) of the finger(s) at the location throughout the PRT treatment procedure until reassessment has occurred.

PRT Clinician Procedure

- The patient is prone with the knee flexed to 90° and the shin supported with either your thigh or a bolster.
- Move the ankle into plantar flexion and marked inversion with your far hand.
- Apply downward compression at the calcaneus with your far hand.

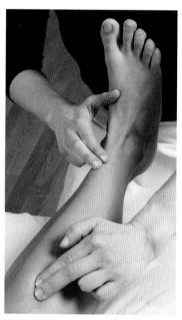

Tibialis anterior muscle palpation procedure.

- Externally rotate the calcaneus with your far hand.
- Corollary tissues treated: Tibialis anterior tendon, extensor digitorum longus

▶ **See video 5.1 for the tibialis anterior muscle PRT procedure.**

Patient Self-Treatment Procedure

- Place the involved side on the opposite thigh.
- Grasp the heel and move the ankle and foot into plantar flexion and marked inversion while feeling for the most relaxed tissue position and also the presence of a fasciculation.
- Once you have obtained the most relaxed position or a strong fasciculation, externally rotate the ankle and then compress it toward the knee by pushing upward against the calcaneus until the fasciculation has subsided or abated.

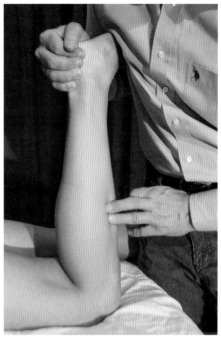

Tibialis anterior muscle PRT clinician procedure.

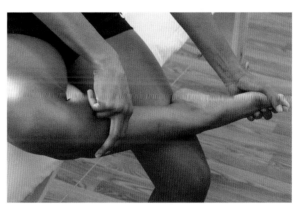

Tibialis anterior muscle patient self-treatment procedure.

Extensor Digitorum Longus Muscle

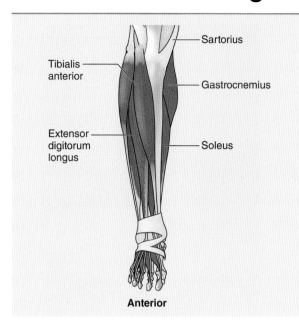

Tibialis anterior

Sartorius

Gastrocnemius

Extensor digitorum longus

Soleus

Anterior

The belly of the extensor digitorum longus is sandwiched between the tibialis anterior and peroneal muscles. The tendon of this muscle bifurcates below the ankle joint to form the peroneus tertius.

Origin: Lateral tibial condyle, proximal medial surface of the fibular shaft, interosseous membrane

Insertion: Second through fifth middle and distal phalanges

Action: Extends the second through fifth toes; assists with ankle dorsiflexion and foot eversion

Innervation: L5-S1 (deep peroneal nerve)

Palpation Procedure

- With the patient supine and the knee flexed, locate the tibialis anterior muscle belly.
- Slide laterally off of the tibialis anterior onto the muscle belly of the extensor digitorum longus. The peroneals are behind or lateral to the extensor digitorum longus.
- While palpating, have the patient extend the lesser toes (second through fifth) against resistance.
- The tendons of this muscle can also be traced superiorly to the muscle belly as well.
- Note the location of any tender points or fasciculatory response of the muscle and its attachments.
- Once you have determined the most dominant tender point or fasciculation (or both), maintain light pressure with the pad(s) of the finger(s) at the location throughout the PRT treatment procedure until reassessment has occurred.

PRT Clinician Procedure

- The patient is prone with the knee flexed to 70 to 90° and the shin supported with either your thigh or a bolster.
- Grasp the calcaneus with your far hand while applying ankle dorsiflexion with your far forearm or torso.
- Extend the toes with the far forearm or torso.
- Move the ankle into eversion with your far hand while applying downward calcaneal compression.

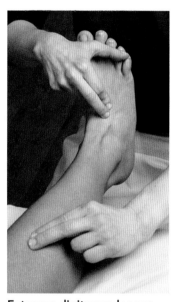

Extensor digitorum longus muscle palpation procedure.

- Externally rotate the tibia with your far hand or torso.
- Corollary tissues treated: Extensor digitorum longus tendon, fibularis muscle and tendons, interosseous membrane

Patient Self-Treatment Procedure

- Place the involved side on the opposite thigh.
- Grasp the heel and move the ankle and foot into dorsiflexion and eversion while feeling for the most relaxed tissue position and also the presence of a fasciculation.
- Once you have attained either the most relaxed position or a strong fasciculation, externally rotate the ankle and then compress it toward the knee by pushing upward against the calcaneus until the fasciculation has subsided or abated.

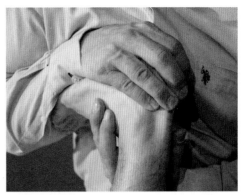

Extensor digitorum longus muscle PRT clinician procedure.

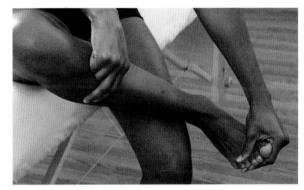

Extensor digitorum longus muscle patient self-treatment procedure.

Anterior Talofibular Ligament

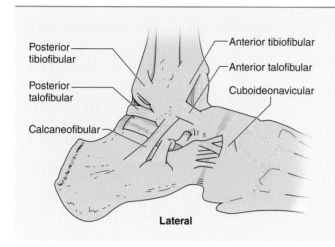

Posterior tibiofibular
Posterior talofibular
Calcaneofibular
Anterior tibiofibular
Anterior talofibular
Cuboideonavicular

Lateral

The anterior talofibular ligament (ATF) is the weakest and one of the most commonly torn lateral collateral ligaments of the ankle. The most common mechanism to tear this ligament is excessive inversion with plantar flexion under a weight-bearing load.

Origin: Anterior surface of the lateral malleolus

Insertion: Lateral neck of the talus

Action: Stabilizes against ankle inversion; prevents anterior luxation of the talus when in a plantar-flexed position

Palpation Procedure

- Because the ATF is a thickening of the ankle's joint capsule, its borders are not readily identifiable, but its location can be ascertained.
- Move anteriorly off the anterior portion of the lateral malleolus toward the neck of the talus.
- Note the location of any tender points or fasciculatory response at the ligament and its origin and attachment.
- Once you have determined the most dominant tender point or fasciculation (or both), maintain light pressure with the pad(s) of the finger(s) at the location throughout the PRT treatment procedure until reassessment has occurred.

PRT Clinician Procedure

- The patient is side-lying on the affected side with the knee flexed.
- Place the lateral ankle joint below a firm bolster to serve as a fulcrum.
- Move the ankle into dorsiflexion with your far hand or your leg and apply a downward force on the calcaneus to produce eversion and a lateral joint glide.
- Apply calcaneal external rotation with your far hand.
- Corollary tissues treated: Calcaneofibular ligament, posterior tibiofibular ligament, peroneal muscles and tendons, extensor digitorum brevis

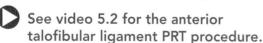 **See video 5.2 for the anterior talofibular ligament PRT procedure.**

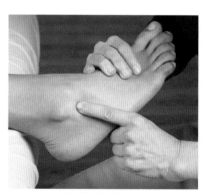

Anterior talofibular ligament palpation procedure.

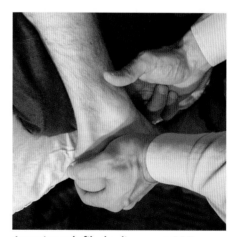

Anterior talofibular ligament PRT clinician procedure.

Deltoid Ligament

The deltoid ligament is composed of four ligaments that fan distally from the medial malleolus to their respective insertion sites denoted by their names: posterior tibiotalar, tibiocalcaneal, tibionavicular, and anterior tibiotalar. Even though the deltoid ligament is located under the flexor retinaculum and flexor tendons, its anterior and posterior fibers can be distinguished. The deltoid ligament is not often injured because of the bony block to eversion created by the inferior fibula shaft.

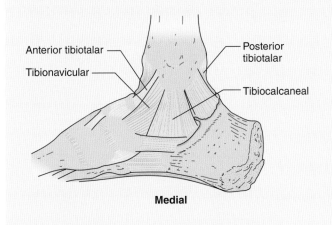

Anterior tibiotalar

Tibionavicular

Posterior tibiotalar

Tibiocalcaneal

Medial

Origin: Anterior and inferior aspects of the medial malleolus

Insertion: Posterior tibiotalar: Medial tubercle

Tibiocalcaneal: Sustentaculum tali of the calcaneus

Tibionavicular navicular and tibiotalar: Anterior medial talar dome

Action: Stabilizes against hindfoot eversion; supports the spring ligament; resists lateral displacement of the talus; prevents external rotation of the talus

Palpation Procedure

- Place the ankle in a neutral and relaxed position.
- Strum across the thickening of the tibiocalcaneal ligament at the junction between the apex of the medial malleolus and sustentaculum tali.
- The posterior and anterior portions of the deltoid ligament are oriented at approximately 45° angles to the tibiocalcaneal ligament and can be felt off the distal portion of the malleolus from where they insert.
- Determine the most dominant tender point or fasciculation (or both) and maintain light pressure with the pad(s) of the finger(s) throughout the treatment until reassessment has occurred.

PRT Clinician Procedure

- The patient is side-lying with the knee flexed. Place the lateral ankle joint below a firm bolster to serve as a fulcrum.
- Place the ankle into dorsiflexion with your far hand and apply a downward force on the calcaneus to produce inversion and a medial joint glide.
- With the far hand apply internal and external rotation to fine-tune.
- Corollary tissues treated: Spring ligament, tibialis posterior, flexor digitorum longus, medial flexor retinaculum, flexor hallucis longus

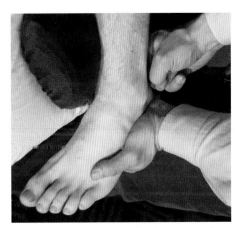

Deltoid ligament PRT clinician procedure.

Tibialis Posterior Muscle and Tendon

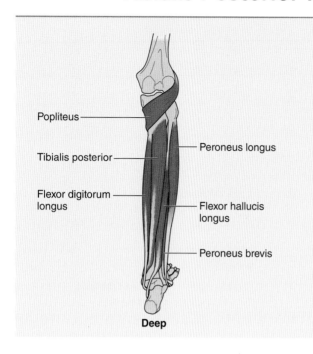

Popliteus

Tibialis posterior

Flexor digitorum longus

Peroneus longus

Flexor hallucis longus

Peroneus brevis

Deep

The tibialis posterior muscle is located in the deep posterior compartment of the lower leg, but its tendon and lower fibers are accessible just behind the medial malleolus. This muscle helps to stabilize the arch during ambulation.

Origin: Posterior surface of the interosseous membrane, proximal two thirds of the posterior lateral shaft of the tibia, medial fibular shaft and head

Insertion: Navicular tuberosity, cuneiform bones, cuboid slip, base of the second through fourth metatarsals

Action: Foot inversion; assists ankle plantar flexion

Innervation: L4-L5 and sometimes S1 (low branches of tibial nerve)

Palpation Procedure

- Place the patient in either a prone or supine knee-flexed position to relax the gastrocnemius and soleus musculature.
- Trace the tendon just medial to the medial malleolus upward along the shaft of the tibia until it dips away under the tibia.
- Continue to palpate superiorly along the tibia's shaft while reaching deep into the space between the tibia and gastrocnemius and soleus musculature.
- Roll the fingers upward against the posterior lateral shaft of the tibia to apply indirect pressure to the posterior tibialis musculature through the pressure exerted on the flexor digitorum longus muscle.
- Note the location of any tender points or fasciculatory response of the muscle and tendon and their attachments.
- Once you have determined the most dominant tender point or fasciculation (or both), maintain light pressure with the pad(s) of the finger(s) at the location throughout the PRT treatment procedure until reassessment has occurred.

PRT Clinician Procedure

- The patient is prone with the knee flexed to approximately 60°.
- Grasp the calcaneus with your far hand with the dorsum of the hand facing outward.

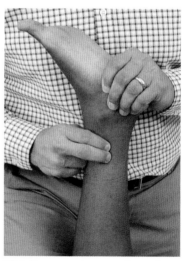

Tibialis posterior muscle and tendon palpation procedure.

- Use the near hand to monitor the lesion.
- Using the calcaneus as a fulcrum, move the lower leg and ankle into marked internal rotation with your far hand.
- Move the ankle into plantar flexion and marked inversion with the far hand.
- Apply cephalad calcaneal compression toward the knee with the far hand.
- Apply internal rotation of the calcaneus for fine-tuning with the far hand.
- Corollary tissues treated: Flexor digitorum longus, flexor hallucis longus, soleus, deltoid ligament complex

See video 5.3 for the tibialis posterior muscle and tendon PRT procedure.

Patient Self-Treatment Procedure

- Place the involved side on the opposite thigh.
- Grasp the heel and forefoot and move the ankle and foot into marked plantar flexion and inversion while feeling for the most relaxed tissue position and also the presence of a fasciculation.
- Once you have obtained either the most relaxed position or a strong fasciculation, invert and internally rotate the ankle and then compress it toward the knee by pushing upward against the calcaneus until the fasciculation has subsided or abated.

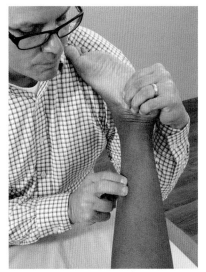

Tibialis posterior muscle and tendon PRT clinician procedure.

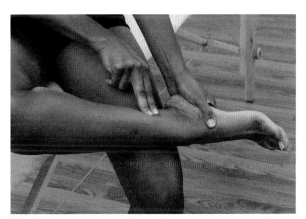

Tibialis posterior muscle and tendon patient self-treatment procedure.

Achilles Tendon

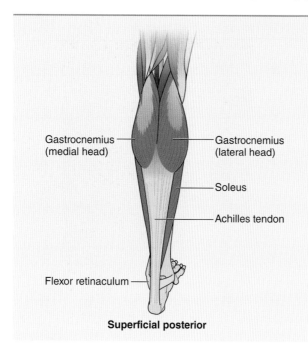

Gastrocnemius (medial head)

Gastrocnemius (lateral head)

Soleus

Achilles tendon

Flexor retinaculum

Superficial posterior

The Achilles tendon, also known as the tendo calcaneus, is formed by the soleus and gastrocnemius musculature and is often a site of irritation in the athletic and recreational population. The broad aponeurosis is flatter at the musculotendinous junction and then becomes more cordlike as it approaches the calcaneus. Therefore, a strumming palpation can be performed to assess its integrity proximally. However, above the heel, a pincing and sliding motion up and down the tendon can be used to assess both the tendon and its sheath for the presence of tissue lesions.

Origin: Inferior fibers of the gastrocnemius and soleus musculature

Insertion: Calcaneus

Action: Plantar flexes and stabilizes the ankle

Palpation Procedure

- The patient should be positioned prone with the knee flexed and ankle bolstered to relax the triceps surae complex.
- Start palpation at the posterior calcaneus and work proximally to the tendinous aspect of the tissue above the heel. Once the tendon is gained, apply light pincing coupled with a sliding motion up and down its sheath and tendon.
- To evaluate the tendon's glide in its sheath, apply slight pressure to both sides of the tendon while the patient plantar flexes the ankle.
- Once the tendon flattens proximally, it can be strummed across its expanse.
- Note the location of any tender points or fasciculatory response of the tendon and its attachments.
- Once you have determined the most dominant tender point or fasciculation (or both), maintain light pressure with the pad(s) of the finger(s) at the location throughout the PRT treatment procedure until reassessment has occurred.

PRT Clinician Procedure

- The patient is prone with the knee flexed to approximately 20 to 30°.
- Place the ankle into marked plantar flexion on your thigh or on a bolster.
- Using the near hand, place one or two fingers over the tender point.

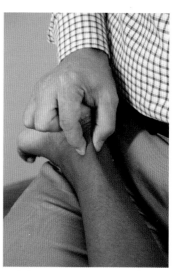

Achilles tendon palpation procedure.

- Use the fingers of your far hand to translate the posterior calcaneal fascia and tendon sheath cephalad while compressing the calcaneus downward.
- Distract the talocrural joint caudally, while simultaneously compressing and rotating the hindfoot downward with the palm of the treatment hand into the talocrural joint. This movement can be facilitated by either pulling the thigh away from the knee or using your far hand.
- Evert or invert the ankle with the far hand based on the location of the lesion.
- Apply calcaneal rotation with the far hand to fine-tune.
- Corollary tissues treated: Gastrocnemius, soleus

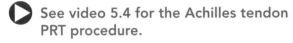 **See video 5.4 for the Achilles tendon PRT procedure.**

Patient Self-Treatment Procedure

- Place the involved ankle on the opposite thigh.
- Move the ankle into maximal plantar flexion.
- Place the fingers over the tender area.
- Compress and rotate the calcaneus upward with the palm while using the thumb and forefinger to translate the fascia or tendon upward.
- Apply eversion, inversion, and rotation to fine-tune the position.
- Find the position of greatest tissue comfort by using the fasciculatory response method.
- Hold the position of comfort until the fasciculation subsides or until three to five minutes have elapsed.

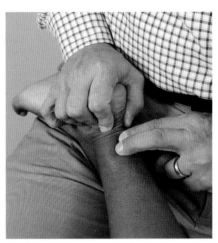

Achilles tendon PRT clinician procedure.

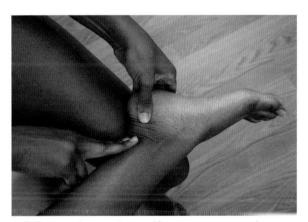

Achilles tendon patient self-treatment procedure.

Soleus

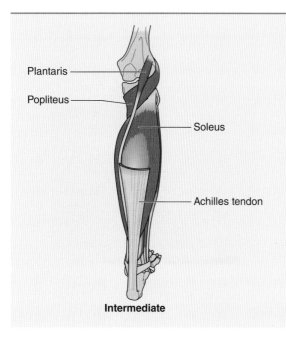

Plantaris

Popliteus

Soleus

Achilles tendon

Intermediate

The soleus lies deep to the gastrocnemius. The muscle is thick and broad but crosses only one joint, the ankle. Its inferior fibers expand beyond the borders of the Achilles tendon and are therefore accessible to palpation; however, deep palpation can be applied between the heads of the gastrocnemius to access the tissue in this location. The soleus primarily functions to prevent anterior translation of the tibia forward during standing, but also stabilizes the ankle during gait. The soleus can be isolated from the gastrocnemius by having the patient plantar flex the ankle while the knee is flexed.

Origin: Posterior fibular head, proximal third of the posterior and medial tibial shaft

Tibial soleal line

Insertion: Calcaneus via the calcaneal tendon

Action: Ankle plantar flexion, foot inversion

Innervation: S1-S2 (tibial nerve)

Palpation Procedure

- The patient should be positioned prone with the knee flexed and the ankle bolstered to relax the triceps surae complex.
- Locate the Achilles tendon and slide the fingers off its borders to locate the lower portions of the soleus.
- While palpating the lower portion of the soleus, have the patient plantar flex the foot to feel its contraction.
- To palpate the deep soleus, press downward between the heads of the gastrocnemius.
- Note the location of any tender points or fasciculatory response of the muscle and its distal attachment site.
- Once you have determined the most dominant tender point or fasciculation (or both), maintain light pressure with the pad(s) of the finger(s) at the location throughout the PRT treatment procedure until reassessment has occurred.

PRT Clinician Procedure

- The patient should be in a prone position.
- Position yourself next to the lower leg in either a seated or standing position.
- Move the knee through flexion and extension to find the location of greatest relaxation, which typically is between 60 and 90°.

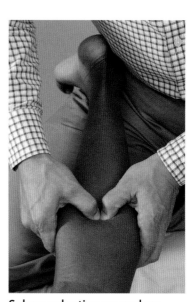

Soleus palpation procedure.

- After finding the knee flexion position, move the ankle through plantar flexion and dorsiflexion with the far hand to find again the greatest position of comfort or fasciculation, or both.
- With the far hand or your torso, apply marked compression of the calcaneus downward, making sure to drop the elbow of the arm applying the compression downward along the line of the tibia to prevent excessive strain on your elbow.
- Apply inversion and eversion of the ankle with the far hand based on the location of the lesion.
- Apply calcaneal rotation with the far hand to fine-tune.
- Corollary tissues treated: Tibialis posterior, flexor digitorum longus, flexor hallucis longus, gastrocnemius, Achilles tendon

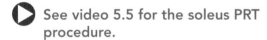 **See video 5.5 for the soleus PRT procedure.**

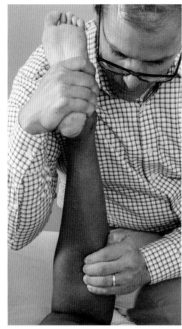

Soleus PRT clinician procedure.

Gastrocnemius

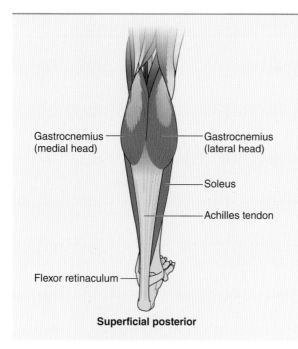

Gastrocnemius (medial head)

Gastrocnemius (lateral head)

Soleus

Achilles tendon

Flexor retinaculum

Superficial posterior

The gastrocnemius is a two-joint muscle that crosses the knee and ankle. Its two heads originate from the femoral condyles and converge distally to form the Achilles tendon. The more robust soleus muscle underneath the gastrocnemius also inserts into the Achilles tendon, and together they form the triceps surae complex. In gait, the gastrocnemius serves an integral role in stabilizing the ankle joint.

Origin: Posterior femoral condyles

Insertion: Calcaneus via the calcaneal tendon; the gastrocnemius fibers insert more laterally at the calcaneus

Action: Ankle plantar flexion; assists knee flexion

Innervation: S1-S2 (tibial nerve)

Palpation Procedure

- The patient should be positioned prone with the knee flexed and ankle bolstered to relax the triceps surae complex.
- Palpate each head individually. Place a stabilizing force upward with one hand on the outside of the lateral head and to the inside for the medial head while palpating upward to their tendinous aspects behind the knee.
- Determine the most dominant tender point or fasciculation (or both) and maintain light pressure with the pad(s) of the finger(s) throughout the treatment until reassessment has occurred.

PRT Clinician Procedure

- The patient is prone with the knee flexed to approximately 20 to 30°.
- Place the ankle into marked plantar flexion in the sulcus of your thigh or on a bolster.
- Using your far hand, evert (for the medial gastrocnemius head) or invert (for the lateral gastrocnemius head) the ankle based on the location of the tender point.
- Using your far hand, distract the talocrural joint caudally while simultaneously compressing and rotating the hindfoot downward into the talocrural joint.
- Apply calcaneal rotation to fine-tune with the far hand.
- Corollary tissues treated: Tibialis posterior, flexor digitorum longus, flexor hallucis longus, soleus, Achilles tendon, gastrocnemius tendons

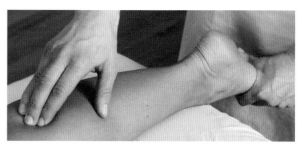

Gastrocnemius palpation procedure.

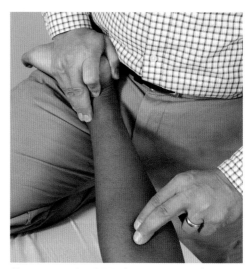

Gastrocnemius PRT clinician procedure.

 See video 5.6 for the gastrocnemius PRT procedure.

Calcaneofibular Ligament

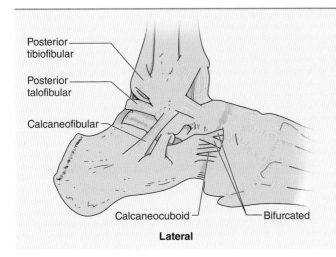

Posterior tibiofibular

Posterior talofibular

Calcaneofibular

Calcaneocuboid

Bifurcated

Lateral

The calcaneofibular ligament is a cordlike extra-articular ligament that crosses both the talocrural and talocalcaneal joints. With more severe inversion ankle sprains, the calcaneofibular ligament is often stressed as a result of a disruption of the anterior talofibular ligament.

Origin: Apex of the lateral malleolus

Insertion: Lateral surface of the calcaneus

Action: Limits ankle inversion; stabilizes the subtalar joint

Palpation Procedure

- Place the ankle in a neutral, relaxed position.
- Locate the tip of the malleolus and slide your fingers off its tip to just underneath the bone. The ligaments fibers are behind the peroneal tubercle, running obliquely toward its insertion on the calcaneus.
- Strum across the ligament's fibers to notice its cordlike nature.
- Note the location of any tender points or fasciculatory response of the ligament and its origin and insertion.
- Once you have determined the most dominant tender point or fasciculation (or both), maintain light pressure with the pad(s) of the finger(s) at the location throughout the PRT treatment procedure until reassessment has occurred.

PRT Clinician Procedure

- The patient is side-lying with the knee flexed.
- Place the medial ankle joint against and below a firm bolster to serve as a fulcrum.
- Using your far hand, place the ankle into dorsiflexion and apply a downward force on the calcaneus to produce a lateral glide while everting the calcaneus.
- Apply calcaneal rotation with your far hand to fine-tune.
- Corollary tissues treated: Anterior talofibular ligament, posterior talofibular ligament, peroneal tendons

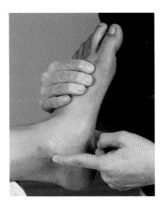

Calcaneofibular ligament palpation procedure.

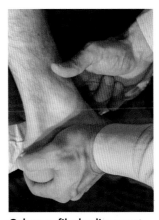

Calcaneofibular ligament PRT clinician procedure.

Peroneus Longus and Brevis

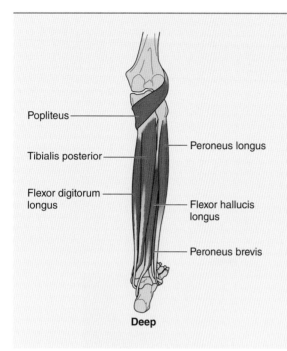

Popliteus

Tibialis posterior

Flexor digitorum longus

Peroneus longus

Flexor hallucis longus

Peroneus brevis

Deep

The peroneal, or fibularis, muscles are commonly strained with inversion ankle sprains in their attempt to resist the roll of the ankle inward. The violent eccentric pull of the tendons on the base of the first metatarsal can often produce an avulsion fracture at this site. The brevis is deep to the longus, but its fibers can be felt on either side of the tendon of the longus at the lower third of the ankle.

Origin: Longus: Fibular head, upper two thirds of the fibular shaft

Brevis: Distal two thirds of the fibular shaft

Insertion: Longus: Lateral plantar base of the first metatarsal and first cuneiform

Brevis: Tuberosity of the fifth metatarsal

Action: Foot eversion; also assists with ankle plantar flexion and supports the longitudinal and transverse arches. The longus also assists to depress the first metatarsal.

Innervation: L5-S1 (superficial peroneal nerve)

Palpation Procedure

- The patient can be either prone or supine with the knee flexed.
- Locate the fibular head, a round bony structure just inferior to the lateral knee joint.
- Dip downward off the fibular head onto the peroneus longus muscle belly in line with the lateral malleolus.
- Strum across the muscle belly into its posterior valley or border between the gastrocnemius and its anterior valley or border of the extensor digitorum longus.
- While strumming, ask the patient to evert the foot to accentuate its location.
- Continue to strum the longus downward to its tendinous aspect.
- Once at the tendinous aspect of the longus, slide your fingers off either side of the tendon onto the muscle belly of the brevis and repeat the strumming procedure for this muscle, working distally to its tendon.
- Note the location of any tender points or fasciculatory response of the muscles and their tendons and attachment sites.
- Once you have determined the most dominant tender point or fasciculation (or both), maintain light pressure with the pad(s) of the finger(s) at the location throughout the PRT treatment procedure until reassessment has occurred.

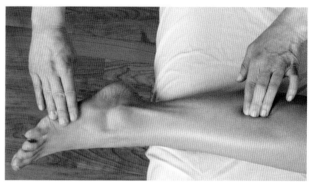

Peroneus longus and brevis palpation procedure.

PRT Clinician Procedure

- The patient is prone with the knee flexed to 90° and the shin supported with either your thigh or a bolster.
- Move the ankle through its range of motion of dorsiflexion and plantar flexion with your far hand to find the optimal treatment position.
- With your far hand, apply marked ankle eversion coupled with heavy calcaneal compression.
- Apply external tibial rotation with your far hand.
- Apply forefoot eversion with your torso for fine-tuning.
- Corollary tissues treated: Peroneal tendons, peroneus tertius, extensor digitorum brevis

▶ **See video 5.7 for the peroneus longus and brevis PRT procedure.**

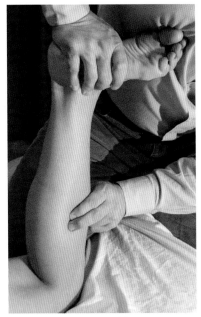

Peroneus longus and brevis PRT clinician procedure.

Medial Tibial Stress Syndrome

Medial tibial stress syndrome, also known as shin splints, is often the result of multiple factors that lead to the development of progressive medial shin pain. Typically, the primary culprits are being female, having less running experience, being overweight, possessing an increased navicular drop (Newman et al. 2013), and having more dynamic pronation (Dowling et al. 2015) through the stance phase of gait. Lack of dynamic hip control may also play a role (Dowling et al. 2015). Prolonged pronation paired with a lack of hip and knee stability and control during gait may place an increased eccentric demand on the medial shin musculature causing the production of somatic dysfunction.

Common Signs and Symptoms

- Pain with walking and stance phase loading during gait that typically increases with use
- Posteromedial tibial point tenderness, particularly over the medial soft tissues
- Pain that subsides with inactivity

Common Differential Diagnoses

- Stress fracture
- Exertional compartment syndrome
- Sciatica
- Muscle strain
- Popliteal artery entrapment
- Deep vein thrombosis (DVT)
- Tumor
- Infection
- Tibial periostitis

Clinician Therapeutic Interventions

- Determine the root of the patient's condition (e.g., faulty biomechanics, training errors, leg length discrepancy, weak hip musculature, surface or shoe alteration).
- Consider requesting an MRI or bone scan to rule out stress fracture if tenderness is localized over the bone.
- Address any insulting factors or conditions, such as increased tibial internal rotation.
- Scan and treat the structures in the order presented in the Treatment Points and

Treatment Points and Sequencing

1. Tibialis posterior and flexor digitorum longus
2. Tibialis anterior
3. Medial gastrocnemius
4. Soleus
5. Popliteus
6. Flexor hallucis brevis
7. Pes anserine
8. Iliotibial band
9. Adductors of the thigh
10. Sacroiliac joint
11. Gluteus medius
12. Psoas

Sequencing box. However, base your treatment sequencing off the most dominant (tender) points first.

- Follow PRT with thermal ultrasound or laser, PNF stretching of the medial and posterior pretibial musculature, and myofascial massage.
- For some patients, KT Tape or shin taping reduces pain during the initial stage of therapy.
- Apply instrumented soft-tissue mobilization (ISTM) if recalcitrant tissue adhesions are present.
- Consider performing a biomechanical evaluation of gait if a training, movement, or biomechanical error is suspected.
- Implement open- and closed-chain strengthening for the intrinsic foot, pretibial and hip, and core muscles to address weaknesses or compensations identified in the gait analysis, with a particular focus on eccentric control of tibial internal rotation.
- Have the patient use temporary or custom orthotics to unload the medial soft tissues during the initial phase of rehabilitation.
- If a walker boot is utilized, address any alteration in gait mechanics it may cause with a temporary lift or orthotic in the non-involved shoe to prevent abnormal joint loading at the non-involved limb, hip, and pelvis.

- Slowly progress the patient to dynamic physical activity through aquatic therapy or with an antigravity assisted running device.

Patient Self-Treatment Interventions

- A continuous low-intensity pulsed ultrasound unit may help.
- Perform self-release of the tibialis posterior on a daily basis or when irritated.
- Perform PNF stretching of the medial pretibial muscles and gastrocnemius soleus complex after exercise on a daily basis. Do not stretch if it produces pain because doing so may result in additional tissue lesions.
- Perform self-massage for five to eight minutes daily after stretching.
- Ice-massage the medial shin when reirritation occurs. Typically, patients with chronic symptoms respond best to heat (e.g., warm whirlpool or Jacuzzi). (*Note:* Consult with the clinician about where you are in the healing process, which will determine whether to apply heat or ice.)

Achilles Tendinopathy (Noninsertional)

Noninsertional Achilles tendon injury, or tendinopathy, is common in athletic and recreational athletes (Peters et al. 2015). According to Murphy, Curry, and Matzkin (2013), runners transitioning from a running shoe to barefoot running may be at more risk for injury than others. Additionally, runners attempting to change their running gait from a heel to midfoot strike pattern may also be susceptible to Achilles tendinopathy. When patients move from a heel to midfoot strike position either through alteration in shoe type or intentionally through gait modification, additional eccentric loading is placed on the Achilles tendon as the heel lowers to the ground (Giandolini et al. 2013). The tendon may simply become irritated when the load placed on it exceeds its extensibility limits or its ability to adapt to the load, which typically occurs from training error (Nielson et al. 2012), pathological biomechanical alterations during the gait cycle, or a sudden shoe or surface change. Although initial insult to the tendon can result in an inflammatory condition known as tendinitis, chronic inflammation of the tendon, or tendinosis, is more often the case. If left untreated, the condition may progress to degeneration of the tendon at its insertion or within the tendon without the classic signs of inflammation that may eventually lead to rupture.

Common Signs and Symptoms

- Pain with walking and toe-off during gait
- Diffuse swelling on the sides of the tendon behind the malleoli
- Point tenderness at the calcaneal insertion site or within the tendon itself

Common Differential Diagnoses

- Calcaneal fracture
- Retrocalcaneal bursitis
- Achilles tendon tear
- Soleus strain
- Haglund's deformity

Clinician Therapeutic Interventions

- Determine the root of the patient's condition (e.g., faulty biomechanics, training errors, leg length discrepancy, surface or shoe alteration).
- Consider requesting a radiograph to rule out Haglund's deformity and calcaneal fracture

Treatment Points and Sequencing

1. Achilles tendon
2. Tibialis posterior
3. Medial gastrocnemius
4. Lateral gastrocnemius
5. Soleus
6. Popliteus
7. Flexor hallucis brevis
8. Plantar interossei and lumbricals
9. Dorsal interossei

if the pain is located at the heel and has been chronic.

- Address any insulting factors or conditions such as excessive heel pressure from tight shoes.
- Scan and treat the structures in the order presented in the Treatment Points and Sequencing box. However, base your treatment sequencing off the most dominant (tender) points first.
- Follow PRT with thermal ultrasound or laser, PNF stretching, and myofascial massage of the Achilles tendon.
- For some patients, the use of KT Tape during the initial stage of rehabilitation reduces pain.
- Consider having the patient use a low-intensity pulsed ultrasound self-adhesive device daily.
- Apply ISTM if recalcitrant tissue adhesions are present.
- Implement an eccentric strengthening protocol as tolerated.
- Consider performing a biomechanical evaluation of gait if a training, movement, or biomechanical error is suspected.
- Implement open- and closed-chain strengthening for the intrinsic foot, pretibial and hip, and core muscles to address weaknesses or compensations identified in the gait analysis.
- Have the patient use temporary or custom orthotics to unload the Achilles tendon if a gait analysis warrants.
- If a walker boot is utilized, address any alteration in gait mechanics it may cause with a temporary lift or orthotic in the non-involved

shoe to prevent abnormal joint loading at the non-involved limb, hip, and pelvis.

- Slowly progress the patient to dynamic physical activity through aquatic therapy or antigravity-assisted running devices.

Patient Self-Treatment Interventions

- Perform self-release on a daily basis or when irritated.
- Perform PNF stretching of the Achilles tendon and gastrocnemius soleus complex after exercise on a daily basis. Do not stretch

if it produces pain because doing so may result in additional tissue lesions.

- Perform self-massage for five to eight minutes daily after stretching.
- Ice-massage the Achilles tendon or insertion site on a stretch when reirritation occurs. Typically, patients with chronic symptoms respond best to heat (e.g., warm whirlpool or Jacuzzi). (*Note:* Consult with the clinician about where you are in the healing process, which will determine whether to apply heat or ice.)

Summary

Because injury to the ankle and lower limb can be a lifelong debilitating event, early management and prevention are paramount. Given that ankle sprain is one of the most common lower-leg injuries seen (Waterman et al. 2010) and has the propensity to result in the development of osteoarthritis (Valderrabano et al. 2006), chronic instability (Doherty et al. 2015), and fibromyalgia (Smith, et al. 2011), this injury may be the most important to treat early with PRT. However, any time pain is associated with an injury, limiting the development of peripheral and centralization sensitization early may mitigate the development of fibromyalgia (Smith et al. 2011) and somatic dysfunction, both of which may affect how the motor system coordinates, initiates, and responds to movement.

According to Bastien and colleagues (2015), even after the healing of a mild ankle sprain, people alter their motor strategy while performing the star excursion balance test. This results in deficient and altered kinematics of the lower leg, knee, and hip, suggesting a reorganization of motor control strategies as a result of the pain and tissue dysfunction experienced during the initial sprain. Moreover, a recurrent sprain may be the result of somatic dysfunction that was not addressed at the time of the initial sprain. As discussed, strengthening the proximal hip musculature may reduce lower-limb injury because the hip is a major driver of control for lower-limb articulations (Dowling et al. 2015). Without adequate control, lower-limb structures may experience additional load and strain. The use of an orthotic by patients with an excessive navicular drop may also limit the load on the lower-extremity articulations (Dowling et al. 2015; Franklyn-Miller et al. 2011). However, initial evidence suggests that correcting training errors may be of the greatest benefit for preventing running-related injury in the active population (Nielson et al. 2012).

Regardless of the injury or patient population, pain and swelling appear to be the most critical healing events to address initially with lower-leg and ankle injuries. Both may be assisted with early PRT or joint manipulation, or both. Identifying strength and balance deficits along with a lack of dynamic foot control should also occur early to allow for the integration of therapeutic measures that can limit their impact on current, recurrent, or future ankle and lower-leg injuries.

CHAPTER 6

Knee and Thigh

After reading this chapter, you should be able to do the following:

❶ Recall the factors that may influence the development of somatic dysfunction at the knee and thigh.

❷ Locate and palpate knee and thigh structures to be treated with positional release therapy (PRT).

❸ Apply PRT techniques to treat the knee and thigh.

❹ Appreciate how common injury conditions such as iliotibial band friction syndrome may be treated based on myofascial lesion patterns.

Knee injury is common among children and young adults (DiFiori et al. 2014; Kraus et al. 2012; Swenson et al. 2013), but it is trending upward in the adult and senior populations (Gage et al. 2012). Between 1999 and 2008 in the United States, 6,664,324 knee injuries were seen in emergency departments, an incidence rate of 2.29 per 1,000. The highest rate of injury (3.83) was among those between 15 and 24 years of age. The 25 to 44 age group presented with the most knee injuries, and those over 64 years of age showed the greatest increase from previous years based on encounters with stairs, ramps, and floors. People younger than 24 were found to incur knee injury primarily during sports and recreation (73%); those over 25, at home (42%). Although the focus in the literature to date has been on knee and thigh injury sustained in the sporting population, particularly among females, the work of Gage and colleagues (2012) revealed no difference in injury rate between the sexes across the life span, and that knee injuries in older people may be as significant as those in the young.

Researchers have pointed to the propensity for knee and thigh injuries incurred during the adolescent years to linger throughout the life span (Foss et al. 2012), potentially disrupting opportunities for scholarships and competitive and recreational play. They may also cause long-term disability, affecting the ability to participate in sports, work, and daily life (DiFiori et al. 2014). Foss and colleagues (2012) tracked 307 American middle school and 112 high school female basketball players over three seasons and found anterior knee pain to be the most prevalent diagnosis (26.6%). Based on these findings and previous reports of anterior knee pain in adolescents, Foss and colleagues (2012) reported that female adolescents diagnosed with anterior knee pain often continue to have symptoms as long as 15 years after the initial diagnosis, and 45% reported a negative effect on daily life.

A previous knee injury has been identified as one of the most significant risk factors for future injury (DiFiori et al. 2014; Murphy, Connolly, and Beynnon 2013). Hewett, Di Stasi, and Myer (2013) found impaired neuromuscular control and abnormal biomechanics to be predictors of initial and future knee injury, and that initial injuries influence these predisposing factors long after resolution of the initial injury. Typically, physical activity improves health; however, vigorous physical activity in the athletic population has been proposed to increase the risk of osteoarthritis (OA) of the knee (Neogi and Zhang 2013). Moreover, both varus and valgus knee malalignment have also been found to increase OA knee risk (Felson et al. 2013), requiring the health care professional to be focused on prevention and the early identification of extrinsic factors that might be mitigated, such as activity level and abnormal biomechanics.

According to a systematic review by Van Gent, Siem, and Middelkoop (2007), U.S. runners demonstrated an incidence rate of running-related injury of 19.4 to 79.3%, and 7 to 50% of these injuries were located at the knee. Crowell and Davis (2011) speculated that the majority of running-related injuries (RRIs) are due to abnormal running gait mechanics that increase lower-extremity loading, and that most RRIs could be mitigated with gait retraining interventions. DiFiori and colleagues (2014) indicated that a significant factor in adolescent injury is improper training (high volume) and possibly burnout from sport specialization. Abnormal gait mechanics coupled with improper training volume may lead to knee and thigh injury if not corrected early in life. With over 27 million adolescents participating in team sports in the United States annually (DiFiori et al. 2014), the high incidence of knee injury, whether acute or attributed to overuse, presents a critical need for developing evidence-based prevention programming.

Between 2005 and 2011 in the United States, 15.1% of high school athletes who were engaged in traditional sports (e.g., football, basketball, soccer, baseball, softball, volleyball, wrestling) incurred knee injuries; the majority (48.2%) were ligament sprains (Swenson et al. 2013). It is estimated that ACL injury in the United States alone may cost upward of $1 billion annually in the form of lost scholarships, rehabilitation, surgery, and lost work time (Smith et al. 2012). Approximately 100,000 ACL injuries occur annually in the United States (Sadohgi, von Keudell, and Vavken 2012), and a disproportionate number occur in the female population. Hip abductor weakness, particularly among females, has been an intensive area of investigation as a cause of ACL injury (Leetun et al. 2004), although the prevailing thought among researchers today is that multiple intrinsic and extrinsic factors are responsible for the increased susceptibility to lower-extremity injury (Murphy et al. 2003; Smith et al. 2012).

Researchers posit that overuse injury among adolescents may be underestimated in terms of prevalence and impact on future injury rates across the life span (DiFiori et al. 2014). As a result, knee or ACL injury prevention programs tailored to the adolescent athletic population, particularly females, have received significant attention in the hope that they might limit the incidence of knee injury (Hewett et al. 2013). However, to date, the literature is mixed on the effectiveness of ACL injury prevention programs. Based on systematic review findings, Grimm and colleagues (2012) found no evidence of a reduction in ACL and knee injury rates among prevention program participants. Michaelidis and Koumantakis (2014) found limited evidence for ACL prevention among females engaged in only soccer and handball, and Noyes and Barber-Westin (2014) reported that three neuromuscular training programs provided a significant reduction in noncontact ACL injuries among adolescent female athletes. However, high compliance with neuromuscular training appears to reduce ACL and acute knee injury rates. Hägglund and colleagues (2013) observed an 88% reduction rate in ACL and acute knee injury rates among youth female Swedish soccer (football) players who demonstrated a high compliance with their neuromuscular training programs compared to controls. The researchers attributed the mixed

ACL and knee injury rates seen in other studies to low program compliance. Is it possible that the high rate of knee injury (initial and recurrent) may be, in part, due to somatic dysfunction?

No studies to date have examined the impact of PRT on orthopedic related injuries to the knee and thigh, but a few have examined its impact on hamstring flexibility. Birmingham and colleagues (2004) were the first to explore whether hamstring flexibility improved with strain counterstrain (SCS) in a healthy population. However, no difference in range of motion was found between the SCS group and the control group. Kaandeepan and colleagues (2011), in contrast, did observe a significant hamstring flexibility improvement with a PRT intervention among healthy females with the sit and reach test. The comparison group that stretched passively also improved. Although increased flexibility has not been shown to reduce injury risk (Herbert and Gabriel 2002), Kaandeepan and colleagues' 2011 study is a promising step in the right direction. Prospective longitudinal studies are needed to validate the assumption that somatic dysfunction may be a factor in knee and thigh injury. Additionally, examinations of the prevalence and impact of somatic dysfunction on a variety of knee and thigh conditions is required.

TREATMENT
Common Anatomical Areas and Conditions for PRT

Anterior Structures
- Patellofemoral pain syndrome
- Osgood-Schlatter disease
- Chondromalacia patella

Medial Structures
- Pes anserine tendinitis
- Meniscal injury

Posterior Structures
- Baker's cyst
- Capsular sprain

Lateral Structures
- Iliotibial band friction syndrome
- Meniscal injury
- Fibular head displacement
- Patellofemoral pain syndrome

Patellar Tendon

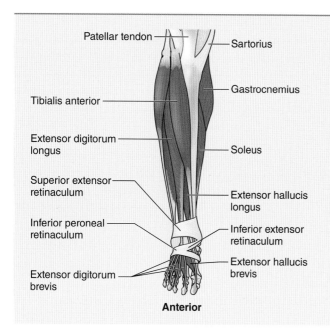

Patellar tendon
Sartorius
Tibialis anterior
Gastrocnemius
Extensor digitorum longus
Soleus
Superior extensor retinaculum
Extensor hallucis longus
Inferior peroneal retinaculum
Inferior extensor retinaculum
Extensor digitorum brevis
Extensor hallucis brevis

Anterior

The patellar tendon, also known as the patellar ligament, is a continuation of the quadriceps tendon that encases the patella. The patellar tendon runs from the inferior pole of the patella to the tibial tuberosity, passing over the anterior joint line of the knee.

Origin: Quadriceps tendon

Insertion: Tibial tuberosity

Action: Provides a mechanical advantage for knee extension and flexion as well as stability of the tibiofemoral joint

Palpation Procedure

- Place the patient in a relaxed supine hip-flexed position.
- Locate the inferior pole of the patella and slide the fingers just inferior to and onto the patellar tendon.
- Strum across the tendon downward to its insertion at the tibial tuberosity.
- Be certain to palpate the medial and lateral borders of the patellar tendon as well as its anterior fibers.
- Note the location of any tender points or fasciculatory response of the tendon and its origin and insertion.
- Once you have determined the most dominant tender point or fasciculation (or both), maintain light pressure with the pad(s) of the finger(s) at the location throughout the PRT treatment procedure until reassessment has occurred.

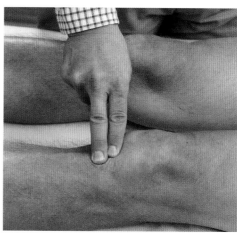

Patellar tendon palpation procedure.

PRT Clinician Procedure

- Place the patient supine.
- Place a bolster or rolled towel under the femur just above knee joint.
- Apply a posterior translational force with your far hand at the distal femur above the patella, being careful not to compress the patella.
- Gently translate the patella inferiorly with your far hand.
- With the far hand, rotate the patella and femur to fine-tune.
- Corollary tissues treated: Quadriceps tendon, patellar retinaculum, joint capsule

▶ **See video 6.1 for the patellar tendon PRT procedure.**

Patient Self-Treatment Procedure

- Sit with the knee extended.
- Place a bolster or rolled towel under the femur above the knee joint.
- Apply a posterior translational force at the distal femur above the patella, being careful not to compress the patella.
- Gently translate the patella inferiorly.
- Rotate the patella and femur to fine-tune.
- Maintain the treatment position until the fasciculatory response abates or for three to five minutes.

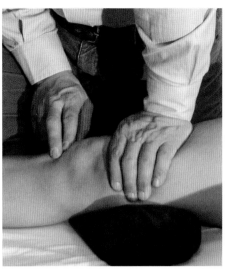

Patellar tendon PRT clinician procedure.

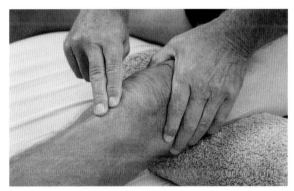

Patellar tendon patient self-treatment procedure.

Quadriceps Tendon

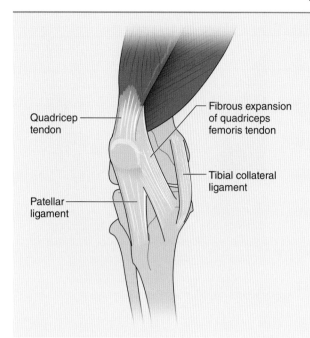

Quadricep tendon

Fibrous expansion of quadriceps femoris tendon

Tibial collateral ligament

Patellar ligament

The quadriceps tendon is a convergence of the inferior fibers of the rectus femoris, vastus medialis, vastus intermedius, and vastus lateralis. Most of the tendon's fibers are formed by the rectus femoris and vastus lateralis. The quadriceps tendon is not as often injured as its cousin the patellar tendon, but it can be a site of irritation due to muscular imbalance between the vastus medialis and vastus lateralis.

Origin: Musculotendinous junction of the quadriceps

Insertion: Superior pole of the patella

Action: Patellar stabilization and transmission of force production to produce and slow knee movement

Palpation Procedure

- Place patient in a short-sit position with the knee fully extended.
- With two fingers, strum across its fibers, noting its distinct borders and medial and lateral depressions.
- Note the location of any tender points or fasciculatory response of the tendon and its origin and insertion.
- Once you have determined the most dominant tender point or fasciculation (or both), maintain light pressure with the pad(s) of the finger(s) at the location throughout the PRT treatment procedure until reassessment has occurred.

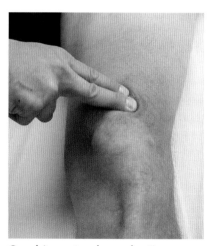

Quadriceps tendon palpation procedure.

PRT Clinician Procedure

- Place the patient supine with the knee extended and the hip flexed to 60°. Place the lower leg on your knee or a bolster.
- With your far hand, apply downward pressure on the tibia below the patella to encourage knee hyperextension.
- Also use your far hand to translate the soft tissue superiorly.
- Rotate the tibia and patella with the far hand to fine-tune.
- Corollary tissues treated: Patella, patellar tendon, quadriceps group

Patient Self-Treatment Procedure

- Place the lower leg and foot on a stool or couch arm.
- Lean forward and place two fingers over the tendon to monitor the fasciculatory response and tissue relaxation.
- Place the palm of the other hand over the tibia below the kneecap and press downward; then translate the tissue up toward the tendon.
- Rotate the tibia and patella to fine-tune.
- Maintain the treatment position until the fasciculatory response abates or for three to five minutes.

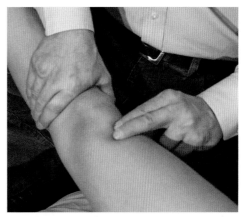

Quadriceps tendon PRT clinician procedure.

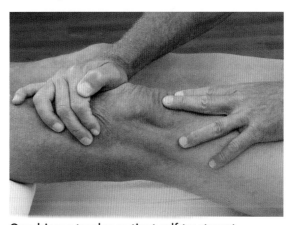

Quadriceps tendon patient self-treatment procedure.

Rectus Femoris

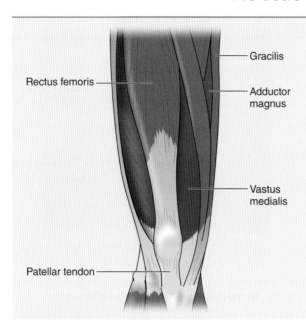

Rectus femoris

Gracilis

Adductor magnus

Vastus medialis

Patellar tendon

The rectus femoris is the only quadriceps muscle that attaches at two joints: the hip and knee. Its superficial fibers are bipennate and its deep fibers are parallel and vertically oriented down the center of the thigh.

Origin: Anterior inferior iliac spine, acetabulum, hip capsule

Insertion: Quadriceps tendon coursing into the patellar tendon to affix to the tibial tuberosity

Action: Knee extension, hip flexion

Innervation: L2-L4 (femoral nerve)

Palpation Procedure

- Place the patient supine with the knee bolstered.
- Follow the tendon's insertion point at the anterior inferior iliac spine to the superior pole of the patella.
- Strum across the fibers. The muscle is approximately two to three fingers in width.
- Resistive hip and knee flexion will make this muscle more pronounced for palpation.
- Note the location of any tender points or fasciculatory response of the muscle and its tendon and respective attachment sites.
- Once you have determined the most dominant tender point or fasciculation (or both), maintain light pressure with the pad(s) of the finger(s) at the location throughout the PRT treatment procedure until reassessment has occurred.

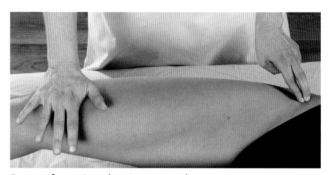

Rectus femoris palpation procedure.

PRT Clinician Procedure

- The patient is supine with the hip flexed and the ankle on your shoulder.
- Using your far hand, apply a posterior pressure at the femur just above the patella to encourage knee hyperextension while moving the quadriceps toward the hip.
- With the far hand, apply rotation to the tissues or femur, or both.
- Compress the femur up toward the hip joint with your body for fine-tuning.
- Corollary tissues treated: Quadriceps tendon, adductors, vasti

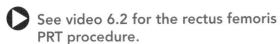 **See video 6.2 for the rectus femoris PRT procedure.**

Patient Self-Treatment Procedure

- Place the lower leg and foot on a stool or couch arm.
- Lean forward and place one or both hands over the femur just above the patella and simultaneously push the femur down and pull the quadriceps toward the hip.
- If possible, monitor the fasciculatory response and tissue relaxation at the site of pain.
- Rotate the femur to fine-tune.
- Maintain the treatment position until the fasciculatory response abates or for three to five minutes.

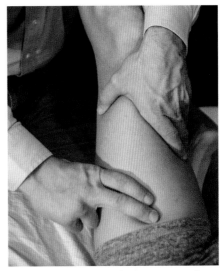

Rectus femoris PRT clinician procedure.

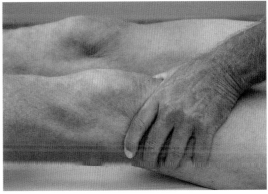

Rectus femoris patient self-treatment procedure.

Patella

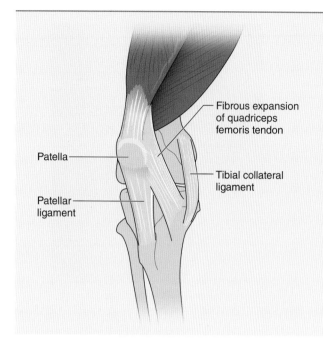

- Fibrous expansion of quadriceps femoris tendon
- Patella
- Tibial collateral ligament
- Patellar ligament

The patella, the largest sesamoid bone in the body, is located within the quadriceps femoris tendon. Its anterior location at the knee allows it to protect the tibiofemoral joint and serve as a fulcrum for the production of joint force and movement. The patella also serves as an attachment site for multiple tissues. Its posterior surface and margins are often sites of irritation when its tracking in the trochlear groove of the knee is abnormal as a result of muscle imbalance, pain, or tissue tightness.

Palpation Procedure

- Place the patient supine in a short-sit position with the knee fully extended.
- Palpate the surface and edges of the patella with light pressure so as not to compress the patella downward.
- Shift and tilt the patella upward in all directions to expose the under margin. Apply light pressure to its undersurfaces.
- Note the location of any tender points or fasciculatory response at or around the structure.
- Once you have determined the most dominant tender point or fasciculation (or both), maintain light pressure with the pad(s) of the finger(s) at the location throughout the PRT treatment procedure until reassessment has occurred.

PRT Clinician Procedure

- The patient is supine in a short-sit position.
- Move the patella toward the tender point with your far hand.
- With the far hand, tilt or rotate the patella to fine-tune.

Patient Self-Treatment Procedure

- Sit against a wall with the knee fully extended.
- Shift, tilt, and rotate the patella toward the area of tenderness to achieve maximal relaxation of the tissue coupled with a rise in the fasciculatory response while keeping the fingers on the area with submaximal pressure.

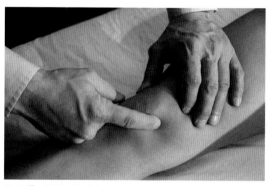

Patella PRT clinician procedure.

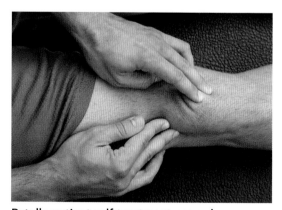

Patella patient self-treatment procedure.

- Maintain the treatment position until the fasciculatory response abates or for three to five minutes.

Medial Collateral Ligament

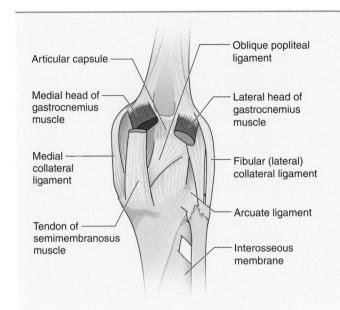

Articular capsule

Medial head of gastrocnemius muscle

Medial collateral ligament

Tendon of semimembranosus muscle

Oblique popliteal ligament

Lateral head of gastrocnemius muscle

Fibular (lateral) collateral ligament

Arcuate ligament

Interosseous membrane

The medial collateral ligament (MCL) is composed of superficial and deep fibers to provide the knee with medial and rotatory stability. Its deep fibers may be torn with meniscal tears because of their direct attachment.

Origin: Posterior aspect of the medial femoral condyle

Insertion: Medial tibial flare 5 cm (2 in.) below the joint line and underneath the pes anserine

Action: Limits valgus and rotatory knee stress

Palpation Procedure

- Place the patient in a knee-flexed seated position to move the iliotibial band posteriorly.
- Move medially off the patellar tendon and toward the medial joint line.
- Strum over the joint line, and then palpate lightly up and down onto the femoral and tibial condyles.
- Note the location of any tender points or fasciculatory response of the ligament and its origin and insertions.
- Once you have determined the most dominant tender point or fasciculation (or both), maintain light pressure with the pad(s) of the finger(s) at the location throughout the PRT treatment procedure until reassessment has occurred.

PRT Clinician Procedure

- The patient is supine.
- Place the patient's knee over your thigh to position it at approximately 30° of flexion.
- Apply a varus force at the knee using your far hand at the ankle.
- Apply marked ankle inversion with your far hand.
- Internally rotate and compress the tibia upward to fine-tune with your far hand.
- Corollary tissues treated: Knee capsule, patellar tendon

▶ See video 6.3 for the MCL PRT procedure.

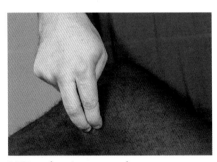

MCL palpation procedure.

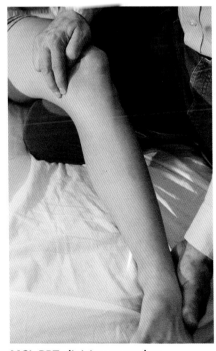

MCL PRT clinician procedure.

Pes Anserine

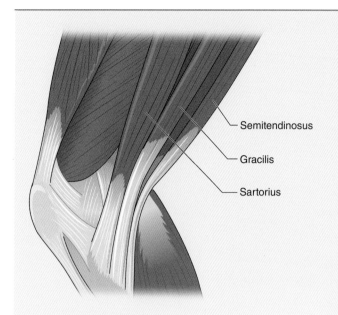

Semitendinosus

Gracilis

Sartorius

The pes anserine is composed of three conjoined tendons (sartorius, gracilis, and semitendinosus) at the medial knee that assist in rotatory control of the knee during gait. Overuse of eccentric hip rotation or lack of eccentric hip rotatory control is often attributed to the development of pes anserine bursitis and tendinopathy. A mnemonic for the orientation of the tendons from anterior to posterior is say (sartorius) grace (gracilis) before tea (semitendinosus).

Origin: Respective musculotendinous junction of the associated musculature

Insertion: Medial to the tibial tuberosity

Action: Provides rotatory control and stability of the knee during gait; assists with hip external rotation and flexion

Palpation Procedure

- The patient is supine.
- Slide the fingers approximately 1 inch (2.5 cm) medially from the tibial tuberosity onto the bony insertion site. On the well-developed patient, the mass of the tendons can be grasped as a group at the medial knee.
- With the pads of the fingers, lightly pin the tendons against the bone while strumming the tendons up and over the bone medial to lateral.
- Be sure to palpate the conjoined tendon from its bony insertion to the individual musculotendinous junction of the respective tendons just above the medial femoral condyle.
- Note the location of any tender points or fasciculatory response of the tendons and their attachment sites.
- Once you have determined the most dominant tender point or fasciculation (or both), maintain light pressure with the pad(s) of the finger(s) at the location throughout the PRT treatment procedure until reassessment has occurred.

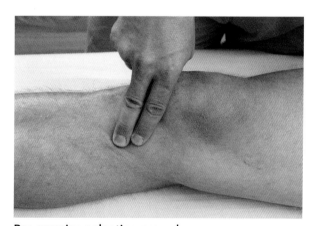

Pes anserine palpation procedure.

PRT Clinician Procedure

- The patient is supine.
- With the knee over the treatment table or your thigh, place the patient into slight hip extension.
- Using your far hand, move the knee into approximately 40 to 60° of flexion.
- With the far hand, move the lower leg into adduction, closing the medial joint line.
- Internally rotate the tibia at the ankle with the far hand.
- Using the far hand, apply marked calcaneal and forefoot inversion.
- Apply tibial traction or upward compression with the far hand for fine-tuning.
- Corollary tissues treated: Medial collateral ligament, posterior tibialis

▶ **See video 6.4 for the pes anserine PRT procedure.**

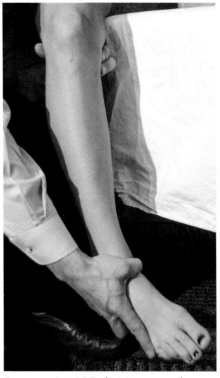

Pes anserine PRT clinician procedure.

Vastus Medialis Oblique

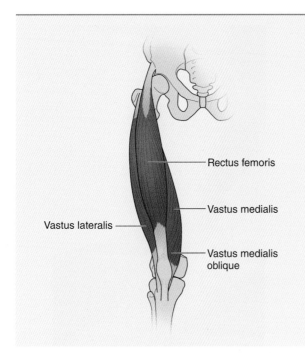

- Rectus femoris
- Vastus medialis
Vastus lateralis
- Vastus medialis oblique

The vastus medialis oblique (VMO) is a small teardrop-looking muscle on the inside of the knee in well-developed people. Its obliquely oriented fibers (50-55°) help to stabilize the patella against the pull of the lateralis. Imbalance between these two muscles has been attributed to patellar maltracking, leading to pain and atrophy.

Origin: Femur, adductor magnus tendon, medial intermuscular septum

Insertion: Patella, medial quadriceps tendon, patellar tendon

Action: Assist with terminal knee extension; stabilizes the patella

Innervation: L2-L4 (femoral nerve)

Palpation Procedure

- Place the patient in a supine short-sit position.
- Place your fingers just superior and medial to the patella over the knee.
- Instruct the patient to extend the knee to feel the contraction of the VMO fibers and also to observe the tracking of the patella.
- Note the location of any tender points or fasciculatory response of the muscle and its attachment site.
- Once you have determined the most dominant tender point or fasciculation (or both), maintain light pressure with the pad(s) of the finger(s) at the location throughout the PRT treatment procedure until reassessment has occurred.

PRT Clinician Procedure

- The patient is supine.
- Place the patient's lower leg on your thigh.
- Grasp above the VMO muscle belly with your near thumb and translate the tissues diagonally toward the inferior lateral knee while using one of the fingers of your near hand to monitor the lesion.
- Apply a posterior force at the superior tibia below the patella with your far hand to encourage hyperextension.

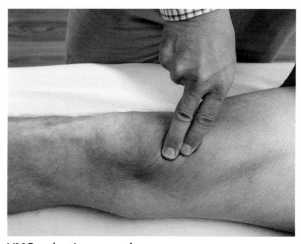

VMO palpation procedure.

- Rotate the tibia with your far hand to fine-tune.
- Corollary tissues treated: Knee capsule, quadriceps tendon, rectus femoris

Patient Self-Treatment Procedure

- Place the lower leg and foot on a stool or couch arm.
- Lean forward and place one hand below the patella at the tibia and the other just superior of the VMO muscle belly.
- Apply downward pressure below the patella while translating the muscle belly diagonally toward the lateral knee.
- Rotate the tibia to fine-tune.
- Monitor the VMO for a fasciculatory response and tissue relaxation at the site of pain.
- Maintain the treatment position until the fasciculatory response abates or for three to five minutes.

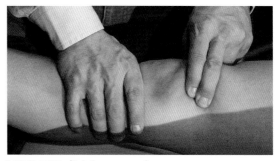

VMO PRT clinician procedure.

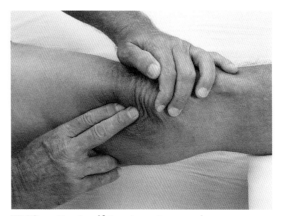

VMO patient self-treatment procedure.

Adductor Group

The adductor group is composed of the adductor magnus, longus, and brevis; the pectineus; and the gracilis. The adductors as a group stabilize the pelvic complex and the lower articulations during locomotion; however, they also produce adduction and assist with hip flexion during open-chain movements.

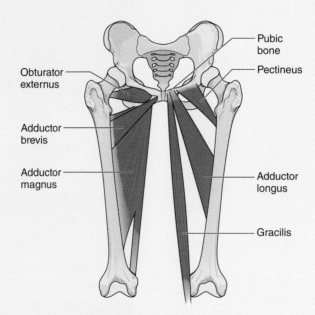

Origin: Adductor magnus: Inferior ramus of the pubis, ischial tuberosity

Adductor longus: Pubic tubercle

Adductor brevis: Inferior ramus of the pubis

Pectineus: Superior ramus of the pubis

Gracilis: Inferior ramus of the pubis

Insertion: Adductor magnus: Linea aspera of the femur, adductor tubercle

Adductor longus: Middle third of the linea aspera medial lip

Adductor brevis: Proximal third of the linea aspera medial lip

Pectineus: Pectineal line of the femur

Gracilis: Medial tibial surface below the tibial condyle, pes anserine

Action: Adductor magnus: Hip adduction, extension (inferior fibers), and flexion (superior fibers); assists with hip rotation

Adductor longus: Hip adduction; assists with hip flexion and rotation

Adductor brevis: Hip adduction and flexion

Pectineus: Hip adduction; assists with hip flexion

Gracilis: Hip adduction, knee flexion; assists with medial knee rotation

Innervation: Adductor magnus: Superior and middle fibers, L2-L4 (obturator nerve); inferior fibers, L2-L4 (sciatic nerve)

Adductor longus: L2-L4 (obturator nerve)

Adductor brevis: L2-L4 (obturator nerve)

Pectineus: L2-L3 (femoral nerve and accessory obturator nerve when present)

Gracilis: L2-L3 (obturator nerve)

Palpation Procedure

- Locate the common adductor tendon at the adductor tubercle of the inferior ramus of the pubis. The tendon is formed by the adductor longus and gracilis and is the largest and most prominent tendon in the medial groin area.
- The pectineus is located lateral and anterior to the common adductor tendon.
- Place the patient in a supine position. The thigh will naturally rotate outward in this position exposing the adductors for palpation.
- Instruct the patient to adduct against resistance to differentiate the adductors' fibers from the vastus medialis musculature.
- Work either from the distal or proximal medial thigh and strum the adductors upward against the femur as a group.
- Note the location of any tender points or fasciculatory response of the muscles and their tendons, origin, and insertions.
- Determine the most dominant tender point or fasciculation (or both) and maintain light pressure with the pad(s) of the finger(s) throughout the treatment until reassessment has occurred.

PRT Clinician Procedure

- The patient is supine.
- Move the limb into straight-leg hip flexion with your far hand to assess where the adductors feel the most relaxed or a fasciculation manifests, and place the limb on either a bolster or your thigh when found. Typically, the more proximal the lesion is, the more hip flexion will be needed.
- Move the limb into adduction with the far hand.
- Apply marked calcaneal and foot inversion with the far hand.
- Apply marked internal rotation of the limb with the far hand.
- Medially translate the quadriceps and fascia toward the lesion with your near hand while using one of the fingers of that hand to monitor the lesion.
- Compress the limb upward with the far hand for fine-tuning.
- Corollary tissues treated: Vastus medialis, sartorius

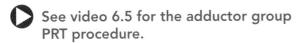 See video 6.5 for the adductor group PRT procedure.

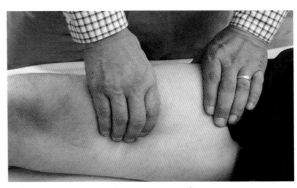

Adductor group palpation procedure.

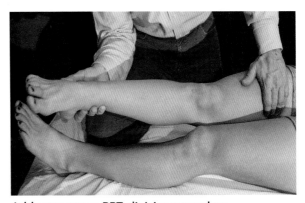

Adductor group PRT clinician procedure.

Patient Self-Treatment Procedure

- Lie supine.
- While palpating the tender area with one hand to assess tissue relaxation and the presence of a fasciculation, cross the involved leg over the other, and rest it on it or within the range of adduction where the greatest position of comfort and tissue fasciculation occurs.
- Internally rotate the leg.

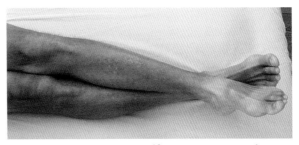

Adductor group patient self-treatment procedure.

Pectineus

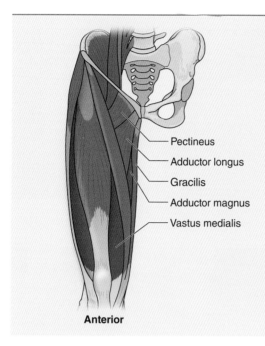

Pectineus
Adductor longus
Gracilis
Adductor magnus
Vastus medialis

Anterior

The pectineus is highlighted in the adductor group because anterior hip pain is often the result of a pectineus lesion rather than from an issue originating from the rectus femoris. A pectineus lesion can present within the muscle belly, but it is often found at its origin on the ramus. However, both are treated with the same PRT procedure.

Origin:	Superior ramus of the pubis
Insertion:	Pectineal line of the femur
Action:	Hip adduction; assists with hip flexion
Innervation:	L2-L3 (femoral nerve and accessory obturator nerve when present)

Palpation Procedure

- Place the patient supine with the hip partially flexed and the knee bolstered.
- Locate the common adductor tendon of the longus and gracilis and move laterally into the soft tissues, where the belly of the pectineus is located.
- With downward pressure, strum the muscle belly of the pectineus; then trace it upward to its tendinous origin on the superior ramus.
- Palpate the superior ramus with light pressure.
- Instruct the patient to adduct the hip during palpation of the pectineus to accentuate its location and tendinous origin.
- Determine the most dominant tender point or fasciculation (or both) and maintain light pressure with the pad(s) of the finger(s) throughout the treatment until reassessment has occurred.

PRT Clinician Procedure

- The patient is supine with the clinician standing at the side of the table of the involved limb.
- Place the patient's noninvolved leg over the involved one, and place both on your thigh. This procedure can also be done with just the involved limb.
- Move the hips into approximately 90° of flexion and, using the far hand, apply adduction while internally rotating the hip.
- Compress the femur downward with your far hand or torso.

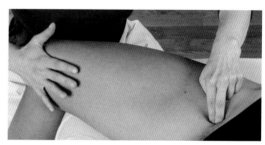

Pectineus palpation procedure.

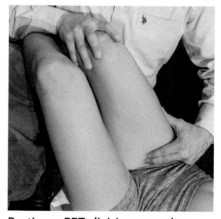

Pectineus PRT clinician procedure.

- Corollary tissues treated: Adductor magnus, psoas, rectus femoris

Patient Self-Treatment Procedure

Use the adductor group patient self-treatment procedure previously described.

Popliteus

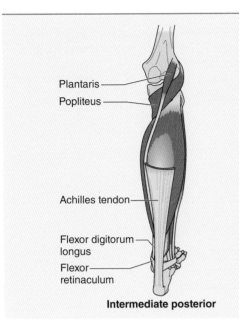

Plantaris

Popliteus

Achilles tendon

Flexor digitorum longus

Flexor retinaculum

Intermediate posterior

The popliteus is considered a weak flexor of the knee, but also an integral muscle during the screw home mechanism, helping the knee to unlock from an extended position. Typically, the muscle is not palpable because of its depth at the popliteal fossa. However, when a popliteal lesion is present, it may be possible to palpate its superior fibers as they course diagonally from the lateral femoral condyle, where the tendon can also be palpated.

Origin: Lateral condyle of the femur, arcuate popliteal ligament, lateral meniscus of the knee

Insertion: Proximal posterior surface of the tibia

Action: Knee flexion, knee internal rotation (proximal attachment fixed), hip external rotation (tibia fixed)

Innervation: L4-S1 (tibial nerve)

Palpation Procedure

- Place the patient in a prone knee-flexed position.
- Locate the inferior lateral femoral condyle and the fibular head.
- Strum the tendon over the posterior aspect of the fibular head as it courses diagonally toward the tibia.
- Trace its line diagonally toward the tibia, orienting the tips of your fingers toward the popliteal fossa.
- With deep pressure, strum your fingers over the hypercontracted popliteus' superior fibers as they pass below the inferior aspect of the posterior tibial condyle.
- Determine the most dominant tender point or fasciculation (or both) and maintain light pressure with the pad(s) of the finger(s) throughout the treatment until reassessment has occurred.

PRT Clinician Procedure

- The patient is prone with the knee flexed.
- Move the knee through flexion and extension; the treatment position is typically at approximately 70 to 90° of knee flexion.
- While grasping the calcaneus with your far hand, apply significant downward compression of the lower limb with either the far hand or your torso.
- Apply internal and external rotation to the tibia with the far hand (internal for medial lesions and external for lateral lesions).

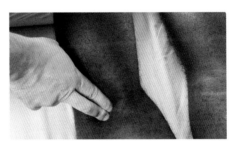

Popliteus palpation procedure.

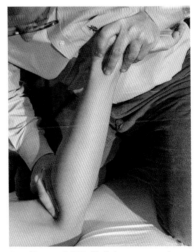

Popliteus PRT clinician procedure.

- Corollary tissues treated: Gastrocnemius, soleus, hamstrings

 See video 6.6 for the popliteus PRT procedure.

Hamstrings

The hamstrings as a group (biceps femoris, semitendinosus, semimembranosus) are typically associated with producing knee flexion and hip extension. However, during the gait cycle, they assist with knee rotation control; therefore, weak hip abductors and rotators may lead to hamstring pathology. If hamstring pathology is implicated, the adductor magnus and sacrotuberous ligament should also be explored because of their communication with the hamstrings' common origin at the ischial tuberosity.

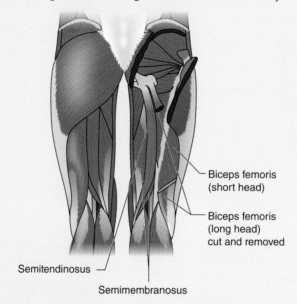

Biceps femoris
(short head)

Biceps femoris
(long head)
cut and removed

Semitendinosus

Semimembranosus

Origin: Long head of the biceps femoris: Ischial tuberosity, sacrotuberous ligament

Short head of the biceps femoris: Linea aspera lateral lip

Semitendinosus: Ischial tuberosity

Semimembranosus: Ischial tuberosity

Insertion: Biceps femoris: Fibular head, lateral tibial condyle via the lamina of the lateral hamstring tendon

Semitendinosus: Proximal medial tibial shaft, pes anserine

Semimenbranosus: Posterior medial tibial condyle

Action: Long head of the biceps femoris: Knee flexion and external rotation, hip extension and external rotation

Short head of the biceps femoris: Knee flexion and external rotation

Semitendinosus: Knee flexion and internal rotation, hip extension; assists with hip internal rotation

Semimembranosus: Knee flexion and internal rotation, hip extension; assists with hip internal rotation

Innervation: L5-S2 (sciatic nerve); all of the hamstrings except the short head of biceps femoris (peroneal branch) share the tibial branch of the sciatic nerve.

Palpation Procedure

- Place the patient prone in a relaxed and supported knee-flexed position.
- Starting at the popliteal fossa, locate the biceps femoris tendon and trace the tendon to the muscle tissue by strumming across its fibers.
- Deeper pressure will be needed as the muscular tissue is gained. The muscular fibers of

the biceps femoris can be isolated by applying pressure with the fingers or thumb of the other hand to the midposterior thigh.

- Continue to apply a deep strumming pressure while moving upward to the ischial tuberosity.
- Apply the technique and approach used for the biceps femoris to isolate the semitendinosus on the medial side of the posterior thigh.

- The tendon of the semimembranosus is difficult to isolate, but the inferior fibers of the muscle lie just lateral to the semitendinosus tendon above the popliteal fossa before they dip deep under the semitendinosus.
- Applying resistive knee flexion can accentuate the hamstrings for palpation.
- Note the location of any tender points or fasciculatory response at the muscle and tendon and their respective origins and insertions.
- Once you have determined the most dominant tender point or fasciculation (or both), maintain light pressure with the pad(s) of the finger(s) at the location throughout the PRT treatment procedure until reassessment has occurred.

PRT Clinician Procedure

- The patient is prone.
- Place the involved limb into hip extension on your thigh or a bolster.
- Typically, the higher the tissue lesion is, the more hip extension will be required.
- Using your far hand, apply hip abduction and internal rotation for the biceps femoris and hip adduction and external rotation for the semitendinosus.
- Once an optimal hip position is found, move the knee through flexion with your far hand. The knee flexion treatment position is typically 60 to 70°.
- Grasp the calcaneus with your far hand to externally rotate the tibia with light downward compression to isolate the biceps femoris and internally rotate the tibia to isolate the semitendinosus.
- Apply a downward translational force to the posterior femur below the gluteal fold with the near hand. At the same time, perform a distal translational movement of the fascia with your near hand toward the knee to accentuate relaxation and the fasciculatory response of the tissue. Use one of the fingers of your near hand to monitor the lesion, if possible.
- Using your far hand, apply marked ankle plantar flexion and big-toe flexion to reduce the strain on the sciatic nerve.
- Corollary tissues treated: Posterior hip capsule, gluteal muscles, sacrotuberous ligament, thoracolumbar fascia

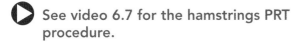 See video 6.7 for the hamstrings PRT procedure.

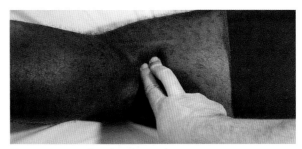

Hamstrings palpation procedure.

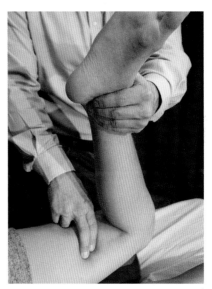

Hamstrings PRT clinician procedure.

Patient Self-Treatment Procedure

- Lie prone with the hip extended and knee flexed.
- Lying on a couch with pillows propped under the femur to accentuate hip flexion and positioning the ankle on the arm of the couch closely replicates the general release position.
- Maintain this position for three to five minutes or apply heat or ice in this position for 20 to 30 minutes to facilitate greater relaxation and pain control.

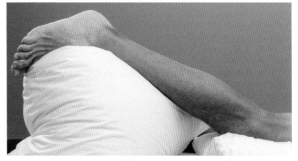

Hamstrings patient self-treatment procedure.

Iliotibial Band

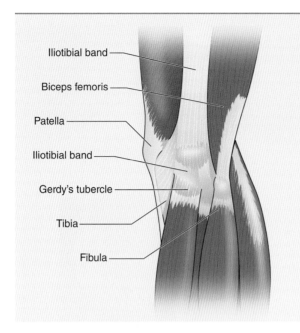

Iliotibial band
Biceps femoris
Patella
Iliotibial band
Gerdy's tubercle
Tibia
Fibula

The iliotibial band, or tract, arises from the gluteal fascia and tensor fasciae latae muscle at the lateral hip. Its vertical fibers become dense as they approach the knee and become cordlike as they cross over the lateral epicondyle of the femur. The lateral epicondyle is often a site of iliotibial band irritation, which has been attributed to increased tension or compression (or both) of the iliotibial band during its movement over this structure when running or squatting.

Origin: Gluteal fascia, tensor fasciae latae

Insertion: Gerdy's tubercle with fascial slip connections to the fibular head and lateral patellar retinaculum

Action: Stabilizes the knee against varus and rotational stress; assists with the screw home mechanism

Palpation Procedure

- Stand on the side of the supine patient that is opposite the band to be palpated.
- With your hands flat, align them over the lateral thigh just below the greater trochanter of the femur.
- Pull the band upward and away from the hamstrings.
- When translating the band upward and across the vastus lateralis, note its movement or lack thereof as well as any pain.
- Continue to palpate in the same manner when approaching the knee; firmer strumming will be needed when assessing the denser cordlike fibers.
- Determine the most dominant tender point or fasciculation (or both) and maintain light pressure with the pad(s) of the finger(s) throughout the treatment until reassessment has occurred.

PRT Clinician Procedure

- The patient is supine.
- Grasp the medial ankle with your far hand to move the hip into approximately 20° of flexion.
- Move the hip through the range of hip abduction with your far hand, noting any tissue resistance from the adductors. If tissue resistance overcomes normal range of motion, release the adductors first.
- Using your far hand, externally rotate the limb.
- Apply marked calcaneal eversion with the far hand.

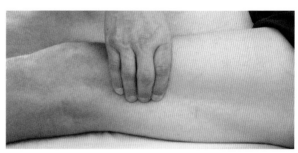

Iliotibial band palpation procedure.

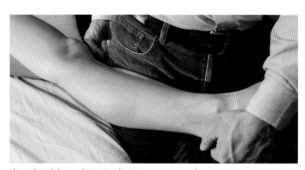

Iliotibial band PRT clinician procedure.

- Place your hip against and below the joint line of the knee as a fulcrum while applying a valgus force to the knee.
- Apply cephalad compression of the limb with the far hand or your body to fine-tune.
- Corollary tissues treated: Gluteus medius, tensor fasciae latae

 See video 6.8 for the iliotibial band PRT procedure.

Lateral Collateral Ligament

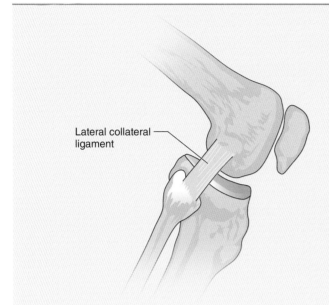

Lateral collateral ligament

The lateral collateral ligament (LCL), also known as the fibular collateral ligament, is the primary restraint against lateral, or varus, stress at the knee. Unlike its cousin the medial collateral ligament, the LCL does not communicate with the knee capsule or lateral meniscus. Therefore, LCL injury is not often associated with lateral meniscal injury; rather, it is associated with hyperextension because the LCL is a secondary restraint to this motion.

Origin: Lateral femoral epicondyle

Insertion: Fibular head

Action: Restraint against varus and internal rotation force at the knee

Palpation Procedure

- If possible, have the patient place the ankle of the involved side on the opposite thigh.
- The LCL will be very prominent as it crosses the lateral joint line of the knee.
- If pain or lack of range of motion inhibits the preceding maneuver, strum across the lateral joint line with the pads of the fingers with the patient in a supine or seated knee-flexed position.
- Note the location of any tender points or fasciculatory response at the ligament and its origin and insertion.
- Once you have determined the most dominant tender point or fasciculation (or both), maintain light pressure with the pad(s) of the finger(s) at the location throughout the PRT treatment procedure until reassessment has occurred.

PRT Clinician Procedure

- The patient is supine.
- Place the knee over your thigh to position the knee at approximately 30° of flexion.
- Using your far hand at the ankle, apply a valgus force at the knee.
- Apply marked calcaneal eversion with your far hand.
- Rotate the tibia and compress it upward for fine-tuning with the far hand.
- Corollary tissues treated: Iliotibial band, peroneals

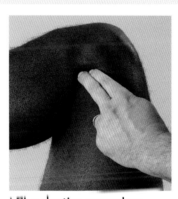

LCL palpation procedure.

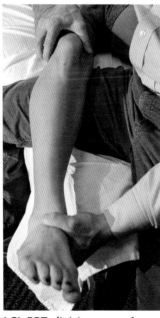

LCL PRT clinician procedure.

Vastus Lateralis

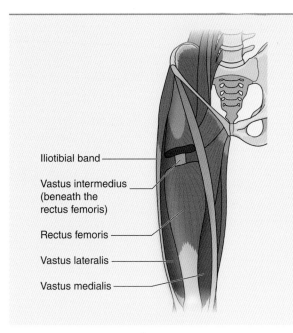

Iliotibial band

Vastus intermedius (beneath the rectus femoris)

Rectus femoris

Vastus lateralis

Vastus medialis

The vastus lateralis, the largest of the quadriceps group, is partially covered by the iliotibial band. Imbalance in the timing and strength of contraction between the lateralis and vastus medialis has often been attributed to the development of patellar maltracking. However, weak hip abductors may also play a primary role.

Origin: Lateral lip of the femoral linea aspera

Insertion: Tibial tuberosity via the quadriceps tendon, ligamentum patellae

Action: Knee extension

Innervation: L2-L4 (femoral nerve)

Palpation Procedure

- The vastus lateralis can be palpated in a supine or side-lying position.
- Locate the iliotibial band and slide your fingers off the band noting the transition into the softer vastus lateralis, both posterior and anterior to the band.
- The patient can actively extend the knee to accentuate the fibers for palpation.
- Note the location of any tender points or fasciculatory response of the muscle and its attachment sites.
- Once you have determined the most dominant tender point or fasciculation (or both), maintain light pressure with the pad(s) of the finger(s) at the location throughout the PRT treatment procedure until reassessment has occurred.

PRT Clinician Procedure

- The patient is supine.
- Place the lower leg on your thigh at approximately 30°.
- Apply a posterior force at the superior tibia below the patella using your far hand to encourage knee hyperextension.
- With your near hand, laterally translate the vastus lateralis muscle belly while monitoring its lesion with the one of the fingers of your near hand.
- With the far hand, apply external limb rotation and a lateral patellar glide for fine-tuning.
- Corollary tissue treated: Iliotibial band

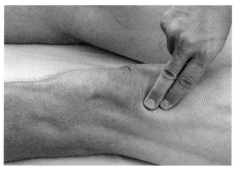

Vastus lateralis palpation procedure.

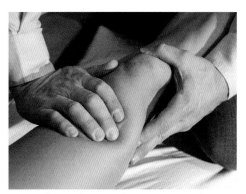

Vastus lateralis PRT clinician procedure.

Patient Self-Treatment Procedure

- Place the lower leg and foot on a stool or couch arm.
- Lean forward and place one hand below the patella at the tibia and the other just above the patella on the vastus lateralis.
- Apply a downward pressure below the patella while translating the muscle belly diagonally away from the patella.
- Externally rotate the limb and glide the patella laterally to fine-tune.
- Monitor the vastus lateralis for a fasciculatory response and tissue relaxation at the site of pain.
- Maintain the treatment position until the fasciculatory response abates or for three to five minutes.

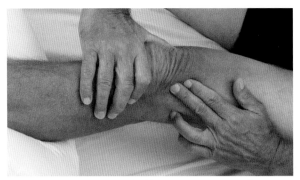

Vastus lateralis patient self-treatment procedure.

Patellar Tendinopathy

Patellar tendinopathy, also known as jumper's knee or patellar tendinitis or grouped with other conditions that cause anterior knee pain, is attributed to the overuse of the patellar tendon (Larsson and Nilsson-Helander 2012). There is no current evidence-based consensus on the optimal treatment of patellar tendinopathy; however, symptomatic treatment coupled with eccentric training has shown promise (Larsson and Nilsson-Helander 2012). Patellar tendinopathy is not an inflammatory condition, but a degenerative condition that results in derangement and weakening of the tendon's fibers (Rodriguez-Merchan 2013). Danielson and colleagues (2008) found that the dorsal paratenon is sympathetically innervated and possesses a blood supply, which provides a rationale for treating this tissue with PRT.

Common Signs and Symptoms

- Patellar tendon pain
- Increased pain with functional activity, particularly running, jumping, and cutting
- Point tenderness of the patellar tendon and, at times, its attachment at the tibial tuberosity

Common Differential Diagnoses

- Osgood-Schlatter disease
- Sinding-Larsen-Johansson disease
- Tibial plateau stress fracture
- Chondromalacia

Clinician Therapeutic Interventions

- Determine the root of the patient's condition (e.g., faulty jumping mechanics, faulty gait biomechanics, training errors, leg length discrepancy, weak hip musculature, surface or shoe alteration).
- Consider requesting an MRI or bone scan to rule out stress fracture if tenderness is localized over the tibial tuberosity or plateau.
- Scan and treat the structures in the order presented in the Treatment Points and Sequencing box. However, you should base your treatment sequencing off the most dominant (tender) points first.
- Follow PRT with thermal ultrasound or laser and PNF stretching of the patellar tendon.

Treatment Points and Sequencing

1. Patellar tendon
2. Pes anserine
3. Iliotibial band
4. Tibialis posterior
5. Popliteus
6. Medial gastrocnemius
7. Tensor fasciae latae
8. Adductors of the thigh
9. Psoas

- Apply eccentric training with a focus on sport- or work-specific demands (or both) in conjunction with PRT and other therapeutic interventions.
- For some patients, KT Tape or the use of a patellar strap or band reduces pain during the initial stage of therapy.
- Apply instrumented soft-tissue mobilization (ISTM) if recalcitrant tissue adhesions are present.
- Consider performing a biomechanical evaluation of jumping mechanics and gait if a training, movement, or biomechanical error is suspected.
- Implement open- and closed-chain strengthening for the intrinsic foot, pretibial and hip, and core muscles to address weaknesses or compensations identified in the biomechanical analysis, with a particular focus on eccentric control of knee flexion and internal tibial rotation.
- Temporary or custom orthotics to unload the patellar tendon may be warranted based on biomechanical evaluation outcomes.

Patient Self-Treatment Interventions

- Self-release the patellar tendon and tibialis posterior on a daily basis or when irritated.
- PNF stretch the patellar tendon after eccentric exercise or on a daily basis. Do not stretch if it produces pain because doing so may result in additional tissue lesions.
- Perform self-massage for five to eight minutes daily after stretching.

Iliotibial Band Friction Syndrome

There is little consensus about what causes the lateral leg and knee pain associated with iliotibial band friction syndrome (Lavine 2010). Initially, pain at or below the lateral femoral condyle was thought to develop from a friction mechanism at the condyle as a result of band tightness. However, evidence points to a compression mechanism at this location and subsequent irritation of the underlying bursae and bone independent of iliotibial band tightness and friction (Lavine 2010). Moreover, intrinsic factors such as overpronation, weak hip abductors, and increased frontal plane movement of the limb, among others, have not been shown to increase the prevalence or risk of this syndrome (Bauer and Duke 2011; Lavine 2010). However, a general consensus is that treating tender and trigger points along the course of the band, or tract, as well as its communicating fascia helps in the treatment of this condition.

Common Signs and Symptoms

- Pain with ambulation, squatting, downhill running, and descending stairs
- Point tenderness at the lateral knee; above, over, or below the lateral femoral condyle; and potentially at Gerdy's tubercle and the fibular head
- Positive Ober's and Noble's test
- Weak hip rotators and abductors
- Increased frontal plane movement of the limb
- Pes planus or cavus

Common Differential Diagnoses

- Stress fracture
- Disc pathology
- Lateral meniscal tear
- Popliteus tendinopathy
- Patellofemoral pain syndrome

Clinician Therapeutic Interventions

- Determine the root of the patient's condition (e.g., faulty biomechanics, training errors, leg length discrepancy, weak hip musculature, surface or shoe alteration).
- Consider requesting an MRI or bone scan to rule out stress fracture if tenderness is localized over the bone.

Treatment Points and Sequencing

1. Iliotibial band at the knee
2. Pes anserine
3. Popliteus
4. Adductor group
5. Adductor magnus
6. Sartorius tendon
7. Gluteus medius
8. Sacroiliac joint
9. Psoas
10. Quadratus lumborum
11. Flexor hallucis brevis

- Scan and treat the structures in the order presented in the Treatment Points and Sequencing box. However, you should base your treatment sequencing off the most dominant (tender) points first.
- Follow PRT with diathermy, laser or thermal ultrasound, PNF stretching of the iliotibial band if tightness exists, and myofascial massage.
- For some patients, KT Tape reduces pain during the initial stage of therapy.
- Apply ISTM if recalcitrant tissue adhesions are present.
- Consider performing a biomechanical gait evaluation if a training or biomechanical error is suspected.
- Implement open- and closed-chain strengthening for the pretibial, hip, and core muscles to address weaknesses or compensations identified in the gait or movement analysis, with a particular focus on the control of abnormal frontal plane movement.
- Have the patient use temporary or custom orthotics to unload the lateral knee tissues during the initial phase of rehabilitation.
- Avoid having the patient run through the pain. The patient should perform only physical activity that is tolerable—ideally with no pain.
- Slowly progress the patient to dynamic physical activity through aquatic therapy or gravity-assisted running devices.

> continued

Iliotibial Band Friction Syndrome *> continued*

- Bursectomy may be warranted if traditional therapeutic interventions fail.

Patient Self-Treatment Interventions

- PNF stretch the iliotibial band and posterior hip musculature if it is tight after exercise or on a daily basis. Do not stretch if it produces pain because doing so may result in additional tissue lesions.
- Perform self-massage or use a foam roll for five to eight minutes daily after stretching.

However, avoid these measures if they cause extreme pain because they may produce additional tissue lesions.

- Apply ice or heat to the affected area to relieve tissue pain and spasm. Typically, patients with chronic symptoms respond best to heat (e.g., warm whirlpool or Jacuzzi). (*Note:* Consult with the clinician about where you are in the healing process, which will determine whether to apply heat or ice.)

Summary

Knee and thigh injury experienced early in life may result in altered neuromuscular control and abnormal biomechanics, predisposing the patient to future injury (Hewett et al. 2013). A multitude of factors have been proposed to predispose a person to knee and thigh injury, such as improper training (DiFiori et al. 2014), altered gait mechanics (Crowell and Davis 2011), and weak hip abductors (Leetun et al. 2004), but somatic dysfunction has not been one of them to date. Han and colleagues (2012) proposed that latent and active myofascial trigger points (MTrPs) may develop in the elbow of children as young as age 4, and Bates and Grunwaldt (1958) found MTrPs in a variety of anatomic locations in children as young as age 3, including the knee and thigh. Given the potential negative impact of osteopathic lesions (trigger and tender points) on strength, range of motion, and neuromuscular control, clinicians should consider a myofascial evaluation or palpatory exam as part of a standard physical in the young and over the life span. Moreover, researchers should examine how osteopathic lesions affect neuromuscular control and biomechanics to ascertain whether they may also be a predisposing factor for knee and thigh injury.

CHAPTER 7

Pelvis

CHAPTER OBJECTIVES

After reading this chapter, you should be able to do the following:

1 State the factors that may influence the development of pelvic somatic dysfunction.

2 Locate and palpate pelvic tissue structures to be treated with positional release therapy (PRT).

3 Apply pelvic PRT techniques.

4 Articulate how common injury conditions such as piriformis syndrome may be treated based on pelvic lesion patterns.

The pelvis serves as the base of support for human locomotion, dissipates forces associated with sport and activities of daily living, and provides a central point of tissue attachment to enable muscular force production (Speicher, Martin, and Desimone 2006). The ilia and their articulations with the sacrum are analogous to a vehicle chassis. Without our chassis, the segments of our body would have no point of attachment, and we would literally go nowhere! Because of the multiple functions of the pelvis and the array of tissues that pass through and attach to it, clinicians are often confounded by somatic dysfunction in this area.

Somatic pelvic dysfunction can ensue from below, within, or above. Compensatory deviations in lower-extremity biomechanical function may cause repetitive loading of pelvic structures; neurological conditions from the lumbar spine above may mimic pelvic conditions; and internally, pelvic floor musculature may be altered as a result of pregnancy, disease conditions, or low back pain (Seidenberg and Bowen 2010). Morelli and Weaver (2005) found that patients presenting with groin pain were afflicted with more than one associated injury condition. Surprisingly, though, only one study (Wong and Schauer-Alvarez 2004) to date has evaluated the impact of strain counterstrain (SCS) on pelvic somatic dysfunction. Based on its potential neurophysiological impact, PRT may decompress neurovascular structures of the hip, invigorate blood flow to tendons, and most important, eliminate or reduce pelvic pain.

Given that so many causes and injury conditions can affect the pelvis, it is not surprising that evaluation, diagnosis, and treatment are so daunting. Moreover, many of the core muscles that provide pelvic stability (e.g., gluteus maximus, erector spinae, rectus abdominis, transverse abdominis, pelvic floor, multifidi) also provide lower-extremity stability and function (Leetun et al. 2004). Leetun and colleagues (2004) examined the lumbopelvic core stability of 80 American female and 60 male basketball and track athletes preseason to determine whether deficits were predictive of lower-extremity injury rates during the competitive season. A regression analysis revealed that hip isometric abduction and external rotation were the only variables of those studied to predict lower-extremity injury status during the season. Even though the authors did not examine functional hip strength, their findings may lend credence to the impact of decreased hip isometric abductor and external strength on the development of lower-extremity injury among female athletes.

Hip abductor weakness, particularly among females, has been an intensive area of investigation as a potential cause of ACL injury. The prevailing consensus among researchers today is that multiple intrinsic and extrinsic factors in combination are responsible for an increased susceptibility to ACL injury. However, one of them may be a lack of lumbopelvic core stability, which could also be attributed to weak hip adductors.

In a retrospective study of 769 Norwegian male amateur soccer players, previous injury and weak adductors were the only variables found to be significant risk factors for groin injury (Engebretsen et al. 2010). Those with a previous history of injury were twice as likely to incur another groin injury, and when weak adductor strength was observed, a fourfold risk existed. Anderson and colleagues (2001) highlighted research indicating the potential role of a muscle imbalance between the adductors and rectus abdominis; they found groin strain to be a potential result of the adductors overpowering weak, delayed, or inactive abdominal muscles. Valent and colleagues (2012) concurred; they posited that an imbalance between these two muscle groups can cause a shearing force at the pubic symphysis, resulting in insertional adductor tendinopathy and referred low back pain.

Given the symbiotic relationship between the pelvis and low back, a lack of core stability often results in low back pain among both sport and occupational athletes. Peate and colleagues (2007) found that a core stability program implemented

Patient Considerations

When working in sensitive anatomical areas such as the pubis, a clinician must explain to the patient the reason for palpating structures in this area and how it will be done, and gain permission to do so before proceeding. Additionally, the parent of a minor should observe and a like-gender colleague should be present during the procedure, whether it be palpation or treatment of these sensitive areas. Patients who are uncomfortable with the palpation or treatment procedure can be instructed to palpate themselves.

among 433 firefighters reduced time lost from work and injury rate to 44 to 62% for lower-extremity and back injuries, respectively. Rupert and colleagues (2009) reported sacroiliac joint pathology to be present in 10 to 27% of chronic low back pain patients. However, until recently, treating nonspecific low back pain with motor control therapy, which may involve training the core musculature, has not been widely supported.

In a 2009 systematic review, Macedo and colleagues found that motor control exercise performed throughout the rehabilitation process was significantly better at resolving low back pain than no intervention. However, it was not better than manual therapy or exercise alone (such as Pilates movements). Gladwell and colleagues (2006) produced significant therapeutic outcomes of pain reduction, sport function, flexibility, and proprio-ception with the application of a six-week Pilates program in a low back pain intervention group compared to controls. However, in a systematic review of Pilates for the treatment of low back pain, Posadzki, Lizis, and Hagner-Derengowska (2011) indicated that the Gladwell study and three others did not possess enough power due to limited subject numbers. Nevertheless, they do appear to show a positive trend of effectiveness in managing low back pain, which has been attributed to improved core stability.

In sum, a multitude of factors may cause pelvic somatic dysfunction. Therefore, it is imperative that clinicians evaluate the origin of the somatic dysfunction, determine modifiable factors that can be corrected, and take into account that pelvic injury conditions may linger as a result of the central role the pelvis plays in sport, work, and life activity.

TREATMENT
Common Anatomical Areas and Conditions for PRT

Anterior Structures
- Muscle strain
- Trochanteric bursitis
- Osteoarthritis
- Athletic pubalgia
- Adductor tendinitis or tendinosis
- Snapping hip
- Anterior innominate rotation

Posterior Structures
- Muscle strain
- Ischial bursitis
- Osteoarthritis
- Piriformis syndrome
- Sacroiliac joint dysfunction
- Sacroiliac joint fixation
- Low back pain
- Posterior innominate rotation

Psoas Major

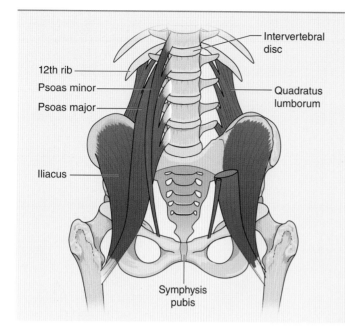

The iliopsoas is composed of both the iliacus and psoas major, which work together to provide hip flexion and stabilization to the low back. However, the psoas major can be partially palpated and differentiated from the iliacus and functions during ambulation to control hip and knee rotation. The psoas minor is frequently absent and is not palpable; therefore, only the psoas major is detailed for palpation and treatment.

Origin: L1-L5 transverse processes, T12-L5 vertebral bodies

Insertion: Lesser trochanter of the femur

Action: Hip flexion with origin fixed, trunk flexion with insertion fixed, hip external rotation, lumbar flexion, lateral trunk flexion to the same side

Innervation: L1-L4 (lumbar plexus)

Palpation Procedure

- Position the patient supine with the knee flexed on either your thigh or a bolster. For a patient with a large amount of adipose tissue or muscle mass, use an exercise ball for positioning.
- The psoas major runs diagonally from the anterior superior iliac spine (ASIS) to the navel. Position your fingers across the fiber orientation diagonally with your fingers stacked over one another.
- Compress downward slowly as the patient exhales, while pushing the rectus abdominis out of the way.
- Strum across the psoas fibers.
- Having the patient flex the hip will aid in palpation of the tissue.
- Note the location of any tender points or fasciculatory response along the muscle.
- Once you have determined the most dominant tender point or fasciculation (or both), maintain light pressure with the pad(s) of the finger(s) at the location throughout the PRT treatment procedure until reassessment has occurred.

PRT Clinician Procedure

- The patient is supine.
- Both of the patient's feet are on your shoulder (video 7.1a) or on an exercise ball (video 7.1b) with the involved ankle on top of the non-involved ankle.

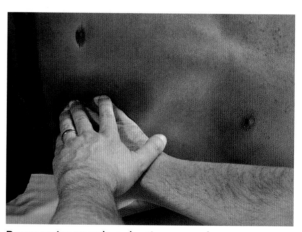

Psoas major muscle palpation procedure.

- The patient's hips are placed in a lateral and flexed position toward the involved hip.
- Move the patient's knees and hips into flexion with your far hand and toward the opposite shoulder or in line with the fibers orientation diagonally.
- Once the flexion position is determined, place your knee or thigh under the pelvis to encourage a posterior pelvic tilt. A bolster or pillow can also be used to bolster the pelvis.
- Using your far hand, move the knees and hips laterally in the frontal plane; then rotate them.
- Once the release is obtained, flex the knees and take the feet to the table. Then bolster the knees into flexion and follow with a palpatory reassessment.
- Corollary tissues treated: Iliacus, rectus abdominis, rectus femoris

▶ **See video 7.1 for the psoas major PRT procedure.**

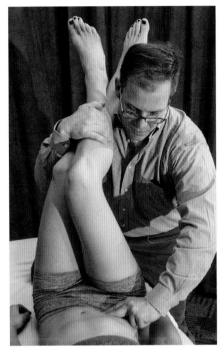

Psoas major PRT clinician procedure.

Rectus Abdominis Muscle: Lower Fibers

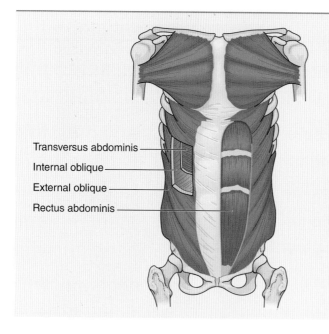

Transversus abdominis
Internal oblique
External oblique
Rectus abdominis

When not covered with a large amount of adipose tissue, the rectus abdominis muscle gives the appearance of a washboard; it is commonly called six-pack abs. The rectus abdominis is often thought to contribute to core stability. However, according to McGill (2007), it plays only a partial role in core stability, but it should be activated along with other core muscles to enhance spinal stabilization or stiffness.

Origin: Pubic crest, pubic symphysis

Insertion: Costal cartilage of ribs 5 through 7, xiphoid process

Action: Flexes the spine; tilts the pelvis posteriorly

Innervation: T7-T12 (ventral rami)

Lower Rectus Abdominis Palpation Procedure

- Place the patient supine with the knees bolstered into flexion.
- While the patient performs a partial sit-up, palpate from the xiphoid process and ribs to the pubic crest.
- Strum across the fibers of the muscle.
- To gain access to the inferior fibers of the rectus and its tendinous origin on the superior pubic crest, position the base of your hand over the umbilicus. The tips of your fingers will now be just above the pubic crest.
- Note the location of any tender points or fasciculatory response along the muscle and its attachment site.
- Once you have determined the most dominant tender point or fasciculation (or both), maintain light pressure with the pad(s) of the finger(s) at the location throughout the PRT treatment procedure until reassessment has occurred.

PRT Clinician Procedure

- Place the patient supine in a supported flexed thoracic position. (Thoracic flexion can be accomplished either by placing a pillow under the upper torso or by elevating the torso with a spit treatment table.)
- Place the ankles on your shoulder or on an exercise ball. Stabilize the ankles with your far hand.

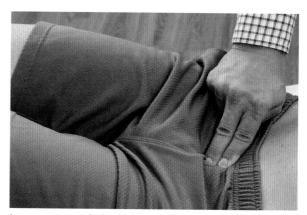

Lower rectus abdominis palpation procedure.

- Using your far hand, move the patient's hips and knees into flexion to encourage thoracic and posterior pelvic tilting.
- Once the optimal pelvic and hip position is attained, bolster the posterior pelvis with either your thigh or a pillow.
- Using your far hand and body, apply hip and femoral rotation for fine-tuning.
- Corollary tissues treated: Hip flexors, obliques

Patient Self-Treatment Procedure

- Lie supine with a pillow under the upper torso and another under the posterior pelvis to encourage posterior tilting.
- Place the ankles on a stable structure such as the arm of a sofa or the edge of a chair to support the knees and hips into flexion.
- During positioning, self-palpate the lower abdominals for the presence of a fasciculatory response and optimal tissue relaxation, which will help you attain the optimal treatment position.
- Maintain the treatment position until the fasciculatory response abates or for three to five minutes.

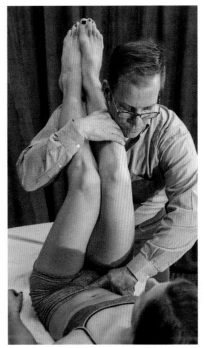

Lower rectus abdominis PRT clinician procedure.

Sartorius Tendon and Muscle

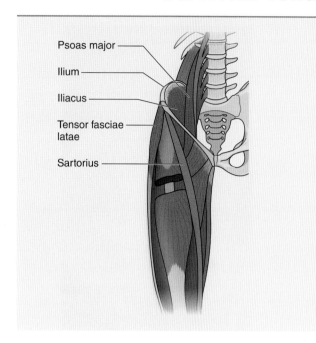

Psoas major
Ilium
Iliacus
Tensor fasciae latae
Sartorius

The sartorius (*sartor* is the Latin term for "tailor") muscle is the longest muscle of the body. It originates from the ASIS and courses obliquely to the posterior femoral condyle to join the gracilis and semitendinosus to form the pes anserine tendon. Its name is associated with the position a tailor might assume when sewing. Even though it is superficial, it can be difficult to isolate, particularly given that it is absent in a small percentage of the population.

Origin: Anterior superior iliac spine

Insertion: Proximal medial surface of the tibial shaft

Action: Hip external rotation, abduction, and flexion; knee flexion and internal rotation

Innervation: L2-L3 (femoral nerve)

Palpation Procedure

- Place the patient in a supine position with the lateral ankle on the opposite shin. This replicates the tailor sitting position or, more recently, the movement often used in the game of Hacky Sack.

- The therapist should resist hip flexion, abduction, and lateral rotation at the ankle or knee to aid in palpation of the structure.

- Moving from the tendinous origin of the sartorius at the ASIS, strum across the tendon to the muscular portion as it courses obliquely across the thigh to the medial knee, where it forms the pes anserine tendon.

- The muscular aspect is only a few fingers wide and is the most superficial of the anterior thigh muscles.

- Note the location of any tender points or fasciculatory response along the muscle or proximal and distal tendon and their attachment sites.

- Once you have determined the most dominant tender point or fasciculation (or both), maintain light pressure with the pad(s) of the finger(s) at the location throughout the PRT treatment procedure until reassessment has occurred.

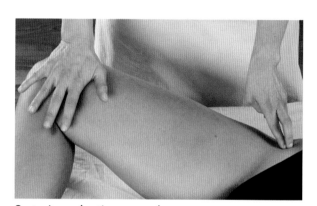

Sartorius palpation procedure.

PRT Clinician Procedure

- Place the patient supine.
- Place your far hand over the involved heel and the patient's knee into your torso.
- Using your far hand, move the hip into marked flexion, external rotation, and abduction while maintaining knee contact with your torso.
- Apply marked calcaneal inversion with the far hand.
- Corollary tissues treated: Iliacus, psoas, tensor fasciae latae, rectus femoris

▶ **See video 7.2 for the sartorius PRT procedure.**

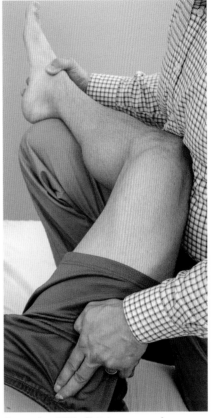

Sartorius PRT clinician procedure.

Rectus Femoris Tendon

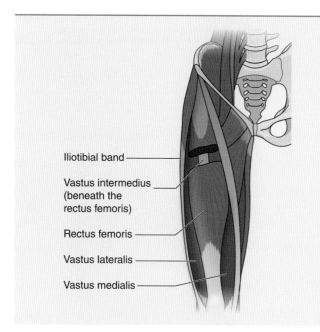

Iliotibial band

Vastus intermedius
(beneath the
rectus femoris)

Rectus femoris

Vastus lateralis

Vastus medialis

The rectus femoris tendon often becomes irritated at its origin site, the anterior inferior iliac spine, when the hip flexor muscles as a group or the rectus femoris muscle itself is strained or overloaded. Particularly in the athletic population, lesions at this tendon often result in a lack of extension at the hip.

Origin: Anterior inferior iliac spine

Action: Assist with hip flexion

Innervation: L4 (femoral nerve); rectus femoris muscle

Palpation Procedure

- The patient should be supine with either a bolster or your thigh under the knee to place the hip in a flexed position.
- Locate the crest of the ilium and trace your fingers downward to the prominent ASIS. Continue downward to the smaller bony prominence of the anterior inferior iliac spine (AIIS).
- The tendon of the rectus femoris is just below the AIIS.
- Strum across the tendon, roughly at the anterior crease of the hip.
- Note the location of any tender points or fasciculatory response along the tendon and its attachment site.
- Once you have determined the most dominant tender point or fasciculation (or both), maintain light pressure with the pad(s) of the finger(s) at the location throughout the PRT treatment procedure until reassessment has occurred.

PRT Clinician Procedure

- Place the patient supine.
- Place the ankles of the patient on your shoulder or on an exercise ball.
- The ankles can be crossed over one another or not based on patient and therapist comfort.

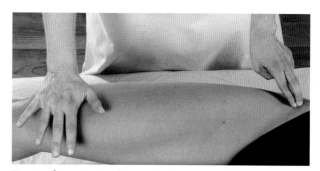

Rectus femoris tendon palpation procedure.

132

- Using your far hand, grasp both knees together while moving the patient's hips into flexion.
- Once the hip flexion position of comfort or fasciculatory response (or both) has been found, apply lateral trunk flexion and femoral internal and external rotation with your far hand to fine-tune the treatment position.
- Corollary tissues treated: Iliacus, pectineus, psoas

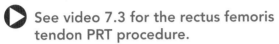 See video 7.3 for the rectus femoris tendon PRT procedure.

Patient Self-Treatment Procedure

- Lie down in front of a couch or chair.
- Place your lower legs on the couch or chair with the knees touching.
- While palpating the rectus femoris tendon, feel for the fasciculatory response of the tissue coupled with its most relaxed position while performing the following motions: hip flexion, lateral trunk flexion, and femoral internal and external rotation.
- Because the hips must remain relaxed during the treatment, support the knees from moving in or out by bolstering them against an immovable object such as a chair or wall.
- Maintain the treatment position until the fasciculatory response abates or for three to five minutes.

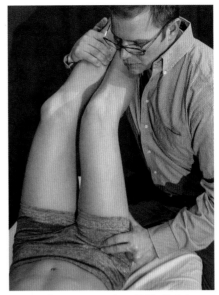

Rectus femoris tendon PRT clinician procedure.

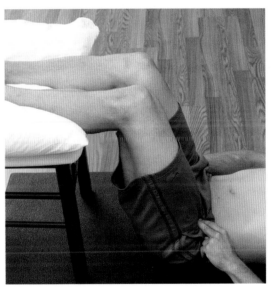

Rectus femoris tendon patient self-treatment procedure.

Iliacus

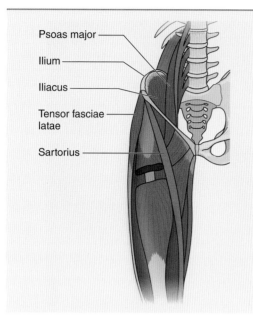

The iliacus is a broad flat muscle that fills the iliac fossa. It converges laterally with the psoas major; the two together are termed the iliopsoas. The iliacus is a hip flexor and contributes to low back stabilization.

Origin:	Superior two thirds of the iliac fossa, inner lip of the iliac crest, anterior sacroiliac and iliolumbar ligaments, lateral sacrum
Insertion:	Lesser trochanter via the psoas major tendon
Action:	Hip flexion with fixed origin; trunk and pelvis flexion with fixed insertion
Innervation:	L2-L3 (femoral nerve)

Palpation Procedure

- Position the patient supine. (A patient with a large amount of adipose tissue can be placed on the contralateral side with the hip and knee flexed to gain access to the iliac fossa.)
- Place either a bolster or your thigh under the patient's knee.
- Locate the iliac crest above its anterior superior iliac spine.
- Ask the patient to exhale; then slowly and gently sink your fingers into the iliac fossa from the lateral crest, moving the superficial abdominal muscles medially.
- Gently strum along the iliac fossa.
- Hip flexion will accentuate the contraction of the iliacus under palpation.
- Determine the most dominant tender point or fasciculation (or both) and maintain light pressure with the pad(s) of the finger(s) throughout the treatment until reassessment has occurred.

PRT Clinician Procedure

- Place both feet of the supine patient on your shoulder or an exercise ball in a butterfly position. The procedure can also be done with a single leg as seen in the sartorius tendon procedure.
- With your far hand, move the hips into flexion allowing the knees to move outward into a butterfly position to attain marked femoral external rotation.
- With your body, fine-tune the positioning by applying femoral abduction, adduction, and rotation.
- Corollary tissues treated: Psoas, rectus femoris, sartorius

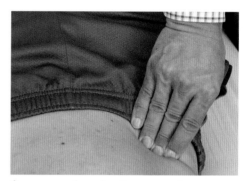

Iliacus muscle palpation procedure.

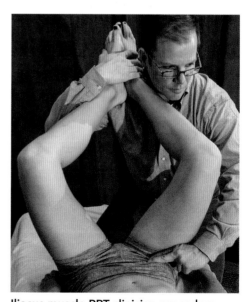

Iliacus muscle PRT clinician procedure.

 See video 7.4 for the iliacus muscle PRT procedure.

Tensor Fasciae Latae

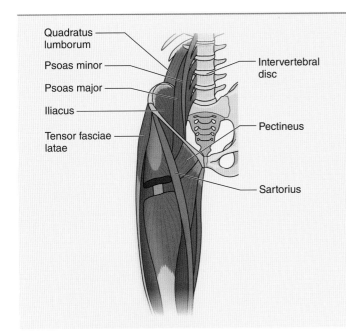

Quadratus lumborum
Psoas minor
Psoas major
Iliacus
Tensor fasciae latae
Intervertebral disc
Pectineus
Sartorius

The tensor fasciae latae, a superficial muscle about two to three fingers wide, is located just inferior and lateral to the ASIS. This muscle communicates with the iliotibial tract and is often a site of restriction when iliotibial band friction syndrome is present.

Origin: Iliac crest, posterior to the ASIS

Insertion: Iliotibial tract (deep and superficial layers)

Action: Hip flexion, internal rotation, and abduction

Innervation: L4-S1 (superior gluteal nerve)

Palpation Procedure

- Position the patient supine with the knee extended.
- Palpate the muscle approximately 1 inch (2.5 cm) below and lateral to the ASIS.
- Ask the patient to internally rotate the leg to feel the muscle contract.
- Strum across the tissues fibers until you feel it blend into the flat, fibrous iliotibial tract.
- Note the location of any tender points or fasciculatory response along the muscle and its sites of attachment.
- Once you have determined the most dominant tender point or fasciculation (or both), maintain light pressure with the pad(s) of the finger(s) at the location throughout the PRT treatment procedure until reassessment has occurred.

PRT Clinician Procedure

- Position the patient supine with the knee and hip flexed.
- Place your far hand over the top of the knee.
- Using the far hand or your body, move the hip into marked flexion with your far hand at the knee.
- Using your far hand, apply internal and external rotation of the hip.
- Apply marked femoral compression downward using either your far hand or your torso.
- Using your body or far hand, fine-tune the position with hip abduction and adduction.
- Corollary tissues treated: Rectus femoris, rectus femoris tendon, iliacus, psoas, iliotibial tract

 See video 7.5 for the tensor fasciae latae PRT procedure.

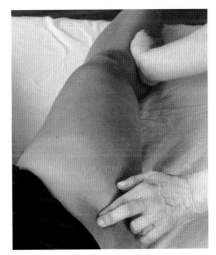

Tensor fasciae latae palpation procedure.

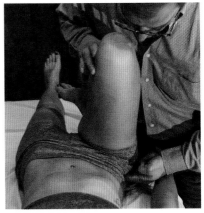

Tensor fasciae latae PRT clinician procedure.

Superior Pubis

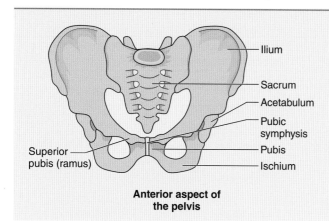

Ilium
Sacrum
Acetabulum
Pubic symphysis
Pubis
Ischium
Superior pubis (ramus)

Anterior aspect of the pelvis

The superior pubis is an important site for several muscular attachments. At the superior aspect of the pubic crest are the pubic tubercles. Each hornlike bony prominence serves as an attachment site for the adductor longus muscle and inguinal ligament as well as the rectus abdominis. Lateral to the pubic tubercles is the superior ramus of the pubis, which is oriented at a 45° angle upward to the ASIS. Lateral to the pubic tubercles lies the origin of the pectineus.

Palpation Procedure

- Place the patient supine and place the knees into flexion using either your knee or a bolster.
- Locate the common adductor tendon (adductor longus and gracilis) at the medial groin (this tendon is the most prominent in the groin and is often visible with resistive adduction). Just under the tendon's attachment on the bone are the pubic tubercles.
- Stack the fingers and hands on one another and move them laterally off the pubic tubercle and superiorly upward onto the superior ramus of the pubis.
- Apply downward pressure and stroke toward the feet to feel the crest of the pubis.
- Palpate across the ramus toward the ASIS.
- Note the location of any tender points or fasciculatory response along the bone.
- Determine the most dominant tender point or fasciculation (or both) and maintain light pressure with the pad(s) of the finger(s) throughout the treatment until reassessment has occurred.

PRT Clinician Procedure

- Place the patient supine.
- Place your far hand over the knee.
- Using your far hand, move the hip and knee into marked flexion.
- Apply downward compression of the femur using either your far hand or your torso while applying femoral rotation (use greater internal rotation for medial tissues and less for lateral tissues).
- Use your far hand to apply adduction and abduction to fine-tune the position.
- Corollary tissues treated: Abdominis, psoas, rectus femoris tendon, tensor fasciae latae

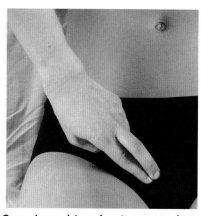

Superior pubis palpation procedure.

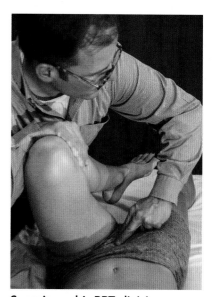

Superior pubis PRT clinician procedure.

Inferior Pubis

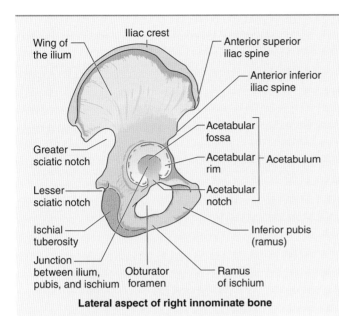

Wing of the ilium

Iliac crest

Anterior superior iliac spine

Anterior inferior iliac spine

Acetabular fossa

Acetabular rim — Acetabulum

Greater sciatic notch

Acetabular notch

Lesser sciatic notch

Ischial tuberosity

Inferior pubis (ramus)

Junction between ilium, pubis, and ischium

Obturator foramen

Ramus of ischium

Lateral aspect of right innominate bone

The inferior pubis is formed by two rami, the inferior ramus of the pubis and the ischial ramus. Both form a bridge (ischiopubic ramus) that connects the pubic crest to the ischial tuberosity. The inferior ramus is an attachment site for the gracilis, adductor brevis, and adductor magnus muscles; the magnus also attaches to the ramus of the ischium. Hamstring and low back injury often produce painful lesions of the adductor magnus at the inferior ramus.

Palpation Procedure

- Place the patient supine with the knees flexed using either your knee or a bolster.
- Locate the common adductor tendon (adductor longus and gracilis) at the medial groin (this tendon is the most prominent in the groin and is often visible with resistive adduction). Just under the tendon's attachment on the bone are the pubic tubercles.
- Palpate the inferior ischium by sliding your fingers inferior and medial to the pubic tubercle.
- Stroke up and down as well as across the inferior ischium, tracing it posteriorly to the ischial ramus.
- Determine the most dominant tender point or fasciculation (or both) and maintain light pressure with the pad(s) of the finger(s) throughout the treatment until reassessment has occurred.

PRT Clinician Procedure

- Place the patient supine with the lower leg on your knee. Placing the patient's lower leg on your knee or thigh or on an exercise ball will position the hip into approximately 90° of flexion.
- Using your far hand, move the hip into flexion, marked adduction, and internal rotation.
- Apply downward femoral compression at the knee using your far hand or your torso.
- This procedure can also be used to treat the tendons and the proximal muscular tissues of the adductor brevis, magnus, and gracilis.
- Corollary tissues treated: Psoas, iliacus, rectus femoris, adductor magnus, adductor longus, gracilis

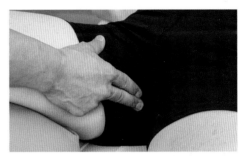

Inferior pubis palpation procedure.

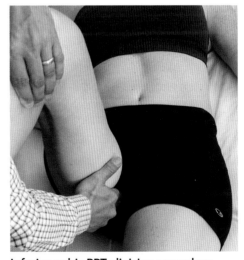

Inferior pubis PRT clinician procedure.

 See video 7.6 for the inferior pubis PRT procedure.

Lateral Rotator Tendons of the Hip

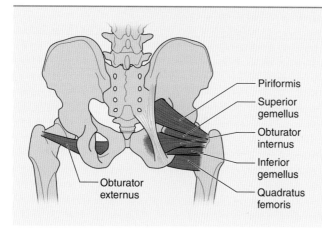

The tendons of the six deep posterior hip muscles (piriformis, quadratus femoris, obturator internus, obturator externus, gemellus superior, and gemellus inferior) share common attachment locations around the greater trochanter. Of the "deep six" muscles, only the piriformis and quadratus femoris are directly palpable; however, the density of their tendons as a group can be discerned with resistive hip external rotation. Because pathology to one or several of the deep rotators often produces lesions at their common attachment location at the greater trochanter, their tendons are grouped for both palpation and treatment.

Palpation Procedure

- Place the patient prone with the knee flexed.
- Locate the mass of the greater trochanter at the lateral leg by moving 4 to 6 inches (10 to 15 cm) inferior to the lateral crest of the ilium.
- Having the patient actively rotate the femur under palpation can help with the location of the greater trochanter.
- Slide your fingers medially and posteriorly off the lateral aspect of the greater trochanter and into the soft tissue just adjacent to the femur, which will now be located over the lateral rotator tendons.
- Ask the patient to externally rotate the hip against your resistance to feel the density of the tendons.
- To feel the tendons, stroke across them with firm pressure.
- Note the location of any tender points or fasciculatory response at the tendons.
- Once you have determined the most dominant tender point or fasciculation (or both), maintain light pressure with the pad(s) of the finger(s) at the location throughout the PRT treatment procedure until reassessment has occurred.

PRT Clinician Procedure

- Place the patient prone with the knee flexed
- Using your far hand, grasp under the patient's knee and move the hip into slight extension.
- Once the extension treatment position is found, move the thigh into a moderate range of abduction with your far hand.

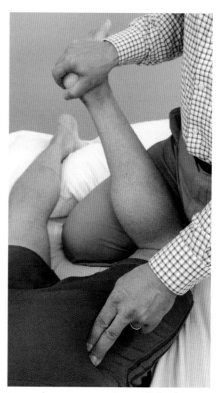

Lateral rotator tendons of the hip palpation procedure.

- Place the patient's thigh on either a bolster or your thigh when the extension and abduction position is determined.
- Using your far hand, apply femoral external rotation.
- For fine-tuning, apply long axis compression with your torso or distraction using your far hand at the popliteal fossa.
- Corollary tissues treated: Gluteus medius, gluteus maximus, gluteus minimus, sacrotuberous ligament, piriformis, erector spinae, thoracolumbar fascia, iliotibial band

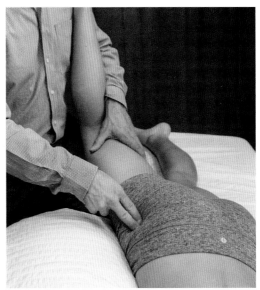

Lateral rotator tendons of the hip PRT clinician procedure.

Piriformis

A hypertonic piriformis muscle may result in compression of the sciatic nerve that is commonly found under the muscle. Compression of the nerve may cause sciatic-like pain, termed piriformis syndrome. However, muscle facilitation may be of cephalad origin, such as with disc or nerve root derangements. In some patients, the sciatic nerve courses through the muscle itself.

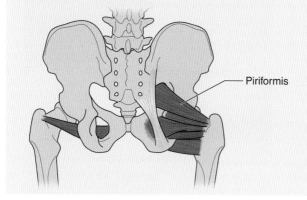

Piriformis

Origin: Anterior surface of the sacrum (first through fourth anterior sacral foramina), sacroiliac joint capsule, pelvic surface of the sacrotuberous ligament, posterior inferior iliac spine

Insertion: Superior medial border of the greater trochanter

Action: Hip external rotation; assists with hip abduction when the hip is flexed

Innervation: S1-S2 (sacral plexus)

Palpation Procedure

- Place the patient prone with the knee flexed.
- Triangulate the location of the piriformis by locating the coccyx and PSIS with the fingers of one hand and the greater trochanter with the other.
- The lines between the fingers form a T, and the piriformis is in line with the stem of the T.
- Orient your palpation fingers toward the iliac crest and strum across the belly of the piriformis toward its origin and insertion.
- The density of the piriformis can be accentuated with resistive hip external rotation.
- Determine the most dominant tender point or fasciculation (or both) and maintain light pressure with the pad(s) of the finger(s) throughout the treatment until reassessment has occurred.

PRT Clinician Procedure

- Place the patient prone at the edge of the treatment table.
- With your far hand, place the ankle on your thigh, and move the hip through flexion and then adduction.
- When the hip flexion and adduction position is found, apply femoral external rotation with the far hand.
- Move your thigh against the patient's thigh to maintain the treatment position and, with your far hand, apply ankle and big-toe flexion coupled with femoral rotation for fine-tuning.
- Corollary tissues treated: Lateral rotator tendons of the hip, iliotibial band, gastrocnemius, soleus, plantar foot structures, quadratus femoris

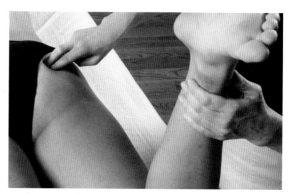

Piriformis palpation procedure.

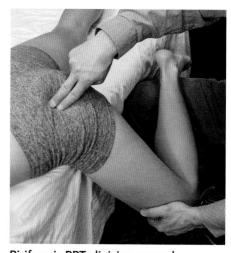

Piriformis PRT clinician procedure.

 See video 7.7 for the piriformis PRT procedure.

Quadratus Femoris

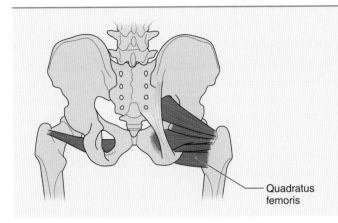

Quadratus femoris

The quadratus femoris is one of the deep six lateral hip rotators. Even though its fibers are flat, it is discernible with deep palpation during resistive hip external rotation.

Origin:	Ischial tuberosity
Insertion:	Intertrochanteric crest, between the lesser and greater trochanters
Action:	Hip external rotation
Innervation:	L5-S1 (lumbar plexus)

Palpation Procedure

- Place the patient prone with the ankles bolstered.
- Locate the distal posterior greater trochanter and ischial tuberosity. The quadratus femoris is between these two landmarks.
- Strum across the quadratus femoris with firm pressure through the inferior gluteus maximus fibers.
- Applying resistive external rotation will accentuate the density of the fibers under the palpation fingers.
- Note the location of any tender points or fasciculatory response along the muscle.
- Once you have determined the most dominant tender point or fasciculation (or both), maintain light pressure with the pad(s) of the finger(s) at the location throughout the PRT treatment procedure until reassessment has occurred.

PRT Clinician Procedure

- Place the patient prone with the knee flexed to 90°.
- Grasp the knee with your far hand and move the hip into extension.
- Once the extension position is determined, place the patient's thigh on your thigh or on a bolster.
- Move the femur into marked internal rotation with your far hand.
- With the far hand, move the femur through abduction and adduction.
- To fine-tune the position, apply hip distraction or compression with your far hand at the posterior knee.
- Corollary tissues treated: Gluteus maximus, gluteus medius, deep hip lateral rotators

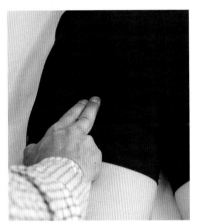

Quadratus femoris palpation procedure.

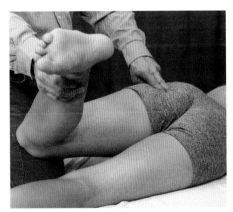

Quadratus femoris PRT clinician procedure.

Sacrotuberous Ligament

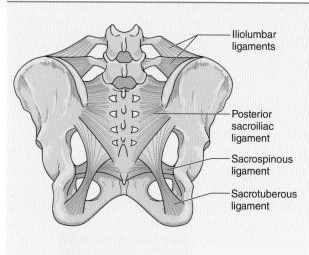

The sacrotuberous ligament is a fan-shaped flat connective tissue that forms the lesser sciatic foramen along with the sacrospinous ligament. Because of its close approximation to posterior neurovascular structures, the sacrotuberous ligament has been implicated as a culprit in the production of perineal pain because of its ability to entrap posterior nerves, such as the pudendal nerve. Additionally, the sacrotuberous ligament is often found to be restricted with hamstring strains because of its contiguous communication with the biceps femoris tendon at the ischium.

Origin: Lower transverse sacral tubercles, inferior sacral margin, coccyx

Insertion: Tuberosity of the ischium

Action: Sacroiliac joint and pelvic stabilization

Palpation Procedure

- Place the patient prone with the ankles bolstered.
- Locate the ischial tuberosity and the inferior margin of the sacrum and coccyx; the sacrotuberous ligament courses between these landmarks.
- Slide off the ischial tuberosity superiorly and strum deeply through the inferior gluteus maximus fibers across the sacrotuberous ligament. The ligament will be approximately 1 inch (2.5 cm) wide and firmly fixed under palpation.
- Note the location of any tender points or fasciculatory response along the ligament and at its attachments.
- Once you have determined the most dominant tender point or fasciculation (or both), maintain light pressure with the pad(s) of the finger(s) at the location throughout the PRT treatment procedure until reassessment has occurred.

PRT Clinician Procedure

- Position the patient prone with a bolster under the ankles to encourage hamstring relaxation.
- Place the thenar eminences of your far hand over the base or most superior aspect of the sacrum with the fingers oriented toward the ischial tuberosity. Place the thenar eminences of your near hand over the ischial tuberosity with its fingers oriented toward the lateral edge of the sacrum.
- Depending on your finger length, the fingers of either hand can be used to monitor the tissue's fasciculatory response and compliance.
- Compress the base of the sacrum downward with your far hand.

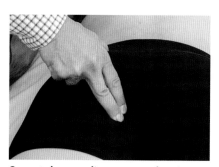

Sacrotuberous ligament palpation procedure.

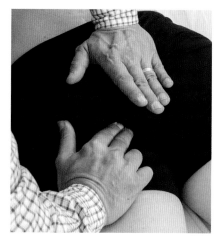

Sacrotuberous ligament PRT clinician procedure.

- Using your near hand and its fingers, translate the inferior tissues upward toward the inferior sacral and coccyx margin.
- Corollary tissues treated: Sacrospinous ligament, iliolumbar ligament, sacroiliac ligaments, biceps femoris

Sacroiliac Joint

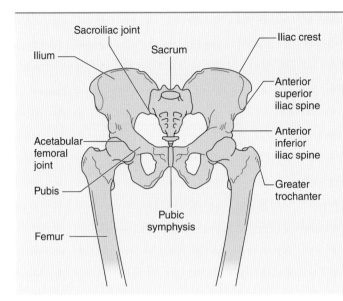

The articulation of the sacrum and ilium forms the sacroiliac (SI) joint. The SI joint is the largest axial joint in the body, but only the anterior third of the joint is synovial; the posterior third is composed primarily of ligamentous and muscular attachments (Cohen 1995). The SI joint provides stability and force transmission and dissipation to the lumbopelvic complex as a result of its complex ligamentous architecture and the attachments of the biceps femoris, gluteus maximus, and piriformis. Disruption and dysfunction of these tissues may result in changes in the joint's movement, approximately 2 to 3° rotation about all three axes (Cohen 1995).

Palpation Procedure

- Place the patient prone with the ankles bolstered to relax the hamstrings and sacrotuberous ligament.
- Wrap both hands around the superior iliac crests with the thumbs pointed toward one another.
- The sacroiliac joints are under the thumb pads. With larger clients, or if your hands are small, you may have to palpate the superior iliac crests downward toward the PSIS where the sacrum articulates with the ilium.
- Apply firm pressure into and along the crescent-shaped SI joint.
- Determine the most dominant tender point or fasciculation (or both) and maintain light pressure with the pad(s) of the finger(s) throughout the treatment until reassessment has occurred.

PRT Clinician Procedure

- Place the patient prone with the knees flexed and ankles supported.
- Place the base of your far hand over the lateral edge of the sacrum on the contralateral side.
- Using a straight arm with the hand affixed under the shoulder, apply downward compression to the lateral edge of the sacrum with the far hand, moving up and down its lateral border to determine the optimal hand placement position that relaxes the joint to the greatest degree or produces the strongest fasciculatory response, or both.
- Once the optimal treatment position is determined, using your far hand, apply rotation of the sacrum toward the involved SI joint coupled

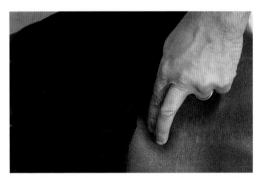

Sacroiliac joint palpation procedure.

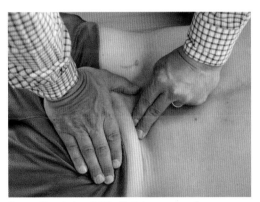

Sacroiliac joint PRT clinician procedure.

with translation of the posterior tissues on the involved side toward the SI joint.
- Corollary tissues treated: Piriformis, sacroiliac ligaments, iliolumbar ligaments, pelvic floor tissues

 See video 7.8 for the sacroiliac joint PRT procedure.

Gluteus Maximus: Superior Fibers

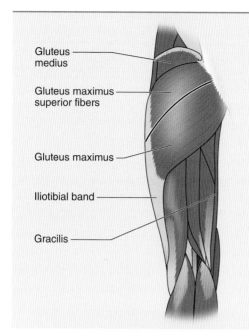

Gluteus medius

Gluteus maximus superior fibers

Gluteus maximus

Iliotibial band

Gracilis

Even though the gluteus maximus is one of the most superficial of the gluteal muscles, it is the most powerful. Its superior and inferior posterior fibers are oriented diagonally, which gives it the ability to propel the body forward and assist with maintaining an upright posture.

Origin: Posterior gluteal line and crest of the ilium, dorsolateral surface of the sacrum, thoracolumbar fascia, sacrotuberous ligament, aponeurosis of gluteus medius

Insertion: Iliotibial tract

Action: Hip extension, external rotation, abduction; knee stabilization

Innervation: L5-S2 (inferior gluteal nerve)

Palpation Procedure

- The patient should be prone with the knee flexed.
- Locate the lateral edge of the sacrum and the posterior superior iliac spine (PSIS) of the ilium.
- Orient your fingers facing the lateral crest of the ilium and stroke across the thick superficial fibers of the superior fibers of the gluteus maximus from the sacrum toward the iliotibial tract.
- Ask the patient to extend the hip with the knee flexed to accentuate the superior fibers' attachment to the iliotibial tract.
- Determine the most dominant tender point or fasciculation (or both) and maintain light pressure with the pad(s) of the finger(s) throughout the treatment until reassessment has occurred.

PRT Clinician Procedure

- Place the patient prone with the knee flexed.
- Using your far hand, grasp the patient's knee and move the hip through extension.
- Once the extension treatment position is found, move the thigh through abduction with your far hand.
- Place the patient's thigh on either a bolster or your thigh when the extension and abduction position is determined.
- Using your far hand, apply femoral external rotation.
- For fine-tuning, apply long axis compression with your torso, or apply distraction using your far hand at the popliteal fossa.

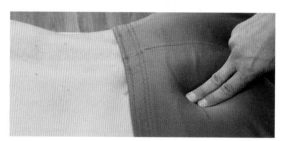

Gluteus maximus (superior fibers) palpation procedure.

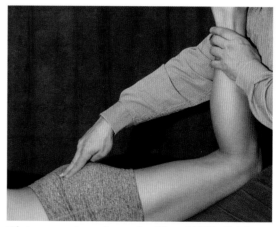

Gluteus maximus (superior fibers) PRT clinician procedure.

- Corollary tissues treated: Gluteus medius, gluteus minimus, sacrotuberous ligament, piriformis, erector spinae, thoracolumbar fascia, iliotibial band

Gluteus Maximus: Inferior Fibers

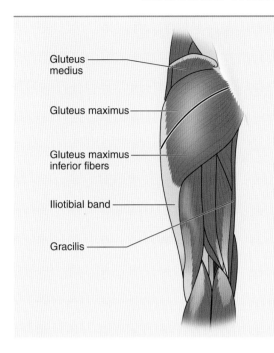

Gluteus medius

Gluteus maximus

Gluteus maximus inferior fibers

Iliotibial band

Gracilis

When adipose tissue is minimal, the inferior fibers of the gluteus maximus may be distinguished during palpation from the superior fibers of the gluteus maximus. Tissue lesions of the inferior fibers are often present when coccyx pain is present.

Origin: Coccyx (lateral surface), dorsolateral inferior surface of the sacrum

Insertion: Gluteal tuberosity of the femur

Action: Hip adduction, extension, and external rotation

Innervation: L5-S2 (inferior gluteal nerve)

Palpation Procedure

- The patient should be prone with the knee flexed.
- Locate the coccyx and lateral inferior edge of the sacrum.
- Orient your fingers facing the lateral crest of the sacrum and stroke across the superficial fibers of the inferior fibers of the gluteus maximus from the lateral surface of the coccyx toward the gluteal tuberosity of the femur.
- The gluteal tuberosity is located on the posterior surface of the femur, below the greater trochanter and close to the level of the gluteal fold.
- Having the patient extend and adduct the hip with the knee flexed will accentuate the density of the inferior fibers' attachment to the gluteal tuberosity.
- Note the location of any tender points or fasciculatory response along the muscle and at its origin.
- Once you have determined the most dominant tender point or fasciculation (or both), maintain light pressure with the pad(s) of the finger(s) at the location throughout the PRT treatment procedure until reassessment has occurred.

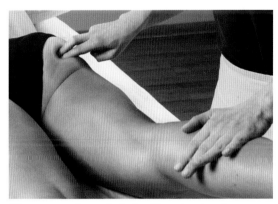

Gluteus maximus (inferior fibers) palpation procedure.

> continued

Gluteus Maximus: Inferior Fibers *> continued*

PRT Clinician Procedure

- Place the patient prone with the knee extended.
- Using your far hand, grasp the patient's knee and move the hip through extension.
- Once the extension treatment position is found, move the thigh through adduction with your far hand.
- Place the patient's thigh on either a bolster or your thigh when the extension and adduction position is determined.
- Using your far hand, apply femoral external rotation.
- Apply long axis compression or distraction with your far hand for fine-tuning.
- Corollary tissues treated: Gluteus medius, gluteus minimus, sacrotuberous ligament, piriformis, erector spinae, thoracolumbar fascia, iliotibial band

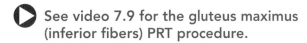 See video 7.9 for the gluteus maximus (inferior fibers) PRT procedure.

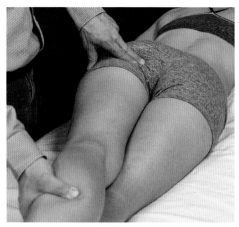

Gluteus maximus (inferior fibers) PRT clinician procedure.

Gluteus Medius

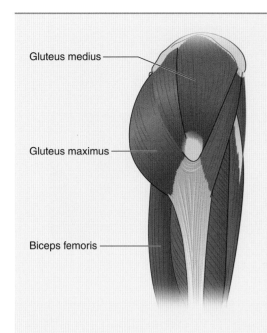

Gluteus medius

Gluteus maximus

Biceps femoris

The fibers of the gluteus medius wrap the ilium from posterior to anterior; the gluteus maximus covers the posterior fibers, and the gluteal aponeurosis covers the anterior fibers. The gluteus medius is an essential muscle in gait. During single-leg stance, it stabilizes the pelvis to keep it from tilting and continues to do so as the opposite leg is moved into the swing phase. The gluteus medius of the stance limb prevents the opposite hip from dropping downward (which is known as gluteus medius sign or gait), indicating stance limb gluteus medius weakness.

Origin: Ilium, gluteal aponeurosis

Insertion: Lateral surface of the greater trochanter

Action: Anterior fibers: Hip internal rotation, hip flexion

Posterior fibers: Hip external rotation, hip extension

All fibers: Hip abduction

Innervation: L4-S1 (gluteal nerve, inferior branch)

Palpation Procedure

- Place the patient prone and the knee into flexion by placing the lower leg on your thigh or on a bolster. Alternately, the patient can be in a side-lying position.
- Locate the posterior iliac crest.
- With your fingers and hands stacked, drop off the posterior iliac crest onto the gluteus maximus, which lies over the posterior fibers of the gluteus medius.
- Using deep palpation, strum across the oblique fibers of the gluteus medius. Lighter pressure will reveal the demarcation of the gluteus maximus fibers. Resistive abduction will enhance the density of the gluteus medius fibers under the gluteus maximus fibers.
- Continue to use the same palpation technique, but move anteriorly around the ilium to the more superficial fibers of the gluteus medius, which do not require as much pressure to palpate.
- Palpate the anterior medial fibers downward to the greater trochanter.
- Note the location of any tender points or fasciculatory response along the muscle.
- Once you have determined the most dominant tender point or fasciculation (or both), maintain light pressure with the pad(s) of the finger(s) at the location throughout the PRT treatment procedure until reassessment has occurred.

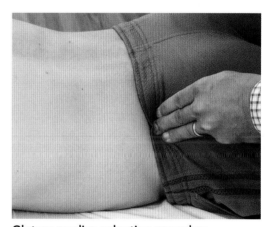

Gluteus medius palpation procedure.

> continued

Gluteus Medius > *continued*

PRT Clinician Procedure

- Place the patient prone with the involved knee flexed.
- Using your far hand, grasp above the knee and bring the leg into extension.
- With the far hand, move the leg into abduction coupled with extension to determine the optimal treatment position.
- Once the optimal combination of extension and abduction is determined, apply external rotation with the far hand.
- Once the optimal treatment position is found, place the patient's thigh on your thigh and brace it against your torso.
- With your torso, apply long axis distraction or compression for fine-tuning.
- Corollary tissues treated: Hamstrings, erector spinae, gluteus maximus, piriformis, quadratus lumborum

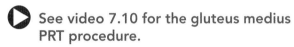 See video 7.10 for the gluteus medius PRT procedure.

Patient Self-Treatment Procedure

- Lie prone.
- Place pillows or a bolster under the thigh to support the limb in a moderate amount of extension. (The arm of a couch under the quadriceps may serve as a good bolster depending on the amount of hip extension available.)
- Move the leg into abduction and external rotation.
- Maintain this position for three to five minutes or apply heat or ice in this position for 20 to 30 minutes to facilitate greater relaxation and pain control.

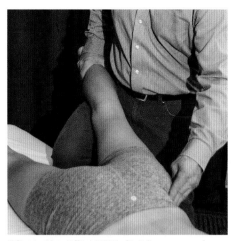

Gluteus medius PRT clinician procedure.

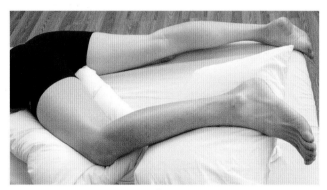

Gluteus medius patient self-treatment procedure.

Adductor Tendinopathy

It is estimated that between 10 and 18% of all injuries worldwide among male soccer players yearly involve groin pain (Engebretsen et al. 2010; Topol, Reeves, and Hassanein 2005). If pain and injury persist, macro- and microscopic tendon changes result in weakening of the tendon and its insertional site (Valent et al. 2012), leading to chronic inflammation. Diagnosis of adductor tendinopathy is often difficult because of the many potential sources of groin pain and the multitude of tissue structures that influence the function of the adductor muscles (Engebretsen et al. 2010). Treatment can also be difficult because of the continued stress and irritation resulting from ongoing athletic activity as well as during activities of daily living. The primary intrinsic risk factors for groin injury have been identified as previous injury and weak hip adductors (Engebretsen et al. 2010; Valent et al. 2012), which may assist in the treatment of persistent adductor tendinopathy. Extrinsic risk factors such as training error, improper footwear, and an irregular playing surface may also be modifiable to aid in the prevention and treatment of adductor groin injury (Valent et al. 2012).

Common Signs and Symptoms

- Pain in the groin, the lower abdomen, or both, particularly at the pubic tubercles
- Pain with stretching of the adductors
- Sharp pain with sprinting, kicking, explosive cutting, and rotating
- Point tenderness over the tendon and its insertion
- Weak groin and abdominal musculature
- Pain with active hip adduction

Common Differential Diagnoses

- Pelvic stress fracture
- Femoral neck stress fracture
- Athletic pubalgia
- Osteitis pubis
- Tendon avulsion
- Symphysis nonunion
- Rectus abdominis tear
- Sports hernia
- Lumbosacral pathology
- Calcific tendinitis
- Facet joint disease
- Lateral hip bursitis

Treatment Points and Sequencing

1. Adductor group
2. Lower abdominis
3. Adductor longus (superior pubis)
4. Adductor magnus (inferior pubis)
5. Sacroiliac joint
6. Quadratus lumborum
7. Gluteus medius
8. Iliopsoas
9. Pes anserine
10. Iliotibial tract
11. Popliteus

- Iliopsoas pathology
- Compression neuropathies

Clinician Therapeutic Interventions

- Confirm the diagnosis with magnetic resonance imaging (MRI). Focal intense marrow edema at the tendon's attachments is often observed with this condition.
- Assess the biomechanics of the patient, particularly load and function at the sacroiliac joints because of their impact on the hip adductors.
- Implement a progressive hip and core strengthening program, particularly for the adductor and abdominal musculature.
- Consider use of aquatic therapy early to facilitate pain-free functional movement and strengthening.
- Use positional release, therapeutic thermal ultrasound, laser, and prolotherapy, as well as other modalities, to help move the tendon out of its chronic inflammatory stage.

Patient Self-Treatment Interventions

- Perform self-release of the adductor group daily.
- Avoid sport activities and ADLs that irritate the tendon until functional strength has been regained.
- Apply thermal modalities to the tendon and its insertion site, if available, to promote blood flow and tissue elasticity. Do not use electric heating pads because of the proximity of the tissue to the genitals.
- Perform nonpainful PNF stretching after physical activity.
- Use a groin wrap or spica cast to limit abduction and provide comfort.

Snapping Hip Syndrome

A patient who complains of a snapping sensation coupled with a sound in the anterior hip may be suffering from snapping hip syndrome. The snapping sensation and sound at the hip are often the result of either an external or internal mechanism (Andersen et al. 2001). Externally, friction may occur at the greater trochanter as a result of the iliotibial band (ITB), anterior border of the gluteus maximus, or posterior portion of the tensor fasciae latae rubbing or snapping over the greater trochanter and its bursae; however, the ITB is considered the most common culprit (Seidenberg and Bowen 2010). The rub of the ITB often occurs during the running motion, which may cause trochanteric bursitis. Internally, the iliopsoas tendon may slip over or catch at the femoral head or iliopectineal eminence when the hip moves from a flexed to an extended position, which may also cause bursitis where it rubs over the bony structures and their respective bursae (Anderson et al. 2001). When nonoperative treatment for both internal and external snapping hip has failed, surgical release or lengthening of the insulting tissues is advocated (Kahn et al. 2013).

Common Signs and Symptoms

- A painful snapping sensation accompanied by a snapping sound at either the anterior or medial hip when moved from flexion to extension
- Point tenderness over the greater trochanter
- Point tenderness of the iliotibial tract or iliopsoas
- A reproduction of snapping with active flexion and abduction into an extended and adducted hip position

Common Differential Diagnoses

- Labral tear
- A loose body in the joint (e.g., acetabular or femoral chondral lesion)
- Femoral head avascular necrosis
- Iliopsoas tendinitis
- Iliotibial band friction syndrome
- Iliopsoas or iliopectineal bursitis

Treatment Points and Sequencing

External Snapping Hip
1. Iliotibial band
2. Adductor group
3. Tensor fasciae latae
4. Gluteus medius
5. Psoas
6. Adductor magnus (inferior pubis)
7. Sacroiliac joint

Internal Snapping Hip
1. Psoas
2. Iliacus
3. Quadratus lumborum
4. Gluteus medius
5. Adductor magnus (inferior pubis)
6. Sacroiliac joint
7. Erector spinae

- Hip subluxation
- Synovial chondromatosis

Clinician Therapeutic Interventions

- Assess and correct the patient's functional movement and biomechanical faults if abnormal loading is occurring to either the iliopsoas or ITB.
- Assess and correct functional pelvic tilt abnormalities, which may cause tightening of the hip flexor tendons.
- Consider advocating relative rest and activity modification until acute symptoms subside.
- Implement a core stabilization and strengthening program to address stabilization and strength deficits.
- Implement a progressive stretching protocol.
- Use PRT prior to joint and soft tissue mobilizations to reduce tissue guarding, relieve pain, and restore resting range of motion.
- Consider using pelvic mobilization to improve pelvic mobility and reduce pain.

- Thermal modalities (e.g., thermal ultrasound, laser) may help move the patient out of a chronic inflammatory state.
- Deep thermal ultrasound may be helpful for iliopsoas tenderness and restriction prior to release and stretching.
- Muscle energy techniques may be helpful to increase range of motion and reduce recalcitrant tissue lesions.
- NSAIDS, cortisone, or surgical interventions may be necessary when traditional treatment has failed.

Patient Self-Treatment Interventions

- Rest and use palliative modalities (e.g., ice and heat) until acute symptoms have resolved.
- Stretch daily after therapeutic or physical activity.
- Use thermal modalities prior to stretching and activity at the greater trochanter if external snapping hip is indicated.
- Use NSAIDs to control pain (after the acute phase), if prescribed by a physician.

Piriformis Syndrome

Piriformis syndrome results from a compression of the sciatic nerve by a hypertonic piriformis muscle (Hopayian et al. 2010). The existence and method of diagnosis of the syndrome remains controversial even though it has been described in the literature for over 75 years, as there is a lack of consensus on a uniform and reliable method of diagnosis, which has thwarted the interpretation and application of study findings (Hopayian et al. 2010). Therefore, the clinical signs and symptoms of the condition should be used to guide diagnosis and treatment until consensus is gained. In agreement with Seidenberg and Bowen (2010), Hopayian and colleagues (2010) found the most common clinical features of piriformis syndrome to be buttock pain, aggravation of sciatica through sitting, greater sciatic notch point tenderness, and increased pain with sitting and maneuvers that increase piriformis muscle tension.

Common Signs and Symptoms

- History of blunt trauma to the posterior hip
- Pain in the sacroiliac joint and posterior hip musculature (piriformis) radiating downward into the inferior buttock, hip, or thigh
- Neurological radiation experienced at rest or with sitting on hard surfaces and with squatting movements
- Point tenderness over the piriformis, greater sciatic notch, sacroiliac joint, and gluteus medius
- Pain with motions that place tension on the piriformis (e.g., passive hip flexion and internal rotation, resistive hip abduction and external rotation)
- Pain with sitting
- Loss of hip internal rotation
- Positive piriformis and Gaenslen's test
- Positive FAIR (flexion, adduction, internal rotation) test
- Lack of hip and knee control during the single-leg reach test

Common Differential Diagnoses

- Hip joint disease
- SI joint dysfunction
- Nerve root irritation or compression
- Lateral intervertebral stenosis
- Lumbar disc pathology
- Sciatica

Treatment Points and Sequencing

1. Piriformis
2. Sacroiliac joint
3. Gluteus medius
4. Erector spinae
5. Quadratus femoris
6. Hamstrings
7. Sartorius
8. Pes anserine
9. Iliotibial tract
10. Adductor group

Clinician Therapeutic Interventions

- Perform a thorough history and biomechanical evaluation to determine why the piriformis muscle is compressing the sciatic nerve.
- Correct any functional movement or biomechanical faults that are increasing load to the posterior hip musculature.
- Release the piriformis and surrounding tissues with PRT.
- Once the tissue is released, slowly introduce stretching of the hip musculature.
- Use a deep thermal modality (e.g., diathermy, ultrasound) prior to the application of stretching.
- Myofascial massage to the piriformis, sacrum, and posterior hip musculature is often helpful in maintaining release of the tissue.
- Implement core and hip strengthening with a focus on hip and knee stabilization during eccentric loading movements.
- Use of an orthosis to limit pronation early in the rehabilitation process may be helpful in mitigating load to the piriformis.

Patient Self-Treatment Interventions

- Avoid compressing the piriformis and sciatic nerve by removing objects from the back pockets (e.g., cell phone, wallet) that may increase compression on the sciatic when sitting. Do not apply ischemic pressure devices to the area such as tennis balls or other massage devices that may increase compression.
- Perform self-release of the posterior hip daily.
- Perform only stretches that do not exacerbate symptoms.
- Apply heat or ice to relieve pain and spasm.

Sacroiliac Joint Dysfunction

Sacroiliac (SI) joint dysfunction has tradition-ally been considered a controversial diagnosis (Seidenberg and Bowen 2010) because of the lack of reliable and valid diagnostics (Rupert et al. 2009; Szadek et al. 2009). SI joint dysfunction has been defined as a lack of voluntary move-ment at the joint (Sharma and Sen 2014). Szadek and colleagues (2009) found select orthopedic tests (e.g., thigh thrust test, compression test, and SI joint stress tests) to show "discriminative power" for the diagnosis of sacroiliac joint pain. However, more work needs to be done to solidify the relationship between these tests and SI joint dysfunction. Sports that require unidirectional repetitive movements such as gymnastics and skating can result in pelvic and rotational shear at the SI joint and may sprain the joint's ligaments and contract surrounding musculature, resulting in impaired movement and function of the SI joint (Cohen 2005; Seidenberg and Bowen 2010). A direct trauma to the pelvis from a fall, car acci-dent, or sudden violent contraction may also result in tearing the joint's surrounding ligaments and tissues, but this is less common (Seidenberg and Bowen 2010).

Common Signs and Symptoms

- Point tenderness over the SI joint (sacral sulcus and PSIS)
- Point tenderness at the posterior hip and low back musculature
- Pain radiating into the buttock, posterolat-eral hip, or low back
- Pain with trunk flexion
- Lack of motor, sensory, or deep tendon reflex
- Positive FABER (flexion, abduction, external rotation) test, piriformis test, or Gaenslen's test
- Positive March test and Gillet test
- Leg length discrepancy
- Innominate upslip or downslip with or with-out rotation

Common Differential Diagnoses

- Lumbar disc pathology
- Piriformis syndrome

Treatment Points and Sequencing
1. Sacroiliac joint
2. Gluteus medius
3. Piriformis
4. Sacrotuberous ligament
5. Biceps femoris
6. Quadratus lumborum
7. Erector spinae
8. Gluteus maximus
9. Psoas (Avoid marked posterior pelvic positioning.)
10. Adductor magus (inferior pubis)

- Gluteus medius strain
- Ankylosing spondylitis
- Reiter's syndrome
- Spondyloarthropathies
- Autoimmune etiologies (if both SI joints are involved)
- Spinal stenosis
- Compression neuropathies

Clinician Therapeutic Interventions

- Perform a thorough clinical and biomechan-ical examination to determine the source of the pain.
- Correct any faulty movement and biome-chanical faults overloading the sacroiliac joint. Leg length discrepancy coupled with weak hip rotators is often seen with this condition.
- If a significant leg length discrepancy is identified, a simple heel lift is *not* advo-cated because the lift may abnormally affect the arthrokinematics of both SI joints and those in the kinetic chain. Therefore, a bilateral custom orthosis correction should be implemented if a leg length discrepancy is modified.
- Release painful contracted tissues first with PRT prior to using direct manipulative tech-niques.

> continued

Sacroiliac Joint Dysfunction *> continued*

- Apply thermal ultrasound or a like modality prior to using direct manipulative techniques.
- Restore normal sacroiliac joint arthrokinematics using muscle energy, joint mobilization, or other manual therapy methods.
- Consider having the patient use an SI belt after the acute phase to promote pain relief and joint stabilization.
- Have the patient avoid movements that produce rotational shear and torsion at the SI joint for four to six weeks, progressing slowly back into these movements once pelvic stabilization has been attained.
- Consider using KT Tape or a similar tape product to provide pain relief.
- Implement a progressive spinal stabilization program.

- Educate the patient about proper ADL movement techniques to reduce stress at the lumbosacral tissues.
- Educate the patient about how to self-mobilize and apply muscle energy to the SI joint to nourish the joint and keep it mobile.

Patient Self-Treatment Interventions

- Avoid movements that cause pain, particularly trunk flexion and rotation.
- Avoid trunk flexion and sit-ups in the initial rehabilitation phase.
- Perform daily SI joint self-mobilization and muscle energy techniques.
- Apply palliative heat and ice as needed.
- Once the joint has stabilized, stretch the posterior muscles after physical or therapeutic exercise.

Summary

Although pelvic somatic dysfunction may appear to be an enigma to both the novice and seasoned practitioner, with close consideration of proximal and distal and intrinsic and extrinsic risk factors, the puzzle may be solved. Given the gravity of potential underlying disease and injury conditions that may mimic pelvic pain, PRT practitioners must be steadfast in their attempt to identify its source. If the causative factors or origin of the pelvic dysfunction are not readily determined, treatment of pelvic somatic dysfunction with PRT will tend to be safer than direct therapies and will yield pain relief, improved strength, and optimally, enhanced function.

CHAPTER 8

Spine

CHAPTER OBJECTIVES

After reading this chapter, you should be able to do the following:

1. Appreciate the factors that may influence the development of somatic dysfunction of spinal tissues.

2. Locate and palpate spinal tissue structures to be treated with positional release therapy (PRT).

3. Apply PRT techniques to spinal tissues affected by somatic dysfunction.

4. Identify how common injury conditions such as thoracic outlet syndrome may be treated based on somatic lesion patterns.

Pain and disability associated with spinal conditions are a common health and economic problem globally. Low back pain is one of the leading causes of disability and work-time loss (Andersson 1999; Hoy et al. 2012; Luo et al. 2004). In 1998 it was estimated that low back pain direct health care expenditures in the United States alone were in excess of $90.7 billion (Luo et al. 2004). Hoy and colleagues (2010) found that low back pain, once thought to be a problem unique to Western countries, is now a global problem that causes a significant burden on all aspects of society.

It is generally accepted that 70 to 85% of people will experience pain and disability related to a spinal condition at some point in life (Andersson 1999). Todd (2011) reported that up to two thirds of people present with degenerative cervical spine disorders in their lifetimes, and the prevalence increases with age. The occurrence of low back pain has also been reported to be greatest in the third decade of life and to be prevalent up to the age of 60 to 65, at which point it gradually declines. The rise and fall of low back pain across the life span has been attributed to a greater work-life demand at middle age, followed by a decrease in the retirement years (Hoy et al. 2010).

Although activity and compressive forces at the spinal tissues are necessary for their nourishment and growth, too much demand may lead to accelerated degeneration and disc derangement (Bartynski et al. 2013). Bartynski and colleagues (2013) proposed that competitive athletes may be more susceptible to disc degeneration and subsequent derangement as a result of increased spinal mechanical compression and strain during the years of competitive activity. Whether athletes are at more risk for spine conditions than nonathletes is still unclear, but Bono (2004) found a greater prevalence of disc degeneration among athletes. However, whether this places them at an increased risk for back pain is uncertain. To date, discography studies have not shown a causal relationship between disc degeneration and disc derangement (Bartynski et al. 2013; Endean et al. 2011), but research with athletes in this area is lacking. However, Livshits and colleagues (2011) did find disc degeneration to be a significant risk factor for low back pain among women.

Additional risk factors for low back pain are increased weight (body mass index); obesity (particularly in women; Shiri et al. 2009); low socioeconomic and educational status (Hoy et al. 2010); genetic predisposition (among women;

Livshits et al. 2011); and psychosocial factors such as increased stress, depression, and work dissatisfaction (Hoy et al. 2010). Although most acute low back pain resolves within three months with little or no intervention irrespective of risk factors, approximately 5% of cases become chronic, which presents unique treatment challenges (Bartynski et al. 2013).

An understanding of the factors that lead to chronicity is lacking at this time, but chronicity may be related to the rate of recurrence. In an examination of low back pain epidemiology between genders and across populations, recurrence within one year ranged approximately between 60 and 80%. The propensity for recurrence increases with age and among females (Hoy et al. 2010). Recurrent episodes of chronic low back pain may propagate somatic dysfunction through a host of dysfunctional neurochemical and structural processes, producing pain generators at multiple neuronal levels (Kuchera 2005). As discussed in chapter 2, persistent chronic pain may result in central sensitization at the second order, resulting in the production of a painful stimulus in the absence of tissue damage. Therefore, when assessing a patient with chronic pain, clinicians must consider potential pain generators and whether multiple factors may be affecting their production and persistence.

Kuchera (2008) recommended that clinicians evaluating patients with chronic pain explore psychosocial (e.g., depression), homeostatic (e.g., increased autonomic activity), and structure-function (biomechanics) issues to develop a multimodal treatment plan (see Kuchera for a full review), which may include the use of PRT. Positional release therapy and strain counterstrain (SCS) have shown promise for reducing acute and chronic spine-related pain (Wong 2012). However, to date, PRT and SCS research has been focused on the cervical area with particular attention on cervicogenic pain, headache, migraine, and temporomandibular dysfunction. Although the review of the effectiveness of SCS for these conditions has been well elucidated by Wong (2011), there is not yet robust support for the use of PRT or SCS for the treatment of acute or chronic nonspecific low back pain over traditional therapies. The lack of support may be related to how PRT and osteopathic therapies are defined.

Some authors consider PRT a manipulative technique that involves the direct and indirect manipulation of tissues (Lewis, Souvlis, and Sterling

2011) and thus group it with joint mobilization, which may result in classification errors in larger systematic studies. For example, in a systematic review and meta-analysis of complementary alternative medicine (CAM) for neck and low back pain, Furlan and colleagues (2011) examined manipulation and mobilization independently, but also in paired fashion, and did not mention the type of mobilization or manipulation. Therefore, terminology may be a confounding factor in determining the efficacy of PRT for the treatment of spine-related pain if it is not identified as PRT and also if it is grouped with other manipulative therapies. Additionally, capturing tissue and neurological changes has traditionally been challenging, as previously discussed. Regardless, the strong evidence of pain reduction and improvement in disability for cervical and cranial conditions observed among SCS and PRT researchers provides a base of support and an impetus for further study of its usefulness in treating a myriad of spinal conditions.

TREATMENT

Common Anatomical Areas and Conditions for PRT

Anterior Structures

- Muscle strain
- Ligament sprain
- Osteoarthritis
- Acquired (acute) torticollis
- Thoracic outlet syndrome
- Whiplash
- Cervicogenic headache
- Cervical fusion
- Disc pathology
- Radiculopathy
- Degenerative disc disease
- Scoliosis

Posterior Structures

- Muscle strain
- Ligament sprain
- Osteoarthritis
- Facet joint syndrome
- Sacroiliac joint dysfunction
- Nonspecific low back pain
- Disc pathology
- Radiculopathy
- Lumbar fusion
- Degenerative disc disease
- Coccydynia
- Scoliosis
- Sciatica
- Spondylolisthesis
- Spondylosis

Sternocleidomastoid

The sternocleidomastoid (SCM) is composed of two large muscular heads at the lateral and anterior aspects of the neck. Both heads merge superiorly at the neck to produce the prominent-looking strap when turning the head side to side. Lesions often develop in the SCM when the head and neck are positioned in a compromised flexed and rotated position during sleep, producing an acute torticollis.

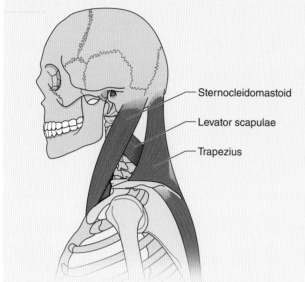

Origin: Sternal (medial) head: Ventral surface of the manubrium

Clavicular (lateral) head: Superior and anterior surface of the medial third of the clavicle

Insertion: Mastoid process of the temporal bone, lateral half of the superior nuchal line at the occiput

Action: Cervical spine flexion (both heads), cervical spine lateral flexion to the same side, cervical spine rotation to the opposite side, capital extension (posterior fibers), sternum elevation with forced inspiration

Innervation: Accessory (XI) nerve

C2-C3 (ventral rami)

Palpation Procedure

- Place the patient in a supine position and sit behind the patient's head.
- Ask the patient to slightly flex and rotate the head to the opposite side to bring out the SCM. Note the V appearance distally formed by the clavicular and sternal heads.
- Lightly pince the midbelly of the SCM between your thumb and forefinger and allow it to roll under your fingers while gently pulling upward. Repeat this procedure moving proximally to the mastoid process and downward along the two heads of the SCM.
- Because the carotid artery passes deep to the SCM, when pincing the tissue, be careful not to impinge the vessel. If you feel a strong rhythmic pulse with your palpation, reposition your fingers and repalpate.
- Note the location of any tender points or fasciculatory response along the muscle and its attachment sites.
- Once you have determined the most dominant tender point or fasciculation (or both), maintain light pressure with the pad(s) of the finger(s) at the location throughout the PRT treatment procedure until reassessment has occurred.

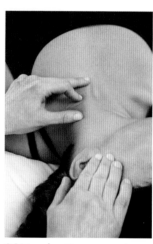

SCM palpation procedure.

PRT Clinician Procedure

- Place the patient supine.
- While palpating the SCM lesion with your near hand, elevate the shoulder of the involved side until a fasciculation is felt or maximal relaxation of the tissue is attained.
- Slide your far hand and arm under the neck and place the palm of the hand on the shoulder of the involved side.
- Using your far forearm, move the cervical spine into flexion.
- After the flexion position of comfort is attained, with the far forearm, rotate the head toward the lesion, and then apply lateral cervical flexion.
- Apply downward shoulder pressure using your far hand to fine-tune the positioning.
- Typically, distally oriented lesions require more cervical flexion than those that are proximally located.
- Corollary tissues treated: Longus colli, anterior rectus capitis, rectus capitis lateralis, hyoids, anterior and middle scalenes

Patient Self-Treatment Procedure

- Identify with your fingers where the SCM is most tender.
- While keeping the palpation fingers on the area of tenderness, place a pillow or folded towel under your head to encourage cervical flexion. Note the amount of cervical flexion that produces the greatest fasciculatory response or level of tissue relaxation, or both.
- Elevate the shoulder on the involved side.
- Laterally flex and rotate your head toward the shoulder on the involved side, noting again the greatest fasciculatory response or tissue relaxation (or both) at which the position should be held.
- Maintain the treatment position until the fasciculatory response abates or for three to five minutes.

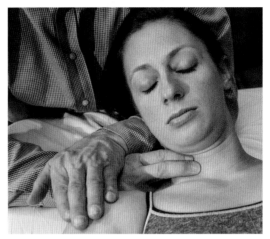

SCM PRT clinician procedure.

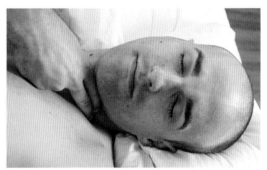

SCM patient self-treatment procedure.

Anterior and Middle Scalenes

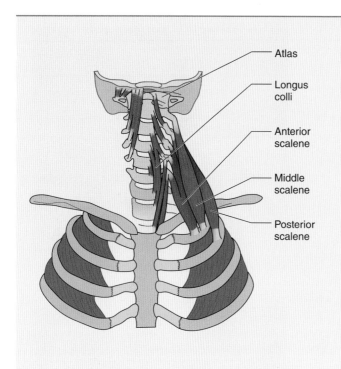

- Atlas
- Longus colli
- Anterior scalene
- Middle scalene
- Posterior scalene

The anterior and middle scalenes share an anatomical significance and are of critical importance when thoracic outlet syndrome (TOS) is suspected. Because the neurovascular bundle (brachial plexus and subclavian artery and vein) of the cervical spine passes between these two muscles, hypertonicity of these muscles can impinge on the bundle and lead to TOS. Therefore, they are grouped here for examination and exploration.

Origin: Anterior: C3-C6 transverse processes

Middle: C2-C7 transverse processes

Insertion: First rib

Action: Cervical flexion, elevation of the first rib during inspiration, cervical rotation to the same side, cervical lateral flexion to the same side

Innervation: C3-C8 (cervical nerves)

Palpation Procedure

- Place the patient in a supine position, and stand behind the patient's head. Position the anterior scalene under the distal lateral margin of the SCM with the middle scalene just behind the SCM.
- Ask the patient to slightly flex and rotate the head to the opposite side and while tucking under the SCM to gain access to the muscular belly of the anterior scalene.
- Gently strum over the anterior scalene following it inferiorly as it disappears under the clavicle.
- Ask the patient to inspire during palpation to feel its contraction.
- Now move laterally off the anterior scalene onto the middle scalene, which will be broader than the anterior scalene.
- Strum across the middle scalene following it as far as you can up and down its fibers.
- Avoid compressing this juncture when palpating these structures because doing so can cause sharp radiating nerve pain as a result of compression of the neurovascular bundle.
- Note the location of any tender points or fasciculatory response along the muscles and their attachment sites.
- Once you have determined the most dominant tender point or fasciculation (or both), maintain

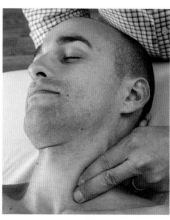

Anterior and middle scalenes palpation procedure.

light pressure with the pad(s) of the finger(s) at the location throughout the PRT treatment procedure until reassessment has occurred.

PRT Clinician Procedure

- Place the patient supine.
- While palpating the scalene lesion with your near hand, elevate the shoulder of the involved with your far hand until a fasciculation is felt or maximal relaxation of the tissue is attained.
- Slide your far hand and arm under the neck and place the palm of your far hand on the shoulder of the involved side.
- Using your far forearm, move the cervical spine into flexion.
- After the flexion position of comfort is attained, rotate the head away from the lesion, and then apply lateral cervical flexion toward the lesion.
- Using your far forearm, attempt to apply slight lateral cranial flexion toward the tender point.
- Apply downward shoulder pressure using your far hand to fine-tune the positioning.
- Typically, distally oriented lesions require more cervical flexion than those proximally located.
- Corollary tissues treated: SCM, longus colli, anterior rectus capitis, rectus capitis lateralis, hyoids

 See video 8.1 for the anterior and middle scalenes PRT procedure.

Patient Self-Treatment Procedure

- The same self-treatment procedure used for the SCM can be applied to the anterior and middle scalenes with one exception. Instead of rotating the head toward the tender tissue or lesion, rotate it away from the lesion.

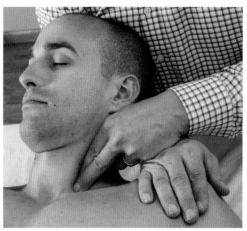

Anterior and middle scalenes PRT clinician procedure.

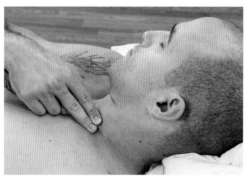

Anterior and middle scalenes patient self-treatment procedure.

Longus Capitis and Longus Colli

The longus capitis and longus colli are grouped here because of their close proximity with one another on the anterior aspect of the cervical vertebrae and also because of the ability to release both with the same PRT procedure. The longus colli possesses three muscular heads that resemble the erector spinae musculature in fiber orientation. Each assists with cervical flexion, but the longus capitis is dedicated to producing capital flexion.

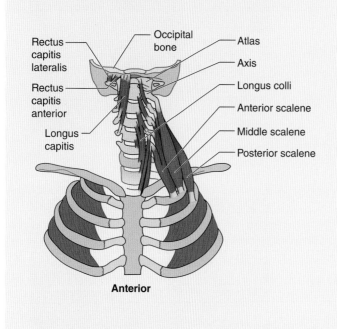

Anterior

Rectus capitis lateralis
Occipital bone
Atlas
Axis
Rectus capitis anterior
Longus colli
Anterior scalene
Longus capitis
Middle scalene
Posterior scalene

Origin: Longus capitis: C3-C6 transverse processes

Longus colli: C3-C5 transverse processes (superior oblique); T1-T3 transverse processes (inferior oblique and vertical portion)

Insertion: Longus capitis: Occiput

Longus colli: Atlas (superior); C5-C6 transverse processes (oblique); C2-C4 anterior vertebral bodies (vertical portion)

Action: Longus capitis: Capital flexion and cervical rotation to the same side

Longus colli: Cervical rotation to the opposite side (oblique), cervical lateral flexion (superior and inferior), cervical flexion (weak)

Innervation: Longus capitis: C1-C3 (ventral rami)

Longus colli: C2-C6 (ventral rami)

Palpation Procedure

- Place the patient prone with the head slightly flexed, and sit at the head of the table.
- Locate the SCM and move medially to find the carotid artery.
- Move the carotid artery out of the way, and then ask the patient to flex the head and neck to make these small, thin muscles palpable.
- Gently roll your index finger over the muscles, which are between the trachea and cervical vertebrae.
- Distinguishing the fasciculatory response of these tissues may be difficult because of their close proximity to the carotid artery; however, the fasciculatory response will be aberrant and will subside when treatment is administered.
- Note the location of any tender points or fasciculatory response along the tissue.
- Once you have determined the most dominant tender point or fasciculation (or both), maintain light pressure with the pad(s) of the finger(s)

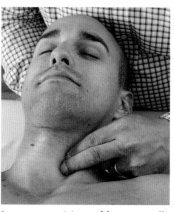

Longus capitis and longus colli palpation procedure.

at the location throughout the PRT treatment procedure until reassessment has occurred.

PRT Clinician Procedure

- Place the patient supine with the head slightly flexed.
- Support the head with your far forearm or hand.
- With your far hand or forearm, flex the neck and head.
- Apply cervical and cranial lateral flexion toward the lesion with the far hand or forearm.
- Apply cervical rotation with the far hand or forearm to fine-tune.
- Corollary tissues treated: Rectus capitis anterior and lateralis, scalenes, SCM, infrahyoids, platysma

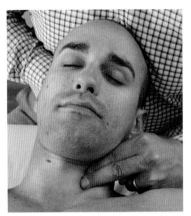

Longus capitis and longus colli PRT clinician procedure.

Patient Self-Treatment Procedure

- In a supine position with the head slightly flexed and supported, use the pads of the fingers of one hand to locate the trachea and carotid artery.
- Move the pads of the fingers either laterally or medially off the carotid artery and onto the longus capitis and longus colli muscles.
- Slightly flex the head to feel these muscles contract under the pads of the fingers.
- Tuck the chin down toward the chest while feeling for a jumpy and irregular fasciculation or twitch of the muscles or the point where they feel most relaxed, or both.
- Laterally flex the head to the side where the tenderness is present.
- Rotate the head slightly to fine-tune the position, and then place a towel or small pillow behind the head to keep it in the position of comfort or where the strongest fasciculatory response is found.
- Maintain the treatment position until the fasciculatory response abates or for three to five minutes.

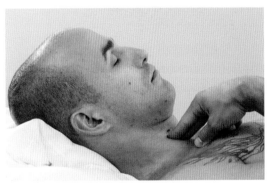

Longus capitis and longus colli patient self-treatment procedure.

Upper Rectus Abdominis

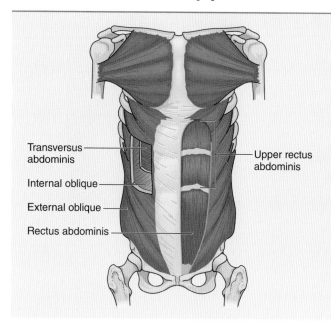

Transversus abdominis

Internal oblique

External oblique

Rectus abdominis

Upper rectus abdominis

When not covered with a large amount of adipose tissue, the rectus abdominis muscle gives the appearance of a washboard; it is commonly called six-pack abs. The rectus abdominis is often thought to contribute to core stability. However, according to McGill (2007), it plays only a partial role in core stability, but it should be activated along with other core musculature to promote spinal stabilization or stiffness.

Origin:	Pubic crest, pubic symphysis
Insertion:	Costal cartilage of ribs 5 through 7, xiphoid process
Action:	Flexes the spine; tilts the pelvis posteriorly
Innervation:	T7-T12 (ventral rami)

Palpation Procedure

- Place the patient supine in a supported flexed thoracic position with the knees bolstered into flexion.
- To help with the visual and tactile identification of the upper rectus abdominis fibers, instruct the patient to perform a partial sit-up.
- With the patient in a flexed and relaxed position, palpate along the costal crest formed by the xiphoid process and ribs downward toward the pubic ramus.
- Strum across the muscle's insertion points on the xiphoid and ribs as well as across the fibers of the muscle.
- Note the location of any tender points or fasciculatory response along the muscle and its attachment to the ribs and xiphoid.
- Once you have determined the most dominant tender point or fasciculation (or both), maintain light pressure with the pad(s) of the finger(s) at the location throughout the PRT treatment procedure until reassessment has occurred.

PRT Clinician Procedure

- Place the patient supine in a supported flexed thoracic position. (Thoracic flexion can be accomplished by either placing a pillow under the upper torso and having the patient lean backward onto your thighs and torso or by using a split treatment table.)
- If the patient has equal tenderness at the right and left upper abdomen, grasp both knees

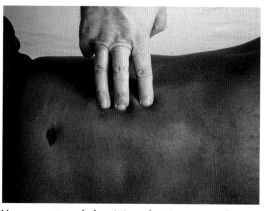

Upper rectus abdominis palpation procedure.

with your far hand and bring them toward the patient's chest to encourage posterior pelvic tilting. If tenderness is focused to one side, grasp the associated knee with your far hand only and move it toward the chest and opposite shoulder in a diagonal pattern.

- If you can support the patient on your thighs and torso, your thighs can be used to accentuate thoracic and lumbar positioning. For right and left upper abdominal tenderness, abduct your thighs to encourage thoracic cage collapse anteriorly as well as lumbar spine flexion. If tenderness is on just one side, say, the right, abduct only your left leg away from the midline of the spine to encourage right-sided thoracic cage collapse. If tenderness is on the left upper abdominis, then move your right thigh outward.
- Apply cervical and thoracic downward pressure from your torso to accentuate tissue relaxation and fine-tune the position.
- Apply femoral internal and external rotation with your far hand for fine-tuning.
- Corollary tissues treated: Hip flexors, obliques, psoas, iliacus, lower abdominals

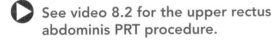 See video 8.2 for the upper rectus abdominis PRT procedure.

Patient Self-Treatment Procedure

- Lie supine with a pillow under the upper torso and another under the posterior pelvis to encourage thoracic flexion and posterior tilting.
- Place your ankles on a stable structure such as the arm of a sofa or the edge of a chair to support the knees and hips into flexion.
- During positioning, self-palpate the upper abdominals for the presence of a fasciculatory response and optimal tissue relaxation, which will guide you in attaining the optimal treatment position.
- Grasp both knees or one knee based on the location of the tenderness and move the knee (or knees) toward the chest, diagonally to the opposite shoulder for one-sided tenderness as described in the clinician procedure.
- Apply hip rotation to fine-tune the position by rotating the knee with your hand(s).
- Maintain the treatment position until the fasciculatory response abates or for three to five minutes.
- This self-treatment position can also be utilized to treat the lower abdominals.

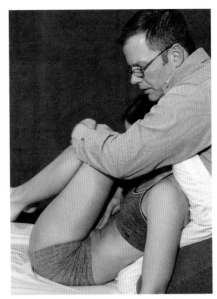

Upper rectus abdominis PRT clinician procedure.

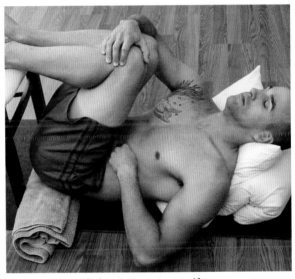

Upper rectus abdominis patient self-treatment procedure.

Intercostals

The intercostal muscles, or spare-rib muscles, are composed of both internal and external fibers that attach to the ribs and their respective costal tissues. The external intercostals are the most superficial, and the internal intercostals are underneath them. The function of the intercostals is debatable, but both are active to one degree or another with both inhalation and exhalation, serving a primary role of assisting with respiration and also stabilizing the rib cage.

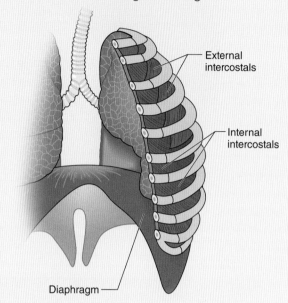

External intercostals

Internal intercostals

Diaphragm

Origin: Ribs 1-11 (Lower border of rib below and costal tubercles)

Insertion: Upper border of the rib below and the sternum via the aponeurosis

Action: External intercostals: Assist the diaphragm with inhalation; rotate the thoracic spine to the opposite side (unilateral); stabilize the rib cage

Internal intercostals: Assist with exhalation; stabilize the rib cage stabilization; 1 through 5 assist with inhalation

Innervation: T1-T11 (intercostal nerves)

Palpation Procedure

- Place the patient supine with the knees bolstered into flexion.
- Start at either the inferior or superior ribs.
- With one or two fingers pads, stroke across the obliquely oriented fibers of the intercostals between the ribs.
- Also stroke over the corresponding rib margins, superior and inferior, working either away from or toward the sternum.
- Instruct the patient to take several slow, deep breaths during palpation to ascertain the quality of rib movement and chest expansion. Compare bilaterally.
- Once the anterior intercostals have been palpated, move the patient into either a side-lying or prone position to continue palpation around the thorax toward the posterior spine.
- When approaching the posterior, palpation of the intercostals can be challenging because of the dense posterior spinal muscles; firmer pressure is required.
- Note the location of any tender points or fasciculatory response along the muscle and its attachment to the ribs.
- Once you have determined the most dominant tender point or fasciculation (or both), maintain

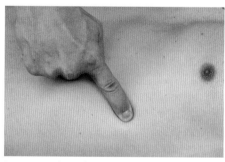

Intercostals palpation procedure.

light pressure with the pad(s) of the finger(s) at the location throughout the PRT treatment procedure until reassessment has occurred.

PRT Clinician Procedure

- The patient is in a seated position on the treatment table or on the floor. If the patient has adequate hip and knee flexibility, position the lower torso in a hook-lying position with the knees stacked, the hips flexed, and the feet and ankles stacked and oriented toward the side to be treated. Patients who cannot obtain this position should place the lower body in a position of maximal comfort.
- Use your near hand to palpate the intercostals. Use your near hand to manipulate the patient's torso during positioning.

- Position yourself behind the patient, kneeling on the treatment table or floor with your knee and thigh supporting the opposite, or contralateral, side of the torso to be treated. The other knee should be in contact with the table or floor.
- Place the patient's contralateral arm and torso on your knee and thigh over a pillow. An exercise ball can be used in place of your knee and thigh either on the treatment table or on the floor.
- Grasp the opposite arm (ipsilateral) with your far hand and bring it across the chest to the pillow, holding it at the bicep area. Place a towel or pillow over your far arm and have the patient laterally flex the head and neck to rest it on the pillow or towel.
- While palpating the anterior intercostals with the fingers of your near hand, move the supporting knee outward from the patient to promote lateral trunk flexion and collapse the ipsilateral rib cage on the side of the lesion.
- Rotate the supporting knee to encourage rotation and flexion of the anterior thorax toward the lesion.
- Once the thorax position of comfort is attained or a fasciculatory response is elicited, encourage further rib and costal compression by applying a downward and anterior compression of the rib cage with the palmar aspect of your near hand.
- Corollary tissues treated: Abdominals, obliques, psoas, diaphragm, hip flexors

 See video 8.3 for the intercostals PRT procedure.

Patient Self-Treatment Procedure

- An exercise ball is needed for self-treatment.
- Position yourself in a seated position on a table, on a bed, or on the floor. If you have adequate hip and knee flexibility, position the lower torso in a hook-lying position, with the knees stacked, the hips flexed, and the feet and ankles stacked and oriented toward the side to be treated.
- Rest your contralateral arm and torso on the exercise ball.
- Rest your arm on the non-affected side on the ball, then place your head on your arm. Use the fingers of your other hand to monitor the tissue fasciculation or relaxation of the tissue.

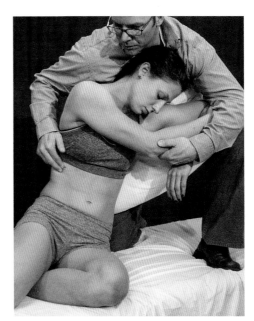

Intercostals PRT clinician procedure.

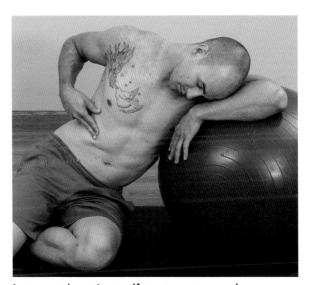

Intercostals patient self-treatment procedure.

- Allow the ball to move outward and away from the tender side, which will promote the treatment side of the torso to collapse, or laterally flex.
- Allow your body to rotate forward on the ball, which will promote anterior thoracic flexion and rotation toward the tender lesion.
- Maintain the treatment position until the fasciculatory response abates or for three to five minutes.

Xiphoid

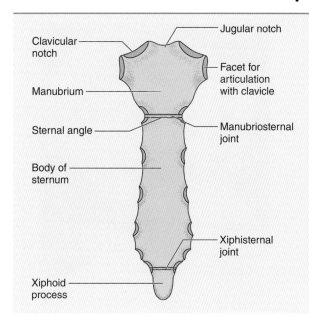

Clavicular notch — Manubrium — Sternal angle — Body of sternum — Xiphoid process

Jugular notch — Facet for articulation with clavicle — Manubriosternal joint — Xiphisternal joint

The xiphoid is a structure of primary importance to evaluate in the presence of spinal, pelvic, or upper-quarter conditions. The xiphoid serves as an attachment site for the abdominal aponeurosis and is a fascial anchor for upper, spinal, and pelvic tissues. Somatic dysfunction often results in lesions at this site that produce significant tenderness and tissue restriction. Because most patients are not aware that they have lesions at this site, gentle palpation is needed when exploring this area to prevent unintentional guarding during palpation and treatment. The xiphoid is typically cartilaginous until the age of 40 and ossifies after this time; thus, greater movement of the xiphoid would be expected in patients under 40 years of age.

Palpation Procedure

- Place the patient in a supine position.
- Locate the sternum and trace it downward to its apex.
- Strum over the anterior and inferior aspects of the xiphoid.
- The xiphoid is often very tender when lesions are present; therefore, use gentle palpation during assessment and treatment to prevent further aggravation.
- Determine the most dominant tender point or fasciculation (or both) and maintain light pressure with the pad(s) of the finger(s) throughout the treatment until reassessment has occurred.

PRT Clinician Procedure

- Place the patient in a recumbent position with the knees flexed and bolstered.
- Position the patient with the torso and head resting against your knees and torso with a pillow between you and the patient, or position the patient on a split treatment table.
- Place the patient's palms behind the head (some call this the arrest position) and position yourself behind the patient if possible. If you can, reach under and through the axilla of the patient to palpate the xiphoid with your near hand.
- Rest the patient's arms and shoulders on your forearms for support and place the fingers of your far hand just below the fingers of your near hand.
- Apply a light cephalad translation of the tissue below the xiphoid while moving the patient into thoracic flexion.

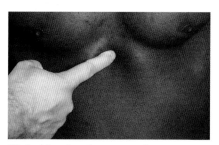

Xiphoid palpation procedure.

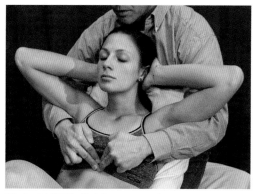

Xiphoid PRT clinician procedure.

- Collapse the upper thoracic cage anteriorly and inward toward the sternum by moving both knees outward and leaning forward to promote kyphotic positioning.
- Rotate the thorax while protracting the shoulder to fine-tune the positioning.
- Corollary tissues treated: Abdominis, obliques, psoas, diaphragm, pectoralis major and minor

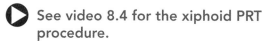 **See video 8.4 for the xiphoid PRT procedure.**

Sternum

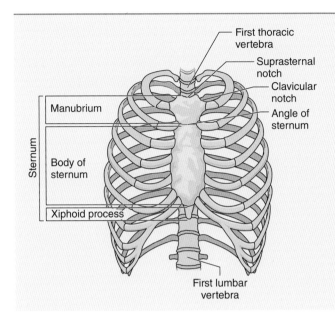

First thoracic
vertebra

Suprasternal
notch

Clavicular
notch

Angle of
sternum

Manubrium

Sternum

Body of
sternum

Xiphoid process

First lumbar
vertebra

The sternum protects the internal organs and is the central attachment point for the ribs and their respective costal cartilage. The manubrium articulates directly with the clavicles and the first and second ribs. The body of the sternum is a major site of attachment for the anterior chest wall muscles and fascia.

Palpation Procedure

- Place the patient in a supine relaxed position with the head slightly flexed.
- Starting at the jugular notch, located at the top of the sternum, stroke across the sternum with the pads of the fingers, moving distally to the xiphoid.
- Explore the lateral margin of the sternum where the ribs articulate with the sternum (this site if often tender in the presence of osteochondritis).
- Note the location of any tender points or fasciculatory response along the bone and its articulation with the abdominal aponeurosis.
- Determine the most dominant tender point or fasciculation (or both) and maintain light pressure with the pad(s) of the finger(s) throughout the treatment until reassessment has occurred.

PRT Clinician Procedure

- Place the patient in a recumbent position, knees flexed, arms relaxed at the sides.
- Position yourself behind the patient, as done in the xiphoid treatment; consider using a split treatment table.
- Place the fingers of your near hand over the sternal lesion.
- With your far hand, grasp either the right or left upper arm of the patient and apply internal rotation and shoulder protraction coupled with distraction. If the patient demonstrates right-sided sternal pain, manipulate the right arm of the patient (vice versa for the left).
- Collapse the upper thoracic cage anteriorly and inward toward the sternum by moving both knees

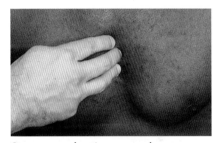

Sternum palpation procedure.

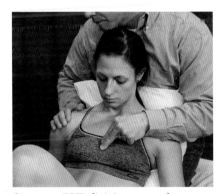

Sternum PRT clinician procedure.

outward and leaning forward to promote kyphotic positioning.
- Rotate the thorax toward the lesion with your body to fine-tune the positioning.
- With the near hand, apply a slight cephalad traction force to the overlying tissue.
- The xiphoid PRT procedure can be used for the sternum when the lesion is centrally located.
- Corollary tissues treated: Pectoralis major and minor, sternocleidomastoid, anterior and middle scalenes, intercostals, rectus abdominis

171

Splenius Capitis

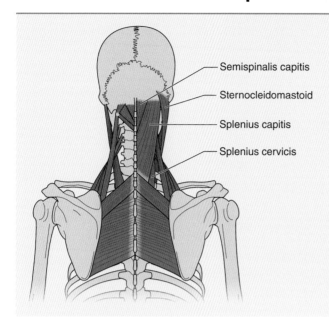

Unlike the other posterior cervical muscles, the splenius capitis runs obliquely in the posterior neck. The majority of the muscle is deep to the trapezius and rhomboids; however, its posterior lateral fibers can be accessed for palpation between the trapezius and levator scapulae muscles.

Origin: Ligamentum nuchae at C3-C7, C7-T4 spinous processes

Insertion: Mastoid process of the temporal bone, lateral third of the superior nuchal line

Action: Capital extension, rotation of the head to the same side, lateral cervical flexion to the same side

Innervation: C3-C6 (cervical nerves); C1-C2 (suboccipital and greater occipital nerves)

Palpation Procedure

- Place the patient supine.
- Locate the mastoid process and slide your fingers inferiorly and medially off this structure onto the fibers of the splenius capitis.
- Move your fingers posteriorly onto the lateral edge of the trapezius and ask the patient to extend the head against the table while rotating it toward the same side, which will produce a contraction of the trapezius fibers.
- Move medially back to the splenius fibers, just off the trapezius. For further orientation, move medially onto the levator scapulae fibers and ask the patient to elevate the shoulder. The splenius capitis fibers do not contract with shoulder elevation, but the levator scapulae fibers will contract with shoulder elevation.
- Strum across the splenius capitis fibers with your fore and middle fingers.
- Determine the most dominant tender point or fasciculation (or both) and maintain light pressure with the pad(s) of the finger(s) throughout the treatment until reassessment has occurred.

PRT Clinician Procedure

- Place the patient supine with the head off the end of the table and cupped in your far hand.
- With your far hand, laterally flex the head and neck toward the lesion, then move the neck into extension.
- With your far hand, apply cervical rotation toward the lesion, then apply cranial lateral flexion toward the lesion.

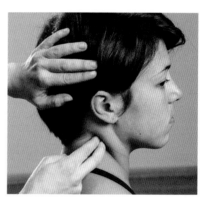

Splenius capitis palpation procedure.

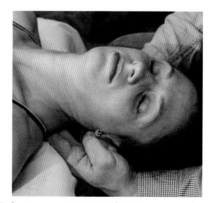

Splenius capitis PRT clinician procedure.

- Corollary tissues treated: Splenius cervicis, upper trapezius, suboccipitals, multifidi, rotatores, levator scapulae, sternocleidomastoid, digastric, longissimus cervicis, spinalis cervicis

Levator Scapulae

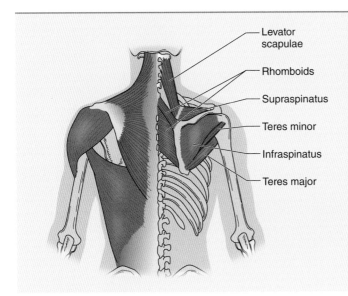

- Levator scapulae
- Rhomboids
- Supraspinatus
- Teres minor
- Infraspinatus
- Teres major

The levator scapulae extends from the superior angle of the scapulae to the transverse processes of C1-C4. Its fibers are deep to the trapezius, but reveal themselves for palpation at the lateral neck, bracketed between the splenius capitis and posterior scalene.

Origin: C1-C4 transverse processes

Insertion: Superior angle of the scapulae

Action: Scapular elevation and abduction, scapular downward rotation, cervical lateral flexion to the same side, cervical rotation to the same side, cervical extension

Innervation: C3-C4 (ventral rami); C5 (dorsal scapular nerve)

Palpation Procedure

- The patient can be prone or supine.
- Locate the lateral border of the trapezius fibers at the lateral neck.
- Slide two fingers forward onto the splenius capitis. Ask the patient to elevate the shoulder. If the fingers are over the splenius capitis, the muscle will not contract with shoulder elevation; if it does contract, the fingers are over the levator scapulae. The levator scapulae muscle is just anterior to the splenius capitis, which on some people is difficult to differentiate from the levator.
- Strum your fingers gently over the levator fibers (they often feel ropelike), which lead superiorly toward the ear and inferiorly toward the scapulae.
- Additionally, the head can be rotated away from the palpation side to accentuate tension at the levator scapulae.
- Determine the most dominant tender point or fasciculation (or both) and maintain light pressure with the pad(s) of the finger(s) throughout the treatment until reassessment has occurred.

PRT Clinician Procedure

- Place the patient supine.
- With your near hand, apply cervical lateral flexion and rotation towards the lesion, then apply slight cranial lateral flexion and rotation.
- With your far hand, grasp the patient's elbow on the involved side. Translate the shoulder toward the head to apply shoulder elevation. Also apply slight shoulder abduction and humeral rotation.

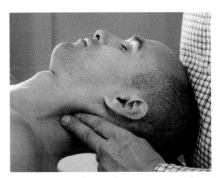

Levator scapulae palpation procedure.

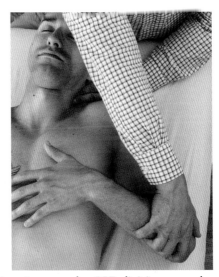

Levator scapulae PRT clinician procedure.

- Corollary tissues treated: Trapezius, sternocleidomastoid, splenius capitis, digastric

 See video 8.5 for the levator scapulae PRT procedure.

Suboccipitals

The suboccipital group is composed of eight individual muscles (rectus capitis posterior major and minor, obliquus capitis superior and inferior, longissimus capitis, splenius capitis, semispinalis capitis, spinalis capitis) at the base of the skull. The muscles course among the atlas, axis, skull, and upper cervical vertebrae. They are primarily responsible for capital extension and rotation and lateral bending of the head. Although they are not discernible individually because of their deep location, the density of their muscle bellies can be felt under palpation.

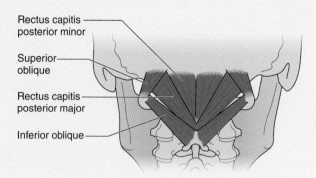

Rectus capitis posterior minor
Superior oblique
Rectus capitis posterior major
Inferior oblique

Origin: Rectus capitis posterior major: Axis spinous process

Rectus capitis posterior minor: Atlas tubercle on the posterior arch

Obliquus capitis superior: Atlas transverse process

Obliquus capitis inferior: Axis spinous process

Longissimus capitis: T1-T5 transverse processes, C4-C7 articular processes

Splenius capitis: Ligamentum nuchae at C3-C7, C7-T4 spinous processes

Semispinalis capitis: C7 and T1-T6 transverse processes, C4-C6 articular processes

Spinalis capitis: C5-C7 and T1-T3 spinous processes

Insertion: Rectus capitis posterior major: Occiput at the lateral portion of the inferior nuchal line

Rectus capitis posterior minor: Occiput at the medial portion of the inferior nuchal line

Obliquus capitis superior: Occiput between the superior and inferior nuchal lines

Obliquus capitis inferior: Atlas

Longissimus capitis: Mastoid process

Splenius capitis: Mastoid process and occiput below the lateral third of the superior nuchal line

Semispinalis capitis: Occiput between the superior and inferior nuchal lines

Spinalis capitis: Occiput between the superior and inferior nuchal lines

Action: Capital extension; head rotation and lateral bending to the same side (as a group)

Innervation: Rectus capitis posterior major: C1 (suboccipital, dorsal rami)

Rectus capitis posterior minor: C1 (suboccipital, dorsal rami)

Obliquus capitis superior: C1 (suboccipital, dorsal rami)

Obliquus capitis inferior: C1 (suboccipital, dorsal rami)

Longissimus capitis: C3-C8 (dorsal rami)

Splenius capitis: C3-C6 (dorsal rami); C1-C2 (suboccipital and greater occipital nerves)

Semispinalis capitis: C2-T1 (dorsal rami and greater occipital nerve)

Spinalis capitis: C3-T1 (dorsal rami)

Palpation Procedure

- Place the patient supine with the neck in slight extension.
- Cup the base of the cranium with both hands.
- Feel the back of the cranium for two bony knobs and C2, the second bony protuberance at the center of the spine. The two knobs are the occiput. The suboccipitals span the region between these landmarks.
- Using your fingertips, apply firm pressure through the overlying tissue to feel the density of the suboccipital muscle bellies.
- Note the location of any tender points or fasciculatory response along the tissues and their attachment sites.
- Once you have determined the most dominant tender point or fasciculation (or both), maintain light pressure with the pad(s) of the finger(s) at the location throughout the PRT treatment procedure until reassessment has occurred.

PRT Clinician Procedure

- Place the patient supine with the head resting on the table.
- With your far hand, move the neck into extension either by moving the patients head off the table or dropping a section of the table.
- Cradle the posterior cranium with your far hand and apply a small upward translational force at the cervical spine with this hand to facilitate capital extension.
- With your far hand, laterally flex the head and neck toward the lesion.
- Rotate the far hand under the cranium to facilitate cranial lateral flexion and rotation for fine-tuning.
- Once the optimal treatment position is attained, place the fingers of your far hand below the lesion and apply a cephalad translational force upward of the tissue.
- Corollary tissues treated: Trapezius, splenius capitis, digastric, levator scapulae, sternocleidomastoid, interspinalis, multifidi, rotatores

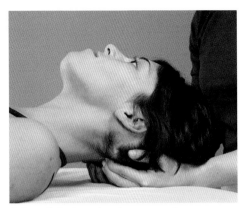

Suboccipitals palpation procedure.

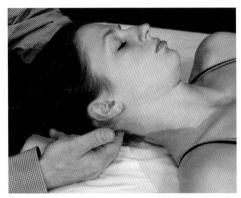

Suboccipitals PRT clinician procedure.

175

Cervical Interspinalis

The cervical interspinalis, like the lumbar interspinalis, is covered by several ligaments and the ligamentum nuchae, which makes direct palpation difficult. However, tenderness between the spinous processes may be an indicator of tissues lesions of the interspinalis as well as its overlying structures. Therefore, PRT may be an effective treatment for somatic dysfunction in this area.

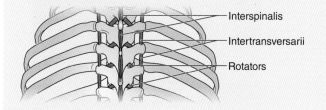

Interspinalis

Intertransversarii

Rotators

Origin and insertion:	C2-T3 spinous processes
Action:	Cervical extension
Innervation:	Respective spinal nerves

Palpation Procedure

- Place the patient supine with the head and neck in slight extension. The patient can also be placed prone for palpation; however, placing the patient supine allows for the use of gravity on the head and neck to assist in the palpation procedure.

- From behind the head, use one or two finger pads to strum in each space between the spinous processes.

- Note the location of any tender points or fasciculatory response along the tissue between the spinous processes.

- Once you have determined the most dominant tender point or fasciculation (or both), maintain light pressure with the pad(s) of the finger(s) at the location throughout the PRT treatment procedure until reassessment has occurred.

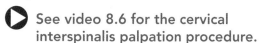 See video 8.6 for the cervical interspinalis palpation procedure.

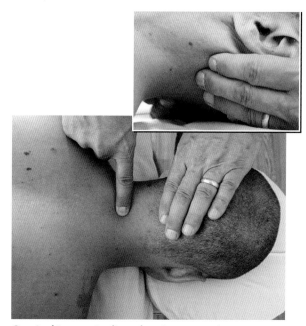

Cervical interspinalis palpation procedure.

PRT Clinician Procedure

- Place the patient supine.

- From behind the head, use the treatment table or your far hand to position the head and neck into marked cervical extension, ideally off the treatment table. If possible, use one or two of the finger pads of your near hand to monitor the lesion's fasciculatory response and treatment position. *Note:* More cervical extension is typically needed for distal lesions than for those located proximally.

- With the palm of your far hand, apply a cephalad translation of the overlying cranial tissue, which will both relax the posterior column tissues and encourage slight cranial extension.

- With your far hand, apply a cephalad translation of the tissues below the lesion. You can also use the fingers of your far hand for palpation rather than for applying translatory force if your fingers are not long enough to reach the tissue lesion. This may be necessary for lesions located at the C6-C7 level.
- With your far hand, apply lateral cervical flexion for lesions that are located more laterally from the midline.
- With your far hand, apply rotation for fine-tuning.
- Corollary tissues treated: Ligamentum nuchae, multifidi, rotatores, spleni musculature, suboccipitals

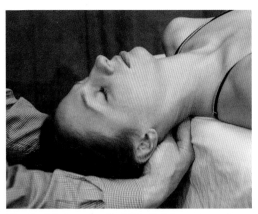

Cervical interspinalis PRT clinician procedure.

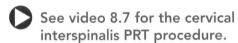 See video 8.7 for the cervical interspinalis PRT procedure.

Patient Self-Treatment Procedure

- Lie supine with a folded bath towel under the upper shoulders to encourage cervical extension.
- Determine where the tender area is and then keep one or two finger pads on the area while actively moving the head through cervical spinal extension and then lateral flexion and rotation while monitoring the lesion.
- Do not hang your head off a table or another structure while applying the PRT patient self-treatment procedure for the interspinalis.
- Maintain the treatment position until the fasciculatory response abates or for three to five minutes.
- This self-treatment procedure can also be utilized for treatment of the suboccipitals.

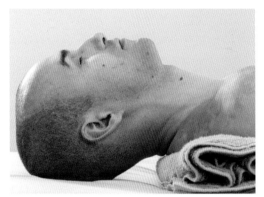

Cervical interspinalis patient self-treatment procedure.

Posterior Scalene

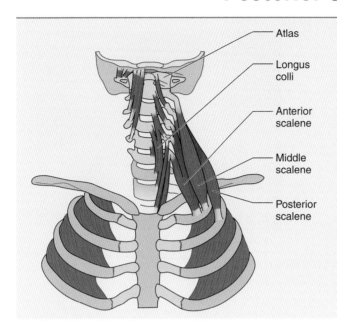

Labels: Atlas, Longus colli, Anterior scalene, Middle scalene, Posterior scalene

The posterior scalene is the smallest of the scalenes and is positioned the deepest of the three in the neck. Because of its size and location, it is often difficult to locate and discern from the middle scalene.

Origin: C4-C6 transverse processes

Insertion: Second rib

Action: Elevation of the second rib during inhalation, lateral cervical flexion to the same side, cervical rotation to the same side, cervical flexion (weak)

Innervation: C6-C8 (ventral rami)

Palpation Procedure

- Position the patient supine, and stand at the head of the table.
- Locate the middle scalene and the levator scapulae muscles at the lateral neck. The posterior scalene is sandwiched between these two muscles.
- Strum across the posterior scalene.
- The posterior scalene can be differentiated from the levator scapulae muscle by having the patient inspire under palpation because the levator will not contract during inspiration. Likewise, you can ask the patient to elevate the shoulder. The posterior scalene should not contract during this movement either.
- Note the location of any tender points or fasciculatory response along the muscle.
- Once you have determined the most dominant tender point or fasciculation (or both), maintain light pressure with the pad(s) of the finger(s) at the location throughout the PRT treatment procedure until reassessment has occurred.

PRT Clinician Procedure

- Place the patient supine, and sit behind the head.
- With your far hand, elevate the shoulder of the involved side toward the lesion.
- With your far hand, move the head into slight cervical extension.
- With your far hand, apply lateral cervical flexion toward the lesion.

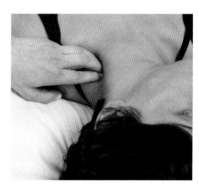

Posterior scalene palpation procedure.

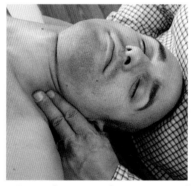

Posterior scalene PRT clinician procedure.

- Apply cervical rotation with your far hand away from or toward the lesion for fine-tuning.
- Corollary tissues treated: Middle scalene, sternocleidomastoid, upper trapezius, suboccipitals, splenius capitis, semispinalis capitis and cervicis, multifidi, rotatores

Posterior Intercostals

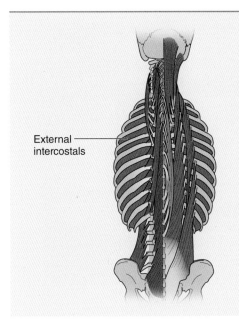

External intercostals

The posterior intercostal muscles can be accessed via palpation, but their identification often requires deeper pressure to overcome the overlying posterior musculature. Treatment with PRT is the same as for the anterior and lateral intercostals with the exception of posterior positioning or manipulation.

Origin: Ribs 1 through 11 (lower border of the rib below the costal tubercles)

Insertion: Upper border of the rib below the sternum via the aponeurosis

Action: External intercostals: Assist the diaphragm with inhalation; rotate the thoracic spine to the opposite side (unilateral); stabilize the rib cage

Internal intercostals: Assist with exhalation; stabilize the rib cage; 1-5 assist with inhalation

Innervation: T1-T11 (intercostal nerves)

Palpation Procedure

- Place the patient prone with the ankles bolstered.
- Start at either the inferior or superior ribs.
- With one or two fingers pads, stroke across the obliquely oriented fibers of the intercostals between each rib.
- Also stroke over the corresponding rib margins, superior and inferior.
- Instruct the patient to take several slow, deep breaths during palpation to ascertain the quality of rib movement and chest expansion. Compare bilaterally.
- Note the location of any tender points or fasciculatory response along the muscle and its attachment to the ribs and xiphoid.
- Once you have determined the most dominant tender point or fasciculation (or both), maintain light pressure with the pad(s) of the finger(s) at the location throughout the PRT treatment procedure until reassessment has occurred.

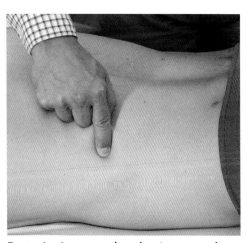

Posterior intercostals palpation procedure.

> continued

Posterior Intercostals > *continued*

PRT Clinician Procedure

- The patient is seated on the treatment table or on the floor. If the patient has adequate hip and knee flexibility, position the lower torso in a hook-lying position with the knees stacked, the hips flexed, and the feet and ankles stacked and oriented toward the side to be treated. Patients who cannot attain this position should place the lower body in a position of maximal comfort.
- Use your near hand to palpate the intercostals. Use your near hand to manipulate the patient's torso during positioning.
- Position yourself behind the patient, kneeling on the treatment table or floor with your knee and thigh supporting the opposite, or contralateral, side of the torso to be treated. The other knee should be in contact with the table or floor.
- Place the patient's contralateral arm and torso on your knee and thigh over a pillow. An exercise ball can be used in place of your knee and thigh either on the treatment table or on the floor.
- With your far hand, grasp the opposite arm (ipsilateral) and bring it across the chest to the pillow, holding the arm at the biceps area. Place a towel or pillow over your arm and have the patient laterally flex the head and neck to rest it on the pillow or towel.
- While palpating the posterior intercostals with the fingers of your near hand, move the supporting knee outward from the patient to promote lateral trunk flexion and collapse the ipsilateral rib cage on the side of the lesion.
- Rotate the supporting knee to encourage rotation and extension of the posterior thorax toward the lesion.
- Once the thorax position of comfort is attained or fasciculatory response is elicited, encourage further rib and costal compression by applying a downward and posterior compression of the rib cage with the palmar aspect of your near hand.
- Corollary tissues treated: Erector spinae, obliques, diaphragm, quadratus lumborum, hip flexors

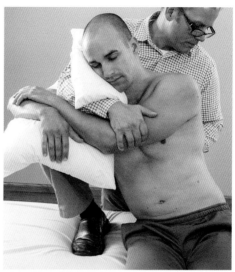

Posterior intercostals PRT clinician procedure.

Thoracic and Cervical Erector Spinae

The musculature of the erector spinae courses from the lumbar region into the upper thoracic and cervical region, where they become less robust under palpation. Most of the thoracic iliocostalis also courses under the scapulae, making it difficult to palpate, but the spinalis and longissimus are ropelike under palpation as they course along the spinal column toward their posterior cranial attachments. The palpation technique described here for the upper thoracic and cervical regions also applies to the lumbar erector spinae group.

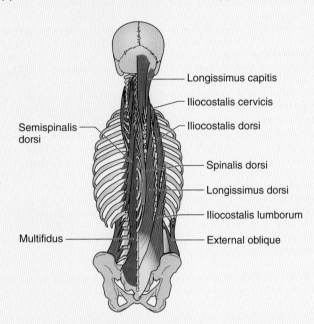

Longissimus capitis

Iliocostalis cervicis

Iliocostalis dorsi

Semispinalis dorsi

Spinalis dorsi

Longissimus dorsi

Iliocostalis lumborum

Multifidus

External oblique

Origin: Spinalis: T11-T12, L1-L2 spinous processes (thoracic), ligamentum nuchae, spinous process of C4-C7 (capitis and cervicis)

Longissimus: L1-L5 transverse processes (thoracic), T1-T5 transverse processes (capitis and cervicis)

Iliocostalis: Ribs 1 through 12 (thoracic and cervicis)

Insertion: Spinalis: T1-T4 (thoracic), mastoid process and occiput (capitis), axis, C2-C3 spinous processes (cervicis)

Longissimus: T1-T12 transverse processes, ribs 2-12 (thoracic), mastoid process (capitis), C2-C6 transverse processes (cervicis)

Iliocostalis: Ribs 1 through 6, C7 transverse process (thoracic), C4-C6 transverse processes (cervicis)

Action: Spinalis: Spinal extension

Longissimus: Spinal extension, lateral flexion to the same side, depression of ribs

Iliocostalis: Spinal extension

Innervation: Spinalis thoracis: T1-T12 (dorsal rami)

Spinalis capitus: C3-T1 (dorsal rami)

Spinalis cervicis: C3-C8 (dorsal rami)

Longissimus thoracis: T1-L1 (dorsal rami)

Longissimus capitis: C3-C8 (dorsal rami)

Longissimus cervicis: C3-T3 (dorsal rami)

Iliocostalis thoracis: T1-T12 (spinal nerves)

Iliocostalis cervicis: C4-T3 (dorsal rami)

> continued

Thoracic and Cervical Erector Spinae > *continued*

Palpation Procedure

- Position the patient prone with the ankles bolstered.
- Start at the lower lumbar spine on the opposite side of the erector group to be palpated.
- With the pads of both hands, find the lateral border of the erector group and strum across their fibers with deep pressure.
- The patient can extend the legs or arms to aid palpation.
- Palpate upward using the same procedure used for the thoracic region. To aid in palpating in this area, ask the patient to extend the spine and head slightly.
- The erector spinae fibers from the scapulae to the head are smaller than those in the lumbar and thoracic regions and do not require as much pressure.
- To demarcate the spinalis fibers, use your thumbs.
- Note the location of any tender points or fasciculatory response along the muscle and its attachments.
- Once you have determined the most dominant tender point or fasciculation (or both), maintain light pressure with the pad(s) of the finger(s) at the location throughout the PRT treatment procedure until reassessment has occurred.

PRT Clinician Procedure

- The patient is prone with the ankles bolstered.
- Position yourself next to the thorax on the side opposite to be treated.
- If possible, elevate the therapy table to waist level or higher for your comfort.
- Use your near hand for palpation with the elbow and forearm positioned diagonally across the back toward the noninvolved hip. Use your near forearm to stabilize the noninvolved rib cage.
- Place your far hand and arm over the opposite shoulder and through the axilla of the patient so that your shoulder is in contact with the patient's shoulder. The anterior aspect of your torso may be in contact with the patient's posterior torso based on table positioning, your size, and the size of the patient.
- Place the palm of your far hand on the posterior aspect of the patient's rib cage.

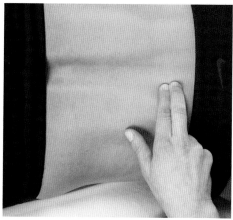

Thoracic and cervical erector spinae palpation procedure.

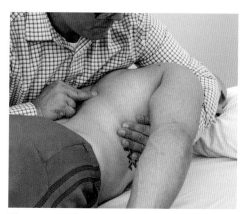

Thoracic and cervical erector spinae PRT clinician procedure (T10-C7).

- While stabilizing the noninvolved side with your forearm, move the thorax and shoulder girdle of the involved side into extension and rotation with your far arm.
- Once extension and rotation positioning are determined, apply elevation and depression to the shoulder girdle of the involved side with the far arm and hand.
- Corollary tissues treated: Rhomboids, middle and lower trapezius, multifidi, rotatores, latissimus dorsi, interspinalis

 See video 8.8 for the thoracic and cervical erector spinae PRT procedure (T10-C7).

Coccyx

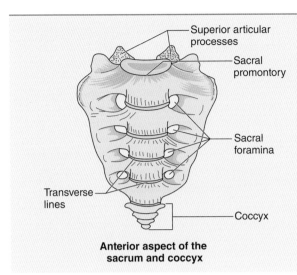

Superior articular processes

Sacral promontory

Sacral foramina

Transverse lines

Coccyx

Anterior aspect of the sacrum and coccyx

Comprising three or four fused bones, the coccyx forms the tail of the sacrum. The coccyx can be injured from an abrupt fall or during birth. Additionally, the coccygeus muscle, which attaches to the lateral aspect of the coccyx, may be affected during injury of the coccyx, which can affect pelvic floor function. Therefore, manipulation of the coccyx may provide relief from pain and somatic dysfunction among patients with pelvic floor disorders.

Palpation Procedure

- Place the patient supine with the ankles bolstered.
- Locate the center of the sacrum and trace down the sacral crest to the level of the gluteal cleft.
- At the top margin of the cleft, you will feel several knobs in close proximity under the fingers. Roll the fingers over the fused coccyx and around its sides to its tip. In some people, the tip is tucked under itself, making palpation of this aspect of the coccyx difficult.
- Note the location of any tender points or fasciculatory response along the bone and its surrounding tissue.
- Once you have determined the most dominant tender point or fasciculation (or both), maintain light pressure with the pad(s) of the finger(s) at the location throughout the PRT treatment procedure until reassessment has occurred.

PRT Clinician Procedure

- Place the patient prone with the knees flexed and ankles supported.
- With the base of your far hand, apply downward pressure to the apex of the sacrum.
- Monitor the lesion with the fingers of your near hand.
- After performing downward pressure, using the far hand, tilt the sacrum from side to side and rotate.
- With your far hand, translate the overlying tissue toward the coccyx.
- Corollary tissue treated: Coccygeus, sacroiliac joints, thoracolumbar fascia, levator ani, piriformis, sacrotuberous ligament, sacrococcygeal ligament

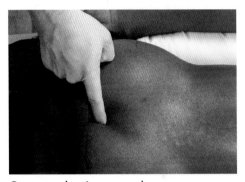

Coccyx palpation procedure.

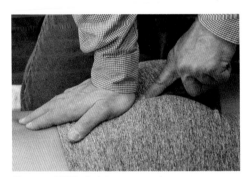

Coccyx PRT clinician procedure.

183

Quadratus Lumborum

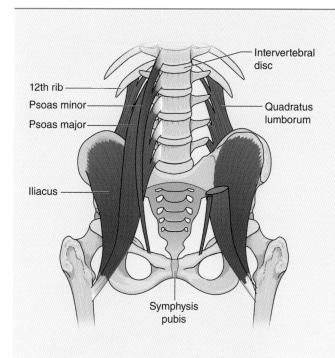

The quadratus lumborum (QL) is buried deep in the abdomen, but it is accessible to palpation at its lateral borders. The QL is encased in the multiple layers of the thoracolumbar fascia and found underneath the erector spinae, but it is situated against the posterior abdominal wall. Because of its articulation with the ilium and lumbar vertebrae, it is a major contributor to the stability of the pelvis and lumbar spine during the single-limb stance phase of the gait cycle.

Origin: Ilium crest, iliolumbar ligament

Insertion: 12th rib (lower border), L1-L4 transverse processes, occasionally the T12 vertebral body

Action: Extension of the lumbar spine, inspiration and exhalation, elevation of the pelvis to the same side, lateral trunk flexion to the same side (pelvis fixed), fixation and depression of the 12th rib

Innervation: T12-L3 (ventral rami)

Palpation Procedure

- Place the patient prone with the ankles bolstered.
- The QL runs between the 12th rib and the crest of the ilium and has attachments to the lumbar transverse processes.
- Because the erector spinae and thoracolumbar fascia lie over the most medial portions of the QL, there are two methods to access the more lateral fibers of this muscle. One is to access the lateral portions by palpating them from the inferior margin of the 12th rib, and the other is to apply deep pressure at the lateral border of the erector spinae.
- If palpating the QL from the 12th rib, roll the pads of your fingers against the inferior margin of the rib and then downward across its vertical fibers as they course down to the ilium.
- If palpating deep to the erector spinae, stand on the side opposite that of the involved tissue and, with firm pressure, strum across the strap-like musculature of the erector spinae at the lumbar spine. With firm strumming pressure, demarcate the lateral border and sink the fingers into the QL, pinning it against the erector spinae and strumming it against the lumbar vertebrae.

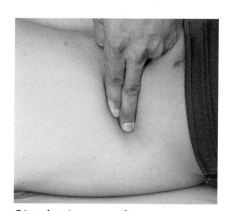

QL palpation procedure.

- Note the location of any tender points or fasciculatory response along the muscle and its articulations (e.g., the 12th rib).
- Once you have determined the most dominant tender point or fasciculation (or both), maintain light pressure with the pad(s) of the finger(s) at the location throughout the PRT treatment procedure until reassessment has occurred.

PRT Clinician Procedure

- Place the patient prone.
- While palpating the QL lesion with your near hand, apply lateral trunk flexion to the involved side by moving both legs with your far hand across the table toward the lesion.
- With your far hand, move the extended limb into extension, abduction, and external rotation.
- Place the patient's thigh on your thigh and brace it against your torso, or use a bolster to stabilize the leg into the optimal treatment position.
- Once the optimal treatment position is obtained, fine-tune it by compressing the limb toward the lesion with your far hand or body.
- Corollary tissues treated: Erector spinae, thoracolumbar fascia, gluteus medius and minimus, gluteus maximus, piriformis, lumbar multifidi, interspinalis, hamstrings

 See video 8.9 for the QL PRT procedure.

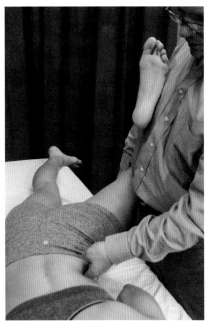

QL PRT clinician procedure.

Lumbar Erector Spinae

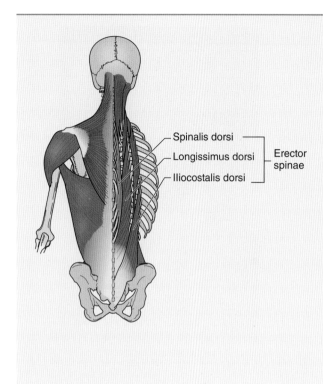

Spinalis dorsi ⎤
Longissimus dorsi ⎬ Erector spinae
Iliocostalis dorsi ⎦

One of the most readily identified muscle groups of the back, the erector spinae courses from the sacrum to the base of the skull. The group is formed by 10 or more muscles with divisions that cover the lumbar, thoracic, and cervical segments of the spine. They are further divided into lateral (iliocostalis cervicis, iliocostalis thoracis, iliocostalis lumborum), intermediate (longissimus capitis, longissimus cervicis, longissimus thoracis), and medial (spinalis capitis, spinalis cervicis, spinalis thoracis) column muscles. Typically, the column muscles are divided into three groups for simple reference: the spinalis, longissimus, and iliocostalis. Distally, the groups converge into the dense thoracolumbar fascia (lumborum ligament) that covers the lumbosacral spine. Above this area, they can be viewed and palpated as a thick muscular column that runs along the spinal column. The PRT technique described here for the lumbar region should follow the palpation procedure outlined previously for the thoracic and cervical erector spinae groups. Anatomical information for the lumbar erector spinae musculature is described previously as well.

Palpation Procedure

See instructions for thoracic and cervical erector spinae palpation procedure.

PRT Clinician Procedure

- Place the patient prone with the ankles bolstered.
- Place a pillow under the upper thorax to the midline.
- The head should be rotated toward the side of the lesion.
- Stand on the side opposite of the lesion.
- With your far hand, grasp the anterior iliac spine of the involved side and rotate the pelvis toward the lesion.
- Gather and translate the gluteal tissues upward on the involved side with the far forearm.
- Flex the hip and knee on the involved side to increase spinal extension.
- Corollary tissues treated: Quadratus lumborum, serratus posterior, multifidi, rotatores, interspinalis, sacroiliac joint

▶ **See video 8.10 for the lumbar erector spinae PRT procedure (L5-T10).**

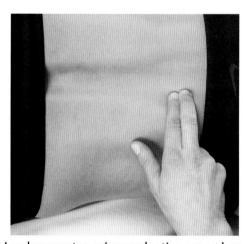

Lumbar erector spinae palpation procedure.

Patient Self-Treatment Procedure

- Lie prone with a pillow under the thorax to the midline and a pillow (sofa size) under the hip on the involved side.

- Increase the relaxation of the involved side by flexing the hip and knee.

- Maintain this position for three to five minutes or apply heat or ice in this position for 20 to 30 minutes to facilitate greater relaxation and pain control.

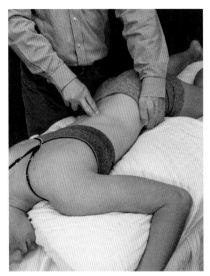

Lumbar erector spinae PRT clinician procedure (L5-T10).

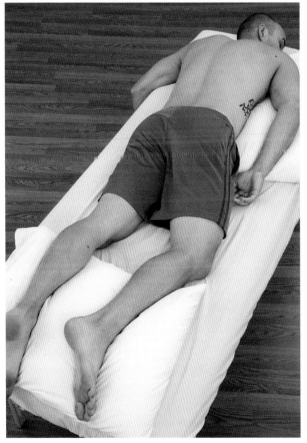

Lumbar erector spinae patient self-treatment procedure.

Lumbar Interspinalis

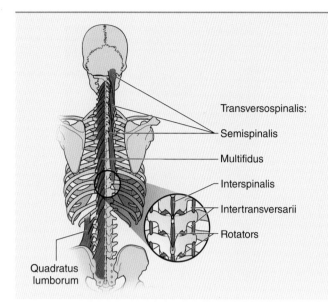

Transversospinalis:

— Semispinalis

— Multifidus

— Interspinalis

— Intertransversarii

— Rotators

Quadratus lumborum

The lumbar interspinalis muscles are located deep in the spaces between the spinous processes. These short muscles are not readily palpable because they are covered by several ligaments including the supraspinous and interspinous as well as the thoracolumbar fascia. When point tenderness exists between the spinous processes, however, both the ligaments and the lumbar interspinalis may be involved. Therefore, PRT may be effective for treating lesions of these tissues.

Origin and insertion: T12- L5 spinous processes

Action: Spinal extension

Innervation: Respective spinal nerves

Palpation Procedure

- Place the patient prone with the ankles bolstered.
- Stack your forefinger and middle finger or use your thumb to apply deep pressure between the spinous processes. Strum across the vertebrae.
- Greater pressure is needed in the lumbar area because of the robust nature of the musculature and ligaments that cover the lumbar vertebrae. A decrease in palpation pressure is needed as the cervical spine is approached because the vertebrae in this area are more readily palpable.
- Note the location of any tender points or fasciculatory response between the spinous processes.
- Once you have determined the most dominant tender point or fasciculation (or both), maintain light pressure with the pad(s) of the finger(s) at the location throughout the PRT treatment procedure until reassessment has occurred.

PRT Clinician Procedure

- Place the patient prone with a pillow under the upper torso to facilitate spinal extension.
- With your far hand, apply marked hip extension.
- With your far hand, adduct and abduct the thigh to fine-tune.
- Corollary tissues treated: Erector spinae, gluteus medius, hamstrings, quadratus lumborum, gluteus maximus

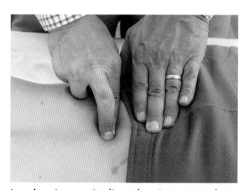

Lumbar interspinalis palpation procedure.

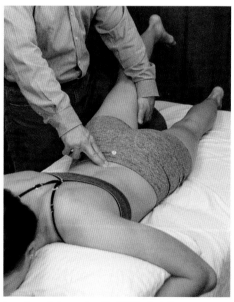

Lumbar interspinalis PRT clinician procedure.

Lumbar Multifidi

The multifidi muscles are deep intrinsics that are found next to the spinous processes from the sacrum to the top of the cervical spine. The multifidi have three heads (superficial, intermediate, and deep) that course obliquely from one vertebra to the next, traversing over two to four vertebrae in most instances. The exceptions are the sacral and lumbar multifidi, which originate from the sacrum, ilium, and posterior sacroiliac ligaments. However, only the lumbar multifidi are accessible for palpation.

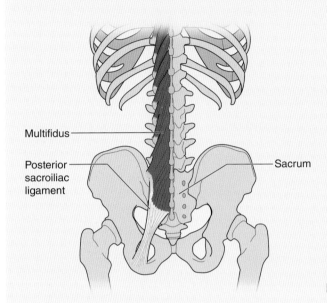

Multifidus

Posterior
sacroiliac
ligament

Sacrum

Origin: Posterior sacrum (as low as the S4 foramen), posterior superior iliac spine and crest, lumborum ligament, posterior sacroiliac ligaments, L1-L5 maxillary processes, T1-T12 transverse processes, C4-C7 articular processes

Insertion: The superficial head runs to the third and fourth vertebrae above its origin. The intermediate head runs to the second or third vertebrae above its origin. The deep head runs between adjacent vertebrae.

Action: Spinal extension, lateral flexion to the same side, rotation to the opposite side

Innervation: Respective spinal nerves

Palpation Procedure

- Place the patient prone with the ankles bolstered.
- Grasp each iliac crest and reach to the center of the spine with your thumbs for the approximate location of the sacroiliac joints.
- Stack and orient your fingers toward the axilla.
- Strum your fingers with firm pressure over the thoracolumbar fascia to feel the density of the lumbar multifidi.
- Note the location of any tender points or fasciculatory response at the muscles' locations.
- Once you have determined the most dominant tender point or fasciculation (or both), maintain light pressure with the pad(s) of the finger(s) at the location throughout the PRT treatment procedure until reassessment has occurred.

PRT Clinician Procedure

- Place the patient prone with the ankles bolstered.
- Follow either the erector spinae or interspinalis procedure for treatment of this tissue.
- Corollary tissues treated: Erector spinae, interspinalis, quadratus lumborum, gluteals, hamstrings

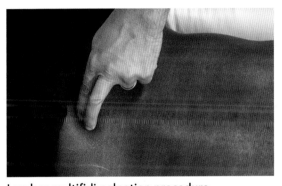

Lumbar multifidi palpation procedure.

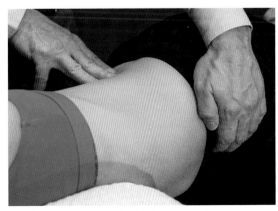

Lumbar multifidi PRT clinician procedure.

Thoracic Outlet Syndrome

Thoracic outlet syndrome (TOS) is often considered a controversial diagnosis in medicine because of a lack of defined objective diagnostic criteria and robust investigation into the effectiveness of its management. TOS is typically classified into three types: vascular (arterial or venous), neurogenic, or a combination of the two (Polvsen et al. 2012). Thoracic outlet syndrome typically occurs when vascular or neural tissues become impinged as they pass through the scalene triangle, costoclavicular space, or subcoracoid space, also known as the cervicothoracobrachial region (Laulan et al. 2011). The primary structures impinged are the brachial plexus, subclavian artery, or subclavian vein—often from hypertonic musculature, fascial restrictions, or an accessory rib. Patients often report shoulder, arm, hand, and cervical pain with or without neurological symptoms. Some also complain of temperature changes in the distal upper extremities. The signs and symptoms of TOS are often difficult to differentiate from those of cervical, shoulder, and upper-extremity disease states (e.g., disc pathology, internal shoulder derangement, carpal tunnel syndrome, shoulder infection). Moreover, conditions such as these often cause muscular and osteopathic lesions resulting in neurovascular compression at the thoracic outlet, clouding where the compression manifests.

Laulan and colleagues (2011) and Belzberg and Dorsi (2012) reported that 95% of TOS cases are the result of neurogenic compression. However, Laulan and colleagues (2011) pointed to four major causes: congenital abnormality, trauma (e.g., whiplash), functional or acquired etiologies (e.g., muscle imbalance in the shoulder or cervical region), and other rare causes (e.g., tumor, osteomyelitis). O'Brien, Ramasunder, and Cox (2011) offered a report of a venous thoracic outlet syndrome in a pediatric patient from a first rib osteochondroma. Although rare, other mechanisms beyond muscular, fascial, and rib compression must be considered when evaluating patients with suspected TOS. Surgical intervention for decompression of the thoracic outlet often involves removal of the first rib and other tissues that appear to be compressing the neurovascular bundle as it passes through the thoracic outlet. However, surgical intervention may not always be the answer, as elucidated by a patient in the *British Medical Journal*, who had

Treatment Points and Sequencing

1. Anterior and middle scalenes
2. Pectoralis minor
3. Subclavius
4. Sternocleidomastoid
5. Levator scapulae
6. Acromioclavicular joint
7. Upper trapezius
8. Serratus anterior
9. Rhomboids

not received relief after seven thoracic decompression surgical interventions (Deane, Giele, and Johnson 2012). Therefore, it behooves clinicians to use PRT to reduce compression of the thoracic outlet in place of surgical decompression, but only after differential diagnoses have been considered.

Common Signs and Symptoms

- Pain and paresthesia in the hand and fingers
- Neck, shoulder, or fascial pain
- Weakness in the upper extremity, particularly in the hand
- Progressive muscular atrophy of the intrinsic muscles of the hand
- Edema of the upper limb
- Pain, paresthesia, and temperature changes when the arms are raised overhead
- Symptoms exacerbated by stress
- Rounded shoulders
- Restricted cervical and shoulder range of motion
- Loss of distal pulses with overhead TOS special tests (vascular)

Common Differential Diagnoses

- Osteomyelitis
- Cervical radiculopathy
- Cervical disc pathology
- Clavicular injury
- Acromioclavicular joint injury
- Pronator teres syndrome
- Thoracic disc injury
- Thoracic discogenic pain syndrome

- Internal shoulder derangement
- Metastatic tumor
- Cubital tunnel syndrome
- Carpal tunnel syndrome
- Brachial plexus injury

Clinician Therapeutic Interventions

- After a thorough orthopedic examination, conduct a postural evaluation to determine whether a postural correction may be helpful.
- Release painful contracted tissues with PRT prior to using direct manipulative techniques.
- Consider first-rib mobilization if other indirect tissue manipulations have been unsuccessful.
- Consider requesting a radiograph if an accessory rib is suspected.
- Evaluate work-related ergonomics as a potential causative factor.
- Have the patient employ stress-reduction measures to reduce somatic triggers.

- Consider neural flossing once painful contracted tissues are released.
- Myofascial massage of the cervical and shoulder musculature may complement PRT as long as it does not invoke reflexive muscular spasm.
- Shoulder girdle, upper-extremity, and cervical strengthening should be focused on gaining postural endurance.

Patient Self-Treatment Interventions

- Regularly stretch the scalenes, upper trapezius, and pectoralis musculature.
- Perform self-release on associated facilitated tissues daily, if possible.
- Avoid overhead activity or work or sport-related movements that produce symptoms.
- Apply palliative modalities to control pain and spasm.
- Perform first-rib mobilizations daily if they produce symptomatic relief.

Acquired Torticollis

Torticollis, which means "twisted neck" in Latin (it is also called wry neck), can arise from both congenital and acquired causes. Acquired torticollis often presents with nuchal rigidity and spasm of the cervical musculature, particularly the sternocleidomastoid. The condition results in neck stiffness, loss of range of motion, and associated pain (Chirurgi and Kahlon 2012). The causes and treatment of congenital torticollis are well documented (Patwardhan et al. 2011; Shankar et al. 2011; Yim et al. 2013), although the mechanisms responsible for the production of acquired torticollis and its effective treatment are yet to be fully elucidated in the literature. However, PRT has shown promise for the treatment of noncomplicated acquired torticollis.

In a case series, Baker and colleagues (2013) examined the clinical effectiveness of PRT on undergraduates with acquired torticollis. Four patients treated over a period of three days with PRT showed a minimal clinically important difference (MCID) for cervical range of motion as well as for pain as rated on the NPRS (numerical pain rating scale) and disablement as rated on the DPA (disablement in the physically active) instrument.

Patients who present with acquired or acute torticollis often report waking up with a stiff neck, being unable to rotate the head to one side or the other, pain in the neck and shoulders, and headache. Per and colleagues (2014) pointed out that head tilt and rotation relative to the cervical spine, or flexion of the cervical spine and head are outward signs of underlying etiologies, not necessarily indicating a specific diagnosis; thus, the clinician must approach the investigation from a multisystem perspective. However, the condition is commonly attributed to contracture of the sternocleidomastoid as a result of the neck being sustained in a compromised position, often during sleep. Contracture of the neck and shoulder musculature may be a result of segmental facilitation due to a pinching of the facet capsule. However, more emergent conditions may also present with similar signs and symptoms.

For example, bacterial meningitis may present as acute torticollis. Chirurgi and Kahlon (2012) reported on a case of bacterial meningitis that presented as acquired torticollis based on the outward clinical signs and symptoms. Only when the patient experienced a syncope episode and was admitted to the emergency room two weeks later was the life-threatening condition of bacterial meningitis discovered. Therefore, it is critical that patients suspected of suffering from acquired torticollis also be screened for other differential diagnoses.

Treatment Points and Sequencing
1. Sternocleidomastoid
2. Digastric
3. Anterior and middle scalenes
4. Levator scapulae at the neck
5. Upper trapezius
6. Pectoralis minor
7. Splenius capitis
8. Interspinalis (cervical)
9. Suboccipitals
10. Infraspinatus
11. Rhomboids
12. Levator scapulae at the shoulder

Common Signs and Symptoms

- Neck pain (stiff neck)
- Spontaneous onset, typically upon waking
- Neck and head tilted and rotated, with possible jaw deviation
- Headache
- Neck and shoulder spasm
- Limited head and neck rotation, typically to one side

Common Differential Diagnoses

- Atlantoaxial rotatory subluxation
- Meningitis
- Infection
- Tumor
- Trauma
- Neck sprain or strain
- Drug reaction
- Psychosocial stress reaction

Clinician Therapeutic Interventions

- After performing a thorough evaluation to rule out differential diagnoses, determine the cervical and shoulder motions that produce pain.
- Apply PRT within the available pain-free range of motion.

- Through a patient history, determine whether other factors could be mitigated (e.g., stress with meditation or counseling).
- Palliative modalities such as moist heat may be helpful prior to the application of intermittent cervical traction.
- Consider using myofascial tissue therapies or massage after the application of PRT.
- Joint mobilizations may be helpful in pain reduction or if a vertebra is luxated. However, be sure to release the tissues prior to mobilization.
- After release, PNF stretching or muscle energy techniques may be helpful to gain range of motion as long as they are performed in a nonpainful manner.

- Laser therapy may be helpful for reducing inflammation of the superficial cervical tissues.

Patient Self-Treatment Interventions

- Perform PRT self-releases daily within a pain-free range of motion.
- Apply palliative modalities as needed.
- Stretch daily within a pain-free range of motion.
- Avoid demanding ADLs (activities of daily living) and work and sport activities until the primary symptoms have subsided.

Chronic Nonspecific Low Back Pain

Chronic low back pain has been identified as a significant problem worldwide. It has significant cost to employers and employees as a result of time lost from work (Hoy et al. 2012) as well as indirect treatment costs (Krismer and Van Tulder 2007). Nonspecific low back pain comprises 90% of low back pain cases, which have no known cause (Krismer and Van Tulder 2007). Kuchera (2008) pointed out that chronic pain often results in "anxiety, depression, and a reduction in quality of life" (p. 33). Without an apparent pain source or cause, treatment is often a challenge for clinicians, and the ambiguous nature of the condition makes it difficult for patients to endure.

In a systematic review of treatment options for nonspecific chronic low back pain, behavioral therapy intervention, exercise therapy, and a multidisciplinary approach that included behavioral therapy were found to have the greatest effect on reducing the intensity of pain and disability (Hoy et al. 2012). However, more traditional therapies such as back schools, low-level laser therapy, patient education, massage, traction, superficial heat and cold, and lumbar supports alone were not found to be effective. The authors of this report, which did not include PRT as an intervention, advocated a multidisciplinary treatment approach coupled with behavioral therapy, which may address some of the anxiety and depression associated with chronic back conditions.

Investigations of the efficacy of PRT as an intervention for both acute and chronic low back pain have been almost nonexistent to date. One randomized trial examined the effectiveness of PRT, or SCS, for the treatment of acute low back pain (Lewis et al. 2011). The authors did not find SCS combined with exercise to be more effective than exercise alone on pain intensity and disability. However, because they used no true control, the findings should be interpreted cautiously. Contrary to these findings, in a case series, Lewis and Flynn (2001) found that pain and disability were reduced in four patients with low back pain who were treated with SCS. Robust study is needed to further investigate the use of PRT for the treatment of nonspecific chronic low back pain both as a stand-alone treatment and within a multidisciplinary approach.

Treatment Points and Sequencing

1. Psoas
2. Iliacus
3. Adductor magnus
4. Inferior ischium
5. Sacroiliac joint
6. Erector spinae
7. Interspinalis
8. Quadratus lumborum
9. Gluteus medius
10. Piriformis
11. Hamstrings

Common Signs and Symptoms

- Dull ache in the low back, buttocks, or legs
- Weakness in the back, hips, or legs
- Localized tingling or numbness
- Pain with activities of daily living (dull or sharp)
- Leg length discrepancy
- Sacroiliac joint fixation
- Innominate rotation
- Pelvic shear

Common Differential Diagnoses

- Scoliosis (functional or congenital)
- Disc disease
- Metabolic bone disease
- Spinal stenosis
- Metastatic disease
- Degenerative facet disease
- Herpes zoster (shingles)
- Spondyloarthropathies
- Osteoporotic compression fracture
- Discogenic pain

Clinician Therapeutic Interventions

- Use behavioral and stress interventions for pain control.
- Integrate PRT with other complimentary therapies.
- Perform a biomechanical analysis to determine whether pathological lower-extremity

biomechanics are placing additional load on the patient's low back.

- Educate the patient about how to perform ADL movements to reduce strain and load on low back tissues.
- Use palliative modalities to control pain and spasm.
- Multiple PRT treatments are often needed to reestablish tissue and neural homeostasis.
- Explore the possibility of the existence of structural faults (e.g., innominate rotation and pelvic shears) and treat accordingly.

- Provide weight reduction strategies if the patient is obese.

Patient Self-Treatment Interventions

- Avoid positions and movements that exacerbate the pain.
- Use palliative modalities to help control the pain and spasm.
- Perform self-release on the low back daily.
- Perform behavioral and stress interventions daily.
- Attempt to stay active within tolerance.

Disc Derangement

Precautions should be taken when treating individuals suspected of having disc derangement because of the potential alteration of disc pressure caused by treatment positioning. Derangement of the disc (e.g., bulging, herniation) may result from either an acute or insidious onset (Bartysnski et al. 2013). However, based on discography study, the presence of disc derangement alone has not been found to be a confirmatory factor for the presence of low back pain. Moreover, degenerative disc changes were found as frequently in symptomatic patients as they were in asymptomatic patients (Bartynski et al. 2013; Endean et al. 2011). Therefore, clinicians should use both physical and diagnostic findings to formulate their treatment plans. However, several factors that increase the risk for disc derangement and the development of low back pain have been identified, including obesity and being overweight (Shiri et al. 2010), genetic predisposition (Livshits et al. 2011), and being female (Bartynski et al. 2013).

When treating symptomatic disc derangement patients with PRT, clinicians should use the concept of centralization or position bias. The concept of centralization or position bias is based on the range of motion or position that does not cause or increase the patient's symptoms. Determining the position bias or area of centralization requires the clinician to move the patient through their available range of motion and various positions (e.g., flexion/extension) to determine where the patient does not experience symptoms. They should also consult diagnostic reports, if available, to learn the type, location, and severity of the disc derangement. For example, a patient may experience radicular symptomology when the leg is positioned at 15° of extension but not between 10 and 15°. In this case, the treatment position bias or zone of centralization would be in the range that does not produce symptoms. A clinician treating a patient with a posterior lateral disc bulge would avoid positioning or manipulating structures in any way that would increase bulging in the posterior lateral direction. My own clinical experience with this patient population has revealed that they often do not tolerate significant range of motion alterations or joint compressions, nor do they tolerate a significant amount of PRT procedures early in their therapy. Therefore, clinicians should use finite and discrim-

Treatment Points and Sequencing

Lumbar
1. Sacroiliac joints*
2. Erector spinae*
3. Interspinalis
4. Quadratus lumborum
5. Adductor magnus
6. Inferior ischium*
7. Psoas*

Thoracic
1. Erector spinae*
2. Sacroiliac joints*
3. Rhomboids*
4. Lower trapezius
5. Xiphoid*
6. Serratus anterior

Cervical
1. Suboccipitals
2. Interspinalis
3. Splenius capitis*
4. Upper trapezius*
5. Pectoralis minor
6. Subclavius
7. Digastric
8. Anterior and middle scalenes*
9. Sternocleidomastoid
10. Rhomboids
11. Levator scapulae at the neck and shoulder*
12. Infraspinatus

inant positioning and avoid large movements or manipulations that would produce significant compressive force at the joints, particularly in the lumbosacral region.

Flexion positioning often aggravates posterior disc bulges; lateral flexion often aggravates posterior lateral disc bulges; and nerve root compressions and extension positioning often aggravate facet joint pathology. Therefore, it is critical to use a centralization approach as a guide for how much manipulation to use during treatment. Additionally, acute patients often can tolerate only three to five PRT procedures in their initial therapy sessions. The treatment points and sequencing followed by an asterisk (*) in the Treatment Points and Sequencing box are considered essential to perform during the acute phase of treatment. However, the selection and sequencing of the treatment will depend on patient assessment, diagnostic findings, and scanning and mapping evaluation findings as well as symptomatic responses during treatment.

Common Signs and Symptoms

- Dermatome and myotome alterations
- Radiculopathy
- Discogenic pain
- Sciatic pain
- Altered deep tendon reflexes
- Allodynia
- Impaired range of motion
- Myofascial pain syndrome
- Pain and sensory changes with neural tension testing
- Leg length discrepancy

Common Differential Diagnoses

- Epidural abscess
- Epidural hemorrhage
- Ankylosing spondylitis
- Multiple myeloma
- Vascular insufficiency
- Caudal equine syndrome
- Arthritis
- Osteoporosis with stress fractures
- Extradural tumors
- Peripheral neuropathy
- Herpes zoster

Clinician Therapeutic Interventions

- If available, request diagnostic reports and images to ascertain the type, extent, and location of the disc derangement.
- Use the concept of centralization or position bias in the application of PRT.
- Use a multimodal treatment approach that incorporates behavioral and stress modification strategies for pain control.
- Use palliative and traditional modalities to limit pain and spasm.
- Provide ADL education to limit mechanical compression and strain at damaged tissues.
- Advocate limited bed rest during the acute phase (one to two days).
- Encourage movement and activity within tolerance.
- Implement a progressive exercise program focusing early on recruitment and stabilization.
- Use PRT prior to joint and neural mobilizations or traction.
- Apply neural mobilizations or flossing as tolerated.

Patient Self-Treatment Interventions

- Use ADL techniques throughout the day.
- Perform applicable self-release techniques daily that do not exacerbate symptoms.
- Consider using home traction or inversion for managing pain and spasm.
- Use palliative modalities to control pain and spasm.
- Limit bed rest to one to two days during the acute phase.
- Use a TENS unit to control pain and spasm as needed or tolerated.
- Perform neural mobilizations or flossing daily as tolerated.

Summary

Pain associated with the cervical and low back region is a significant global problem that affects upwards of 85% of the population, resulting in a significant societal financial burden. Evidence of the efficacy of PRT for the treatment of spinal conditions is emerging. Although the current body of research has focused on the use of PRT for the cervical spine and head, interest is mounting in its application in the lumbar and thoracic regions for a variety of ailments. Using PRT with people suffering from acute pain related to spinal injury may reduce the formation of central sensitization, somatic dysfunction, autonomic nervous system dysfunction, and associated psychosocial issues such as depression, disability, and lost work time. If researchers and clinicians can integrate PRT into a multimodal treatment plan to reduce pain, disability, and time lost from work and physical activity, the implications for society as a whole would be undoubtedly rewarding.

CHAPTER 9

Shoulder

CHAPTER OBJECTIVES

After reading this chapter, you should be able to do the following:

1. Recall the factors that may influence the development of somatic dysfunction at the shoulder.

2. Locate and palpate shoulder structures to be treated with positional release therapy (PRT).

3. Apply PRT techniques to shoulders affected by somatic dysfunction.

4. Ascertain how somatic lesion patterns in the shoulder girdle may affect the development of common shoulder conditions such as impingement syndrome.

The prevalence of upper-quarter injury among the athletic and working populations has been proposed to be as significant as that of lower-quarter and spinal conditions (Ootes, Lambers, and Ring 2012). Fernandez-de-las Penas and colleagues (2012) reported that arm pain was only second to back pain as a cause of work-related illness. Even though the majority of upper-extremity injuries occur at home, sports injuries are becoming a significant contributor, particularly among adolescents.

Gottschalk and Andrish (2011) found that U.S. high school athletes sustain upwards of 2 million injuries a year and that the leading reason for a visit to the pediatrician's office was sport-related injury. One of the most prevalent injuries among adolescents has been upper-extremity fracture (Gottschalak and Andrish 2011; Sytema et al. 2010). Sytema and colleagues' 2010 study revealed a high rate of upper-extremity fracture among adolescents, which is in agreement with other studies that attribute adolescent upper-extremity fracture to immature skeletal growth, making the upper extremity vulnerable when falling on the outstretched arm. In their study, the sports with the highest risk for fall (horse riding, speedskating, skiing, snowboarding, and school sports such as soccer) demonstrated the most upper-extremity fractures, and individual sports had an increased risk over team sports. Although sport-related trauma is a primary culprit in upper-extremity injury, repetitive movements may also result in microtrauma, chronic pain, and osteopathic lesions in both athletes and workers.

In a systematic review of risk factors for upper-extremity work-related musculoskeletal disorders (WRMDs) among computer users, Andersen and colleagues (2011) could not establish a strong link for any of Da Costa and Vieira's (2009) reported WRMD risk factors among computer users, such as heavy physical work and lifting, excessive repetition, awkward postures, smoking, high body mass index, high psychosocial work demands, and the presence of comorbidities. The only risk factor that was moderately associated with upper-extremity acute and transient pain was excessive mouse use. Additionally, Andersen and colleagues (2011) also did not find any upper-quarter disease or injury to be related to computer work and found only a preventive effect when a workstation and ergonomic intervention were combined, but this association was small.

Although these studies differ in their risk factor findings for WRMD, the authors of both indicated that the findings should be interpreted with caution because of the low methodological quality of the workplace studies examined. Regardless of the risk factors that affect WRMDs, a pattern of somatic dysfunction appears to exist in both white- and blue-collar workers.

A significant number of myofascial trigger points (MTrPs) are often assumed to manifest in manual laborers, which may be associated with heavy physical work or lifting. However, other risk factors identified by Da Costa and Vieira (2010) such as excessive repetitive tasks and awkward postures may also be factors for both manual and office workers. In a study examining referred pain from MTrPs in the head, neck, shoulder, and arm among blue-collar and white-collar workers, Fernandez-de-las-Penas and colleagues (2012) did not find any significant differences in the location or amount of both active and latent MTrPs between these groups. The authors found the most common areas for MTrPs for both groups to be in the upper trapezius, levator scapulae, and extensor carpi radialis brevis muscles. The areas producing the most referred pain were the pectoralis major, infraspinatus, upper trapezius, and scalenes. Treatment of upper-quarter lesions in these areas with the use of dry needling has received a significant amount of attention in the literature.

In a systematic review and meta-analysis, Kietrys and colleagues (2013) did not find dry needling to be more effective than any other therapeutic interventions for the treatment of upper-quarter active MTrPs in patients with myofascial pain syndrome. They did find that it was more effective at reducing immediate pain over sham or placebo treatments.

To date, no high-quality studies have investigated the use of PRT for the reduction of upper-quarter pain in the workplace population. However, Jacobson and colleagues (1989) provided an early theory for the use of PRT for shoulder somatic dysfunction, which they termed the circulatory model. The authors proposed that when the arm is passively manipulated above shoulder level, vascular vessels within the muscle regain circulation as a result of reduced tension on the muscle and perfusion of the tissue; pain subsequently decreases. The authors based their proposition on a previous study (Rathbun and Macnab 1970) of cadaver shoulders injected with a micro-opaque suspension. When the arm was at its side, the injected solution did not fill the supraspinatus vessels; when the arm was raised into passive abduction, complete perfusion occurred. The findings of this study coupled with clinical observations of patients unable to relax during upright PRT treatments resulted in placing patients with upper-quarter somatic dysfunction in a prone or supine position for treatment, when possible. Patients involuntarily contract the shoulder and sometimes the entire upper extremity when treated in a seated position. Moreover, treating the upper quarter in a seated position may limit perfusion of the tissues because of involuntary muscular stabilization of the shoulder girdle and extremity. Therefore, because of the potential impact on circulatory flow based on shoulder position, overhead athletes deserve special consideration.

The shoulder is inherently an unstable joint that relies on its contractile and noncontractile tissues for stabilization. Injury to the shoulder among athletes may occur in the presence of fatigue, weakness, range of motion deficits, overuse, or previous injury (Sytema et al. 2010). In an examination of 246 U.S. high school baseball and softball players, Shanley and colleagues (2011) found that subjects with internal rotation deficits of greater than 25° in the dominant throwing arm were four or five times more likely to suffer an upper-quarter injury during the season. Baseball players were most likely to suffer from glenohumeral internal rotation deficit (GIRD), but both groups suffered shoulder and elbow injuries. However, shoulder and elbow injuries were most prevalent among the baseball players. Swimmers have also been found to have a high rate of shoulder injury. Wanivenhaus and colleagues (2012) reported a prevalence of shoulder injury among swimmers of between 40 and 90%, which they attributed primarily to fatigue of the rotator cuff, upper back, and pectoral musculature.

Rotator cuff fatigue results in less dynamic stabilization of the humeral head during the arc motion of swimming, which may also lead to microtrauma of the tissues, shoulder impingement, and thoracic outlet syndrome (Wanivenhaus et al. 2012). Shoulder girdle somatic dysfunction, whether driven by active or latent osteopathic lesions, impairs range of motion, strength, and scapulothoracic rhythm (Lucas, Polus, and Rich 2004). This may inhibit the rotator cuff's ability to stabilize the humeral head in the glenoid fossa, resulting in impingement of the supraspinatus tendon at the subacromial arch (Ebaugh, Spinelli, and Schmitz 2011).

The majority of research involving PRT has largely focused on reducing immediate pain; functional improvement has received limited attention. One test that shows promise for capturing functional upper-quarter closed-chain improvement among athletes and possibly injured workers is the Y Balance Test. Westrick and colleagues (2012) found it to be a reliable test of upper-quarter closed-kinetic-chain function in a healthy collegiate population. Additionally, the authors found no difference between dominant and nondominant limbs, which indicates that it may serve as a useful tool for assessing injury in the upper extremity (i.e., the noninjured limb can serve as the normal reference limb).

Given that the number of upper-quarter ambulatory surgeries in the United States increased from 380,000 in 1983 to 1 million in 2006 (Jain et al. 2014), more definitive assessment methods for upper-quarter injury risk are needed as well as functional performance measures. PRT may be an excellent intervention to not only decrease pain and improve range of motion and strength deficits, but also enhance functional performance, which for most athletes and workers is the most critical aspect of their lives.

TREATMENT
Common Anatomical Areas and Conditions for PRT

- Muscle strain
- Ligament sprain
- Osteoarthritis
- Thoracic outlet syndrome
- Disc pathology
- Radiculopathy

- Shoulder impingement
- Frozen shoulder
- Dislocation (postrelocation)
- Scapular dyskinesis
- Tendinosis

Trapezius: Upper Fibers

The trapezius is composed of three muscle groups: upper, middle, and lower. The flat superficial fibers of the three groups span from the base of the head to the bottom of the thoracic cage. The upper fibers travel from the occiput laterally to the clavicle; the middle fibers travel horizontally from the thoracic vertebrae to the scapula and acromion; and the lower fibers course upward laterally from the thoracic vertebrae to the spine of the scapulae. The trapezius fibers, particularly the upper fibers, are frequent sites of lesions because of their role as a force couple with other intrinsic muscles of the shoulder and cervical spine.

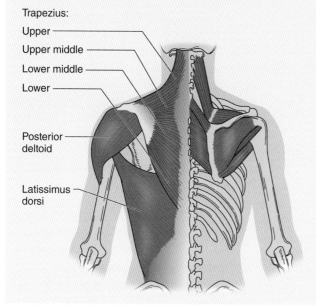

Trapezius:
Upper
Upper middle
Lower middle
Lower

Posterior deltoid

Latissimus dorsi

Origin: Occiput, medial third of the superior nuchal line

Insertion: Clavicle (posterior lateral third)

Action: Scapular stabilization and rotation, shoulder and scapular elevation (shoulder shrug), head rotation to the opposite side, capital extension, cervical extension, cervical lateral flexion

Innervation: Accessory (XI) nerve

Palpation Procedure

- Place the patient prone, and stand or sit facing the patient.
- Grasp the upper trapezius gently with your near hand, much like grasping a hamburger, to demarcate the upper trapezius fibers from the middle trapezius fibers, which course superficially over the superior scapulae.
- Palpate from the clavicular attachment site to the occiput.
- Stack your forefinger and middle finger and strum with firm pressure from a posterior to anterior direction using the clavicle as a base against which to apply pressure.
- Once the trapezius bends at the neckline, orient your fingers perpendicular to the cervical spine and decrease the palpation pressure while strumming the superficial fibers medial to lateral.
- Note the location of any tender points or fasciculatory response along the muscle and its attachments.
- Determine the most dominant tender point or fasciculation (or both) and maintain light pressure with the pad(s) of the finger(s) throughout the treatment until reassessment has occurred.

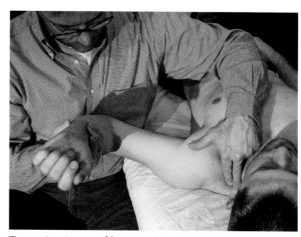

Trapezius (upper fibers) palpation procedure.

PRT Clinician Procedure

- The patient is supine, and you are either seated or standing.
- Move the head into lateral flexion toward the lesion; then apply capital lateral flexion and rotation toward the lesion.
- With your far hand, place the patient's elbow into the proximal sternum or abdomen.
- Then, with your far hand, grasp the anterior aspect of the flexed elbow, which at this time is typically at 90° of flexion.
- Move the patient's involved arm with your far hand into flexion. The position of comfort is typically found at approximately 90 to 120°.
- Once the flexion position is found by either eliciting the fasciculatory response or determining optimal tissue relaxation, move the arm through horizontal adduction and abduction with the far hand. Then apply humeral rotation with the far hand, typically marked external rotation.
- With your far hand at the patient's elbow, apply distraction and compression to facilitate optimal joint and tissue relaxation.
- With the thenar aspect of your near hand, apply a light inferior glide to the humerus.
- Corollary tissues treated: Sternocleidomastoid, splenius capitis, cervical spleni, levator scapulae, cervical multifidi, rotatores

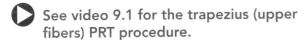 See video 9.1 for the trapezius (upper fibers) PRT procedure.

Patient Self-Treatment Procedure

- Lie supine. A sofa is an ideal place to perform this self-release.
- Use your opposite hand to monitor the tissue for the fasciculatory response and tissue positioning to fine-tune the treatment position.
- Place your head and neck in a laterally flexed position with your chin pointed toward the involved shoulder.
- Support the elbow at 90 to 120° of shoulder flexion with the elbow slightly flexed and the hand relaxed on the sofa or pillows. Also move the arm into slight external rotation. The elbow should be supported against the back of a sofa or bolstered in the treatment position with pillows.
- Maintain the treatment position until the fasciculatory response abates or for three to five minutes.

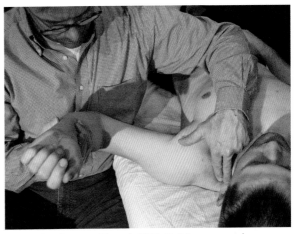

Trapezius (upper fibers) PRT clinician procedure.

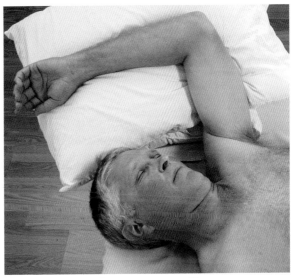

Trapezius (upper fibers) patient self-treatment procedure.

Subclavius

The subclavius is found where its name dictates, under the clavicle. It is a slender muscle running between the first rib and the clavicle, deep to the pectoralis major, which can make its palpation challenging. The subclavius serves the vital function of stabilizing the sternoclavicular joint and assisting respiration; therefore, lesions of this muscle are often present when scalene, sternocleidomastoid, and trapezius lesions are also present. Additionally, lesions of this tissue also frequently disturb the normal arthrokinematics of the sternoclavicular joint.

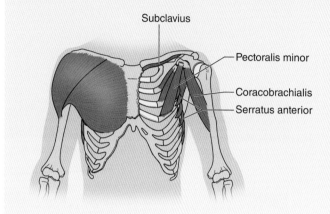

Origin: First rib and cartilage

Insertion: Clavicle (inferior third surface)

Action: Assists shoulder depression; stabilizes the sternoclavicular joint by moving the clavicle forward during shoulder motion; elevates the first rib during inhalation

Innervation: C5-C6 (subclavian nerve arising from the brachial plexus)

Palpation Procedure

- Place the patient in either a side-lying or supine position.
- With the elbow flexed, position the patient's involved arm in slight horizontal adduction.
- Using your thumb or fingers, curl them under the clavicle, strumming up and down the length of the clavicle.
- Note the location of any tender points or fasciculatory response along the muscle.
- Determine the most dominant tender point or fasciculation (or both) and maintain light pressure with the pad(s) of the finger(s) throughout the treatment until reassessment has occurred.

PRT Clinician Procedure

- Place the patient in a supine position.
- Grasp the patient's wrist with the far hand and pull the involved limb across the patient's body toward the patient's opposite hip.
- With the far hand, move the arm up and down the patient's opposite flank while keeping the limb extended. Typically, the treatment position is found just above the iliac crest of the opposite hip.
- Apply limb distraction with internal limb rotation with the far hand.
- Corollary tissues treated: Pectoralis minor and major
- Alternate position: If the patient can't tolerate limb distraction, place the patient in a side-lying position. Grasp the posterior shoulder and move

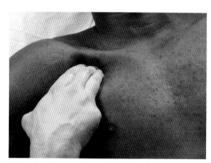

Subclavius palpation procedure.

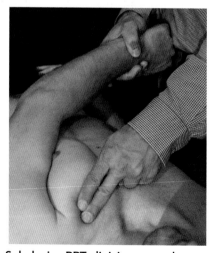

Subclavius PRT clinician procedure.

it into a protracted, adducted position with the far hand. Fine-tune with scapular depression or elevation and rotation with the far hand.

Anterior Acromioclavicular Joint

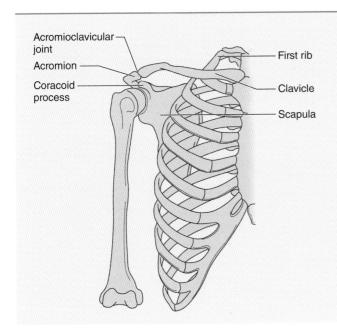

Acromioclavicular joint
Acromion
Coracoid process
First rib
Clavicle
Scapula

The articulation between the acromion of the scapula and the acromial end of the clavicle forms the acromioclavicular (AC) joint. The AC joint is often a site of irritation in the presence of rotator cuff weakness. Lesions at this joint can be found either at its anterior or posterior aspects.

Palpation Procedure

- Place the patient supine or in a seated position.
- Trace the clavicle to its lateral tip until you feel a small valley; this is the AC joint.
- Just lateral and posterior to the valley is the acromion. Explore the joint from anterior to posterior.
- Note the location of any tender points or fasciculatory response at the joint articulation.
- Once you have determined the most dominant tender point or fasciculation (or both), maintain light pressure with the pad(s) of the finger(s) at the location throughout the PRT treatment procedure until reassessment has occurred.

PRT Clinician Procedure

- The straight-arm PRT procedure used for the subclavius can be used to treat the anterior aspect of the AC joint, with one exception: the diagonal arm position across the body should be placed at the level of the anterior inferior iliac spine or lower.
- Corollary tissues treated: Subclavius, pectoralis minor and major

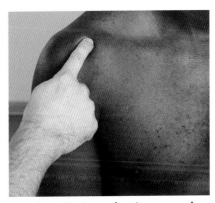

Anterior AC joint palpation procedure.

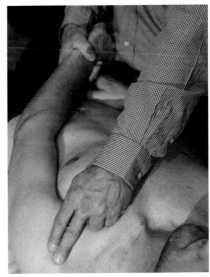

Anterior AC joint PRT clinician procedure.

Deltoid

The fibers of the deltoid are composed of three separate groups: the anterior, middle, and posterior. The broad triangular multipennate fibers of the deltoid cover most of the shoulder, working primary to abduct the arm. The deltoid also serves as a force couple to the intrinsic rotator cuff musculature.

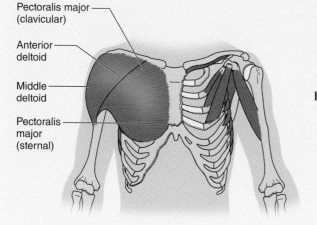

Pectoralis major (clavicular)

Anterior deltoid

Middle deltoid

Pectoralis major (sternal)

Origin: Anterior: Lateral third of the clavicle

Middle: Scapula (acromion, lateral superior surface)

Posterior: Scapula (lower posterior border of the scapular spine)

Insertion: Deltoid tuberosity

Action: Anterior fibers: Shoulder flexion, internal rotation, and horizontal adduction

Middle fibers (primarily): Shoulder abduction

Posterior fibers: Shoulder extension, external rotation, and horizontal abduction

Innervation: C5-C6 (axillary nerve)

Palpation Procedure

- Place the patient supine or in a seated position.
- Start at the anterior crease of the shoulder just below the clavicle.
- The anterior fibers of the deltoid are located just lateral to the tendon of the long head of the biceps.
- Using either your thumb or fingers, stroke perpendicularly across the anterior fibers until you feel a distinct separation at the most lateral aspect of the shoulder, where the middle fibers are found. Continue to move posteriorly across the middle fibers to the next valley, where the posterior fibers begin.
- Distinct, firm pressure is needed to demarcate the fiber groups.
- Explore the fibers from their proximal insertions to their common distal insertion at the deltoid tuberosity.
- Note the location of any tender points or fasciculatory response at the muscle and its sites of attachment.
- Once you have determined the most dominant tender point or fasciculation (or both), maintain light pressure with the pad(s) of the finger(s) at the location throughout the PRT treatment procedure until reassessment has occurred.

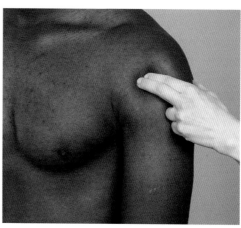

Deltoid palpation procedure.

PRT Clinician Procedure

- The patient is supine.
- Using your far hand, grasp the patient's elbow and move the patient's arm, with the elbow in a relaxed flexed position (approximately 90 to 100°).
- Then move the arm into horizontal adduction (middle fibers only) with the far hand.
- Apply humeral distraction or compression with your far hand; then a slight inferior humeral glide with your near hand.
- Apply humeral rotation with the far hand for fine-tuning.
- Corollary tissues treated: Pectoralis minor, coracobrachialis, long head of the biceps tendon, middle deltoid

Patient Self-Treatment Procedure

- Lie supine. A sofa is an ideal place to perform this self-release.
- Support the elbow at 90° of shoulder flexion with the elbow relaxed. The elbow should be supported against the back of a sofa or bolstered in the treatment position with pillows.
- Use the opposite hand to monitor the tissue for the fasciculatory response and tissue positioning once bolstered to fine-tune the treatment position.
- Maintain the treatment position until the fasciculatory response abates or for three to five minutes.

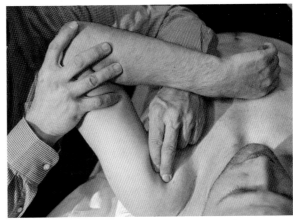

Deltoid (anterior and middle fibers) PRT clinician procedure.

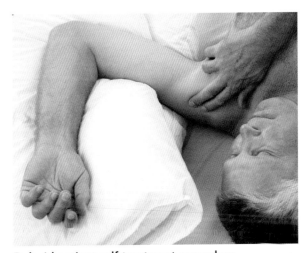

Deltoid patient self-treatment procedure.

Biceps Brachii Long Head Tendon

The biceps brachii is composed of two muscle bellies, the long and short heads. The tendon of the long head is more cylindrical than the tendon of the short head and can be easily located at the anterior crease of the shoulder. Lesions of the tendon of the long head of the biceps brachii are often present in conjunction with conditions of the shoulder such as impingement syndrome, rotator cuff weakness, and instability. Lesions at this tendon may be present when these shoulder conditions manifest because the tendon and muscle reverse their role from a secondary to primary shoulder stabilizer and mover, which may cause excessive eccentric load to the tendon–muscle complex.

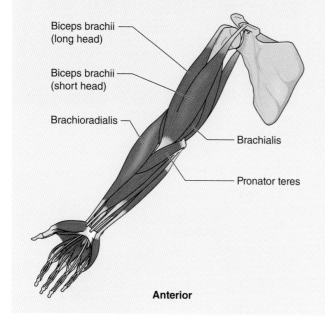

Biceps brachii (long head)

Biceps brachii (short head)

Brachioradialis

Brachialis

Pronator teres

Anterior

Origin: Supraglenoid tubercle, glenohumeral capsule

Insertion: Radial tuberosity, bicipital aponeurosis

Action: Elbow flexion and supination, stabilization and depression of the humeral head into the glenoid fossa with deltoid contraction

Innervation: C5-C6 (musculocutaneous nerve)

Palpation Procedure

- Place the patient supine with the elbow flexed and forearm supported.
- Place two fingers at the anterior crease of the shoulder, perpendicular to the tendon of the long head of the biceps. The long head of the biceps is located in the intertubercular groove of the humerus, just lateral to the anterior crease of the shoulder.
- Resistive elbow flexion with supination will make the tendon under palpation more prominent.
- Strum lightly over the long head of the tendon.
- Note the location of any tender points or fasciculatory response at the tendon.
- Once you have determined the most dominant tender point or fasciculation (or both), maintain light pressure with the pad(s) of the finger(s) at the location throughout the PRT treatment procedure until reassessment has occurred.

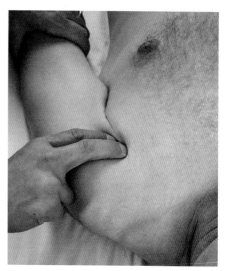

Biceps brachii (long head tendon) palpation procedure.

PRT Clinician Procedure

- Place the patient supine.
- Using your far hand, grasp the patient's elbow and move the arm through shoulder flexion to approximately 90 to 120°.
- Move the arm through horizontal adduction with the far hand.
- With your far hand, rotate the forearm into a supinated position.
- Apply humeral distraction and compression with your far hand.
- Corollary tissues treated: Biceps brachii, brachialis, anterior and middle deltoids

 See video 9.2 for the biceps brachii (long head tendon) PRT procedure.

Patient Self-Treatment Procedure

- Lie supine.
- Use the opposite hand to monitor the tissue for the fasciculatory response and tissue positioning once bolstered to fine-tune the treatment position.
- Place the dorsum of the hand on the involved side on the forehead with the elbow flexed and shoulder at approximately 90°.
- The elbow and shoulder should be either bolstered or placed against the back of a sofa or another immovable object.
- Maintain the treatment position until the fasciculatory response abates or for three to five minutes.

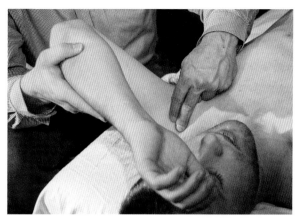

Biceps brachii (long head tendon) PRT clinician procedure.

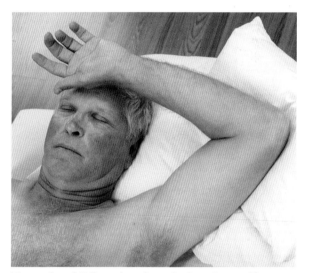

Biceps brachii (long head tendon) patient self-treatment procedure.

Biceps Brachii Short Head Tendon

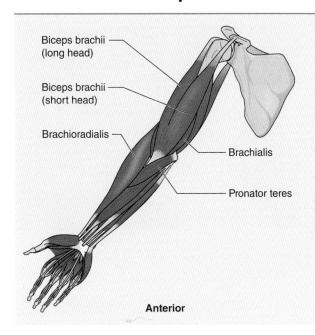

- Biceps brachii (long head)
- Biceps brachii (short head)
- Brachioradialis
- Brachialis
- Pronator teres

Anterior

The biceps brachii short head tendon originates from the apex of the coracoid process and traverses inferiorly next to the long head merging distally to form the bicipital aponeurosis. Unlike the long head of the biceps, the short head does not play a major role in the stabilization of the humeral head with deltoid contraction. Typically, the coracoid process is sensitive to palpation; therefore, light palpation of the tendon's origin is necessary to limit guarding from overpressure.

Origin: Coracoid process of the scapula

Insertion: Radial tuberosity, bicipital aponeurosis

Action: Elbow flexion and supination

Innervation: C5-C6 (musculocutaneous nerve)

Palpation Procedure

- Place the patient supine with the elbow flexed and forearm supported.
- Locate the clavicle and trace it over to the anterior crease of the shoulder. The coracoid process is just below the inferior margin of the clavicle, just medial to the anterior crease of the shoulder.
- Lightly apply a circular pressure to feel the coracoid process.
- Move distally off the coracoid process, orienting your fingers perpendicular to the short head tendon of the biceps brachii.
- Strum lightly over the short head tendon, which is medial to the long head tendon.
- Resistive elbow flexion with supination will make the tendon under palpation more prominent.
- Determine the most dominant tender point or fasciculation (or both) and maintain light pressure with the pad(s) of the finger(s) throughout the treatment until reassessment has occurred.

PRT Clinician Procedure

- Place the patient supine.
- With your far hand, grasp the patient's elbow, positioning it at 90°, then move the arm into approximately 90 to 100° of shoulder flexion.
- Using your far hand, move the arm into a 90/90 horizontal adduction position, then rotate the forearm into a supinated position.
- Apply humeral distraction and compression using your far hand or your torso if just applying compression.

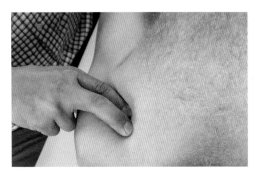

Biceps brachii (short head tendon) palpation procedure.

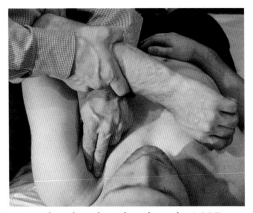

Biceps brachii (short head tendon) PRT clinician procedure.

- Apply humeral and forearm rotation for fine-tuning with the far hand.
- Corollary tissues treated: Biceps brachii, brachialis, anterior and middle deltoids

Subscapularis

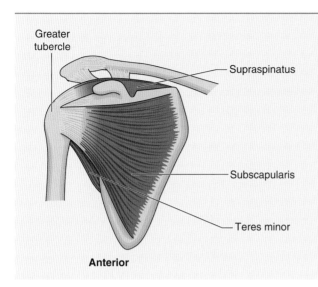

Greater tubercle
Supraspinatus
Subscapularis
Teres minor

Anterior

The subscapularis is the largest of the rotator cuff muscles, covering the anterior surface of the scapulae. It is also the only rotator cuff muscle to medially rotate the arm because of its insertion site at the lesser tubercle of the humerus.

Origin: Scapular fossa

Insertion: Lesser tubercle of the humerus, glenohumeral joint capsule

Action: Shoulder internal rotation, glenohumeral joint stabilization

Innervation: C5-C6 (upper and lower subscapular nerves)

Palpation Procedure

- Place the patient in a side-lying position.
- Flex the shoulder to approximately 70 to 90° and apply distraction anteriorly to pull the scapula off the chest wall.
- While holding the arm, use your thumb or fingers to explore the inferior lateral margin of the scapula. While attempting to locate the inferior lateral surface of the scapulae, move under the latissimus dorsi and teres major during palpation.
- Once your fingers or thumb are on the subscapular fossa, instruct the patient to internally rotate the arm to accentuate the subscapularis for palpation. Only the inferior margin of the subscapularis will be accessible to palpation.
- Alternately, the patient can be palpated supine. When palpating supine, the arm and elbow should be in a supported 90/90 flexed position; apply slight distraction at the elbow.
- Note the location of any tender points or fasciculatory response at the muscle.
- Once you have determined the most dominant tender point or fasciculation (or both), maintain light pressure with the pad(s) of the finger(s) at the location throughout the PRT treatment procedure until reassessment has occurred.

PRT Clinician Procedure

- Place the patient supine.
- With your far hand, grasp the arm above the elbow.
- Using your far hand, move the shoulder into approximately 30° of extension and abduction.

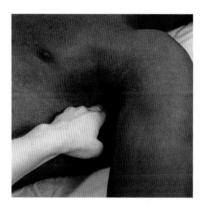

Subscapularis palpation procedure.

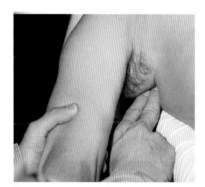

Subscapularis PRT clinician procedure.

- Apply humeral internal rotation with your far hand.
- Using your far hand, apply humeral distraction or compression.
- Corollary tissues treated: Latissimus dorsi, serratus anterior, teres major

Serratus Anterior

The majority of the serratus anterior is not accessible to palpation because of its coverage by the scapulae, latissimus dorsi, and pectoralis major. However, as its fibers extend anteriorly around the thorax, its axillary fibers are accessible to palpation. Traditionally in therapy, the serratus anterior is dubbed the punching muscle because it assists in the protraction of the scapula when reaching forward. It also stabilizes the scapula against the chest wall to prevent winging and works with the upper and lower trapezius in a force couple to facilitate upward scapular rotation.

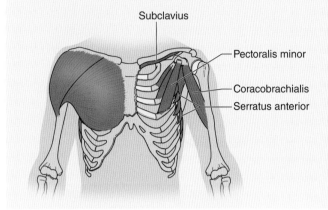

Subclavius
Pectoralis minor
Coracobrachialis
Serratus anterior

Origin: Ribs 1 through 8 (often 9 and 10 also)

Insertion: Scapula (ventral surface at vertebral border)

Action: Scapular abduction, upward rotation, and depression; stabilizes the scapulae against the thoracic wall

Innervation: C5-C7 (long thoracic nerve)

Palpation Procedure
- Place the patient supine or in a seated position.
- The axillary fibers of the serratus anterior are located between the margins of the pectoralis major and latissimus dorsi.
- Place your fingers within the axillary region on the rib cage, just underneath the lower margin of the pectoralis major.
- Orient your fingers perpendicular to the fibers of the serratus anterior or lay them across the ribs, pointing toward the head.
- The serratus anterior musculature has a soft speed-bump feel as you strum across their fibers.
- To accentuate palpation of the muscle, have the patient punch the arm toward the ceiling against your resistance while palpating.
- Note the location of any tender points or fasciculatory response at the muscle.
- Once you have determined the most dominant tender point or fasciculation (or both), maintain light pressure with the pad(s) of the finger(s) at the location throughout the PRT treatment procedure until reassessment has occurred.

PRT Clinician Procedure
- The patient is supine with the knees bolstered.
- While palpating the serratus anterior with the near hand, grasp the patient's wrist with your far hand and move the arm into approximately 20 degrees of shoulder flexion.

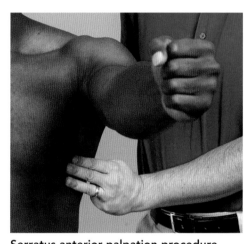

Serratus anterior palpation procedure.

- Using the far hand, move the arm through adduction and abduction. Typically, the treatment position of the arm is found either at the side of the patient's torso or in slight adduction over the ipsilateral anterior hip.
- With the far hand, apply marked distraction of the arm downwards towards to the ipsilateral hip.
- With the far hand, apply internal rotation to the arm.
- Fine-tune with application of wrist extension or flexion with the far hand.
- Corollary tissues treated: Teres major, latissimus dorsi, obliques, diaphragm, intercostals

 See video 9.3 for the serratus anterior PRT procedure.

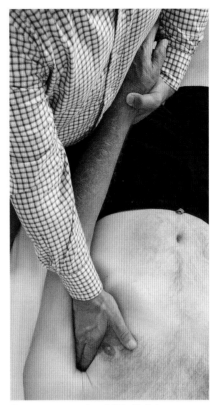

Serratus anterior PRT clinician procedure.

Pectoralis Minor

The pectoralis minor lies on the upper thorax underneath the pectoralis major. The fibers of the pectoralis minor are oriented perpendicular to those of the pectoralis major and course inferiorly from the coracoid process to their rib attachments to form the anterior wall of the axillary region. Because the neurovascular bundle of the neck and shoulder pass under the pectoralis minor, lesions of the pectoralis minor can result in neurovascular compression, which may facilitate the development of thoracic outlet syndrome.

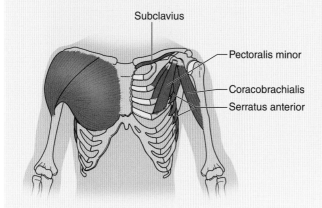

Origin:	Ribs 3 through 5
Insertion:	Coracoid process of the scapulae (medial and superior surface)
Action:	Scapular protraction and abduction, rib elevation during forced inspiration (when scapula is fixed), scapular depression
Innervation:	C5-T1 (medial and lateral pectoral nerves)

Palpation Procedure

- Position the patient supine.
- The pectoralis minor can be palpated indirectly through application of deep palpation across its fibers, but over and through the anterior aspect of the pectoralis major. This palpation procedure is less painful than accessing the pectoralis minor under the pectoralis major which is also detailed below.
- To palpate the pectoralis minor directly, abduct the arm to expose the axillary region.
- Gently slide your fingers under the lateral border of the pectoralis minor and onto the anterior chest wall.
- While palpating inward, you will feel the lateral border of the pectoralis minor. Move your fingers inward and down in a strumming fashion to feel the fibers of the pectoralis minor. Be careful to use gentle pressure when utilizing this palpation method because it is often very painful.
- To accentuate palpation of the muscle, ask the patient to depress the shoulder during palpation.
- Patients with a large amount of breast tissue can be positioned in a side-lying position to move the tissue and the pectoralis major off the anterior chest wall. The palpation procedure in this position is the same as described earlier.
- Note the location of any tender points or fasciculatory response at the muscle.

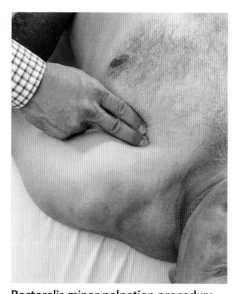

Pectoralis minor palpation procedure.

- Once you have determined the most dominant tender point or fasciculation (or both), maintain light pressure with the pad(s) of the finger(s) at the location throughout the PRT treatment procedure until reassessment has occurred.

PRT Clinician Procedure

- The treatment is similar to that used for the subclavius, with the exception of often applying a greater amount of humeral distraction and internal rotation.
- Place the patient in a supine position.
- Grasp the patient's wrist with the far hand and pull the involved limb across the body toward the opposite hip.
- With the far hand, move the arm up and down the patient's opposite flank while keeping the limb extended.
- Apply significant limb distraction with marked internal limb rotation with the far hand.
- Alternate position:
  - Place patients who can't tolerate limb distraction in a side-lying position.
  - With the far hand, grasp the posterior shoulder and move it into a protracted, adducted position.
  - Using the far hand, fine-tune with scapular depression or elevation and rotation.
- Corollary tissues treated: Pectoralis major, subclavius, AC joint

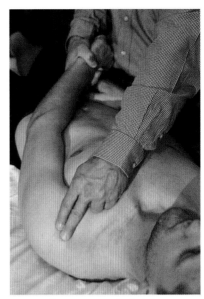

Pectoralis minor PRT clinician procedure.

Pectoralis Major

The fibers of the pectoralis major are separated into two major divisions: the clavicular (upper) portion and the sternocostal (middle and lower) portion. The two divisions form part of the anterior axillary wall. Fibers from both divisions converge into a common tendon to insert on the humerus.

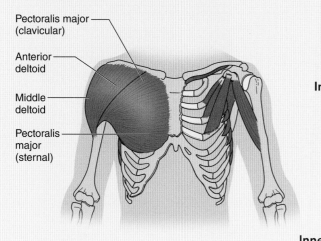

Pectoralis major (clavicular)

Anterior deltoid

Middle deltoid

Pectoralis major (sternal)

Origin: Clavicular fibers: Clavicle (sternal half)

Sternocostal fibers: Sternum (anterior surface), ribs 1 through 6, 2 through 6 rib cartilage, aponeurosis of obliquus externus abdominis

Insertion: Greater tubercle of the humerus

Action: All fibers: Shoulder adduction, internal rotation, horizontal adduction; thorax elevation during forced inspiration (with both extremities fixed)

Clavicular fibers: Shoulder internal rotation, flexion

Sternocostal fibers: Shoulder extension

Innervation: Clavicular fibers: C5-C7 (lateral pectoral nerve)

Sternocostal fibers: C6-T1 (medial and lateral pectoral nerves)

Palpation Procedure

When palpating the pectoralis major of women, it is advisable to palpate around the breast tissue, not directly through it. Because many women feel uncomfortable with palpation in this area, explain why palpation in this area is needed and how it will be done before proceeding. Most important, gain consent from the patient before performing the palpation procedure. The two methods for moving the breast tissue away from the chest wall to gain access to the pectoralis major and other chest wall muscles are to (1) place the patient in a side-lying position, which will facilitate the breast tissue to fall away from the chest wall, or (2) have the patient manually move the breast tissue medially.

In the side-lying position:

- Support the arm at the elbow while slightly flexing the shoulder upward.
- Apply slight distraction to the shoulder at the elbow.
- The pectoralis major can be grasped with the thumb underneath its inferior border while the fingers above are in position to strum across the clavicular and sternocostal fibers.
- During palpation, passively flex and extend the shoulder to accentuate the upper and lower fibers.

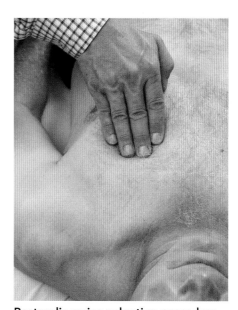

Pectoralis major palpation procedure.

In a supine position:

- Slightly abduct the shoulder.
- Locate the inferior medial clavicle and lateral surface of the sternum. From this location, drop your fingers off the bony structures and onto the clavicular fibers.
- Orient your fingers perpendicular to the fibers and strum across them toward their common tendon at the coracoid process.
- Continue to explore the middle and inferior sternocostal fibers in the same way you explored the clavicular fibers.
- Ask the patient to internally rotate the shoulder to accentuate palpation of the muscle fibers.

For both positions:

- Note the location of any tender points or fasciculatory response at the muscle.
- Once you have determined the most dominant tender point or fasciculation (or both), maintain light pressure with the pad(s) of the finger(s) at the location throughout the PRT treatment procedure until reassessment has occurred.

PRT Clinician Procedure

- Place the patient supine.
- Using the far hand, grasp the patient's wrist with your dominant hand.
- For the clavicular fibers, pull the arm across the chest above the nipple line.
- For the sternal fibers, pull the arm diagonally across the chest at or below the nipple line.
- With your far hand, apply humeral distraction and internal rotation.
- Corollary tissues treated: AC joint, pectoralis minor, sternalis, sternocostal joint, serratus anterior

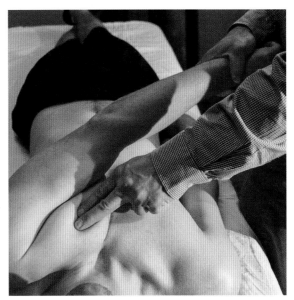

Pectoralis major PRT clinician procedure.

Supraspinatus

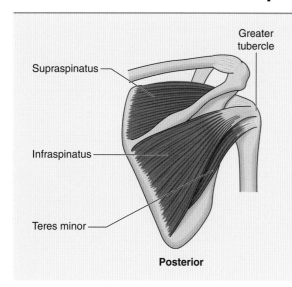

Posterior

Greater tubercle
Supraspinatus
Infraspinatus
Teres minor

The supraspinatus is one of the four rotator cuff muscles, which form the acronym SITS (supraspinatus, infraspinatus, teres minor, subscapularis). The muscle occupies the entire supraspinous fossa, traversing under the acromion as a tendon to insert on the greater tubercle of the humerus. A common method to place more emphasis on the supraspinatus during muscle testing is to use the empty can orthopedic special test.

Origin:	Supraspinous fossa of the scapula
Insertion:	Humerus (greater tubercle)
Action:	Shoulder abduction, shoulder external rotation, humeral head stabilization in the glenoid fossa
Innervation:	C5-C6 (suprascapular nerve)

Palpation Procedure

- To promote relaxation of the shoulder girdle, palpate while the patient is in a supine position, but you can also perform the palpation with the patient seated if necessary.
- Locate the spine of the scapula, then, using one or two fingers, strum the fibers of the supraspinatus either against or away from it, demarcating the fibers of the supraspinatus that run parallel to the scapular plane.
- Follow the belly of the supraspinatus as it courses under the acromion. When the tendinous aspect is reached, strum over the fibrous tendon.
- To accentuate this muscle, instruct the patient to abduct or externally rotate the humerus (or do both) during palpation.
- Note the location of any tender points or fasciculatory response at the muscle, the tendon, or the supraspinatus attachment at the humeral head.
- Determine the most dominant tender point or fasciculation (or both) and maintain light pressure with the pad(s) of the finger(s) throughout the treatment until reassessment has occurred.

PRT Clinician Procedure

- Place the patient supine and, with your far hand, move the shoulder into flexion and abduction while supporting the elbow with your far hand or torso.
- The supraspinatus is typically most relaxed at 120° of abduction, with a greater amount of horizontal adduction positioning needed than the infraspinatus PRT procedure.

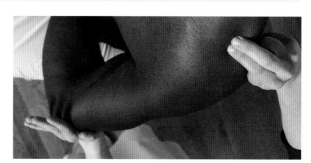

Supraspinatus palpation procedure.

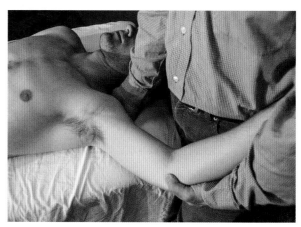

Supraspinatus PRT clinician procedure.

- With your far hand, apply external rotation.
- Apply humeral distraction or compression with your far hand or torso to promote relaxation.
- If possible, use the thenar aspect of your near hand to apply an inferior glide to the humerus to facilitate further relaxation.
- Corollary tissues treated: Infraspinatus, upper trapezius, middle deltoid, teres minor

Infraspinatus

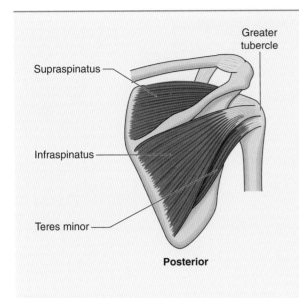

Supraspinatus

Greater tubercle

Infraspinatus

Teres minor

Posterior

The infraspinatus, the *I* in the SITS acronym for the rotator cuff group, also assists the other rotator cuff muscles to stabilize the humeral head in the glenoid fossa, particularly during overhead movements. The infraspinatus is composed of three distinct muscle bellies that can be palpated individually. The infraspinatus occupies most of the infraspinous scapular fossa, but its tendon, unlike that of the supraspinatus, does not traverse under the acromion. Rather, it crosses over the lateral border of the scapular spine to attach to the humerus. Lesions of the infraspinatus are common when rotator cuff weakness or impingement is present.

Origin: Scapula (infraspinous fossa)

Insertion: Humerus (greater tubercle)

Action: Shoulder external rotation, humeral head stabilization in the glenoid fossa

Innervation: C5-C6 (suprascapular nerve)

Palpation Procedure

- Place the patient prone or supine.
- Locate the spine of the scapula.
- Using one or two fingers, strum the upper fibers of the infraspinatus upwards against the spine of the scapula and for the middle and inferior fibers, pin and strum them against the scapula. With the patient supine, gravity and the weight of the thorax can be used to facilitate palpation of the infraspinatus against the scapula.
- Follow the belly of the infraspinatus as it courses over the lateral border of the scapula.
- To accentuate this muscle, instruct the patient to externally rotate the humerus during palpation.
- Note the location of any tender points or fasciculatory response at the muscle, the tendon, or its attachments.
- Once you have determined the most dominant tender point or fasciculation (or both), maintain light pressure with the pad(s) of the finger(s) at the location throughout the PRT treatment procedure until reassessment has occurred.

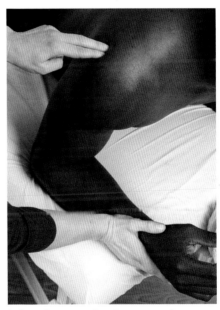

Infraspinatus palpation procedure.

> continued

Infraspinatus > *continued*

PRT Clinician Procedure

- Place the patient supine.
- With your far hand, move the shoulder into flexion and abduction while supporting the elbow with your far hand or torso.
- Typically, the infraspinatus requires minimal horizontal adduction positioning, unlike the supraspinatus.
- The infraspinatus is typically most relaxed at 100 to 120°.
- With your far hand, apply external rotation.
- Apply humeral distraction or compression with your far hand or torso to promote relaxation.
- If possible, use the thenar aspect of your near hand to apply an inferior glide to the humerus to facilitate further relaxation.
- Corollary tissues treated: Supraspinatus, upper trapezius, middle deltoid, teres minor

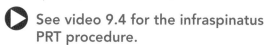 See video 9.4 for the infraspinatus PRT procedure.

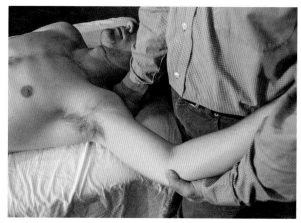

Infraspinatus PRT clinician procedure.

Teres Minor

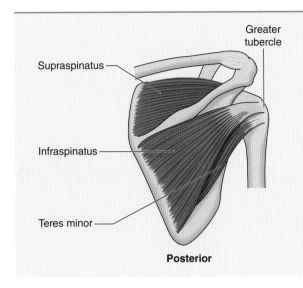

Greater tubercle

Supraspinatus

Infraspinatus

Teres minor

Posterior

The last of the three rotator cuff muscles to produce external shoulder rotation, the teres minor lies directly medial to its cousin, the teres major, and inferior to the infraspinatus. This small cylindrical muscle is located along the upper lateral edge of the scapula.

Origin: Scapula (proximal two thirds of the dorsal axillary border)

Insertion: Humerus (greater tubercle)

Action: Shoulder external rotation, humeral head stabilization in the glenoid fossa, shoulder adduction (weak)

Innervation: C5-C6 (axillary nerve)

Palpation Procedure

- Place the patient prone or supine.
- Locate the lateral axillary border of the scapula.
- Strum across the upper lateral axillary border of the scapula to locate the muscle belly of the teres minor, which can be grasped between the fingers at the axilla much like a hamburger.
- During palpation, instruct the patient to externally and internally rotate the arm to help you differentiate between the teres minor and teres major. The teres minor will contract with external rotation but not internal rotation.
- Note the location of any tender points or fasciculatory response at the muscle, tendon, or its attachments.
- Once you have determined the most dominant tender point or fasciculation (or both), maintain light pressure with the pad(s) of the finger(s) at the location throughout the PRT treatment procedure until reassessment has occurred.

PRT Clinician Procedure

- The patient can be treated in either a supine or a prone position.
- With your far hand, support the shoulder at the forearm and elbow. The elbow can also be supported on your knee.
- With your far hand, move the shoulder into approximately 20 to 30° of extension.
- Apply marked external rotation with your far hand.
- Apply humeral compression or distraction with your far hand to create further relaxation.
- Corollary tissues treated: Infraspinatus, supraspinatus, subscapularis, posterior deltoid

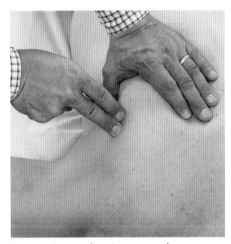

Teres minor palpation procedure.

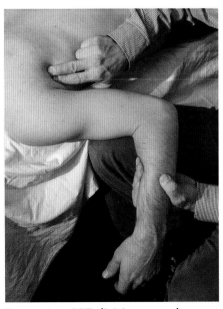

Teres minor PRT clinician procedure.

Teres Major

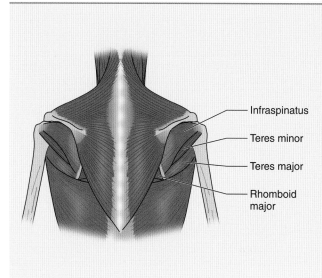

Infraspinatus

Teres minor

Teres major

Rhomboid major

Even though the teres major and teres minor share a name, the teres major is not considered a rotator cuff muscle. The teres major rotates the arm internally, whereas the teres minor rotates the arm externally. The teres major is oriented along the lateral border of the scapula, and its tendon lies behind the latissimus dorsi (the tendons of both converge for a brief period). Because of its anatomical relationship and similar muscle action, the teres major functions as a synergist with the latissimus dorsi.

Origin: Scapula (dorsal surface)

Insertion: Humerus (lesser tubercle)

Action: Shoulder internal rotation, adduction, and extension

Innervation: C5-C6 (lower subscapular nerve)

Palpation Procedure

- Place the patient prone or supine.
- Locate the lateral border of the scapula.
- Grasp the lateral border of the scapula with your thumbs and fingers much like you would a hamburger, and strum the teres major against the dorsal lateral surface of the scapula.
- Follow the fibers proximally as they converge with the latissimus dorsi at the axillary region.
- To accentuate the palpation of this muscle, have the patient internally rotate the arm.
- Note the location of any tender points or fasciculatory response at the muscle, tendon, or its attachments.
- Once you have determined the most dominant tender point or fasciculation (or both), maintain light pressure with the pad(s) of the finger(s) at the location throughout the PRT treatment procedure until reassessment has occurred.

PRT Clinician Procedure

- The patient can be treated in either a supine or a prone position.
- With your far hand, support the shoulder at the forearm and elbow. The elbow can also be supported on your knee.
- With your far hand, move the shoulder into approximately 20 to 30° of extension.
- Apply marked internal rotation with your far hand.
- Apply humeral compression or distraction with your far hand to promote further relaxation.
- Corollary tissues treated: Latissimus dorsi, subscapularis, posterior deltoid

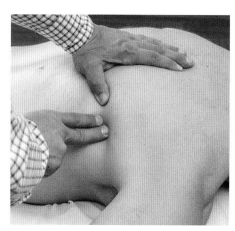

Teres major palpation procedure.

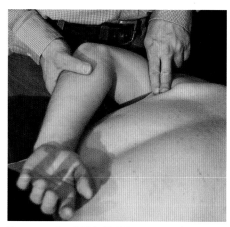

Teres major PRT clinician procedure.

Latissimus Dorsi

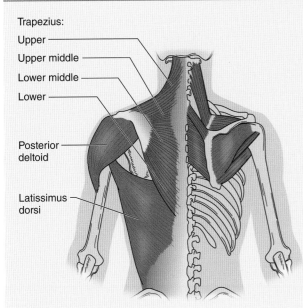

Trapezius:
Upper
Upper middle
Lower middle
Lower

Posterior deltoid

Latissimus dorsi

The superficial and thin fibers of the latissimus dorsi, one of the broadest muscles in the body, ascend from the low back to cover the posterior thorax to the axilla. The winglike appearance of the back formed during a bodybuilding pose is produced from the contraction of the latissimus dorsi. The superior fibers are almost horizontal, but as they pass over the scapulae, they move into a more vertical orientation distally.

Origin: T6-T12 spinous processes, L1-L5 spinous processes via the thoraco-lumbar fascia, ribs 9 through 12, posterior third of the ilium, supraspinous ligament

Insertion: Humerus (intertubercular groove)

Action: Shoulder extension, adduction, and internal rotation; spine hyperextension; pelvis elevation with arms fixed

Innervation: C6-C8 (thoracodorsal nerve)

Palpation Procedure

- Place the patient prone.
- Locate the lateral border of the scapula.
- Grasp the fibers of the latissimus dorsi and teres major at the lateral border of the scapula and roll them between the fingers to feel the demarcation between them. The most lateral fibers are those of the latissimus dorsi. Trace the fibers superiorly and inferiorly.
- To accentuate the muscle, ask the patient to extend the arm toward the feet against resistance.
- Note the location of any tender points or fasciculatory response at the muscle, tendon, or its attachments.
- Once you have determined the most dominant tender point or fasciculation (or both), maintain light pressure with the pad(s) of the finger(s) at the location throughout the PRT treatment procedure until reassessment has occurred.

PRT Clinician Procedure

- The patient can be either prone or supine.
- With your far hand, place the arm in approximately 30° of extension.
- Adduct and abduct the arm with your far hand until you feel the fasciculatory response or maximal relaxation, or both.
- Using your far hand, apply humeral internal rotation.
- Apply humeral distraction or compression by grasping above the wrist with the far hand.

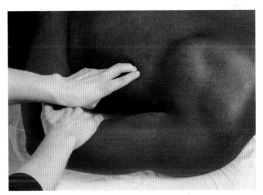

Latissimus dorsi palpation procedure.

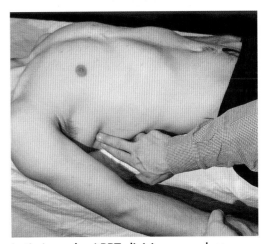

Latissimus dorsi PRT clinician procedure.

- Corollary tissues treated: Teres major, lower trapezius

223

Posterior Acromioclavicular Joint

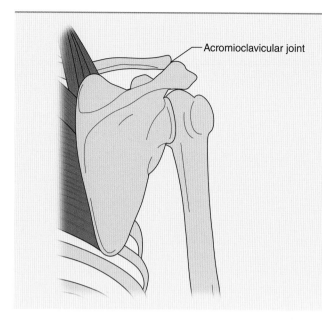

Acromioclavicular joint

The articulation between the posterior aspect of the acromion of the scapula and the acromial end of the clavicle forms the posterior acromioclavicular (AC) joint. The posterior AC joint is often a site of irritation in the presence of rotator cuff tear and weakness. Lesions at this joint can be found at either its anterior or posterior aspects.

Palpation Procedure

- Place the patient prone.
- Trace the clavicle to its lateral tip until you feel a small valley, which is the AC joint.
- Just lateral and posterior to the valley is the acromion. Explore the joint from its anterior to its posterior joint line.
- Note the location of any tender points or fasciculatory response at the joint articulation.
- Once you have determined the most dominant tender point or fasciculation (or both), maintain light pressure with the pad(s) of the finger(s) at the location throughout the PRT treatment procedure until reassessment has occurred.

PRT Clinician Procedure

- Place the patient prone.
- Stand on the side opposite the side of the shoulder to be treated.
- Using your far hand, move the arm into extension and adduction while applying humeral distraction across the body to the patient's opposite hip.
- Apply internal humeral rotation with your far hand above the patient's wrist.
- Corollary tissues treated: Inferior trapezius, serratus posterior, rhomboids

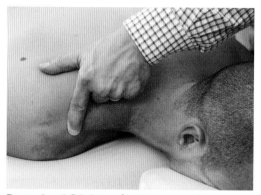

Posterior AC joint palpation procedure.

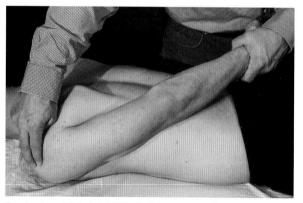

Posterior AC joint PRT clinician procedure.

Trapezius: Lower Fibers

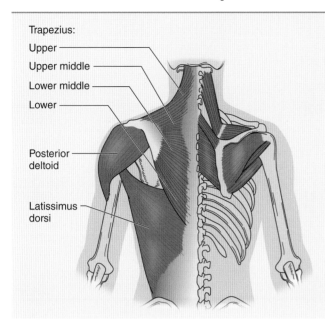

Trapezius:
Upper
Upper middle
Lower middle
Lower

Posterior deltoid

Latissimus dorsi

The trapezius is composed of three muscle groups, upper, middle, and lower. The lower fibers course upward laterally from the thoracic vertebrae to the spine of the scapula. The lower fibers work in concert with the upper fibers to produce scapular depression.

Origin:	T6-T12 spinous processes, supra-spinous ligaments
Insertion:	Scapular spine
Action:	Scapular adduction, depression, and upward rotation
Innervation:	C3-C4 (cervical plexus) with contribution from the accessory (XI) nerve

Palpation Procedure

- Place the patient prone.
- Locate the lower border of the scapular spine and the T12 spinous process. The lower fibers of the trapezius course between these two locations.
- Because the lower fibers of the trapezius are superficial and thin, ask the patient to raise the arms in a superman position to bring out their density under palpation.
- Strum lightly across the lower fibers with the palpation fibers oriented toward the opposite scapula.
- Note the location of any tender points or fasciculatory response at the muscle and its attachments.
- Once you have determined the most dominant tender point or fasciculation (or both), maintain light pressure with the pad(s) of the finger(s) at the location throughout the PRT treatment procedure until reassessment has occurred.

PRT Clinician Procedure

- Place the patient in a prone position with the head and neck in slight extension, if possible.
- Stand on the opposite side to be treated.
- Use the posterior AC joint PRT clinician procedure, but apply marked humeral distraction with the far hand.
- Alternatively, grasp the shoulder with your far hand and apply shoulder depression, retraction, and medial rotation.

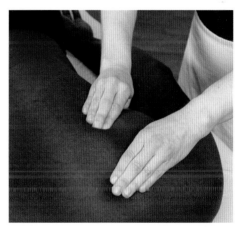

Trapezius (lower fibers) palpation procedure.

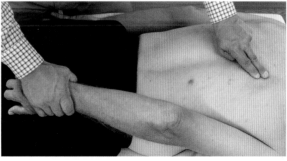

Trapezius (lower fibers) PRT clinician procedure.

- Corollary tissues treated: Posterior AC joint, latissimus dorsi, serratus posterior, thoracic erector spinae, rhomboid major

Rhomboid Minor

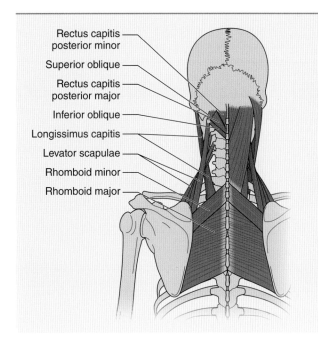

Rectus capitis posterior minor
Superior oblique
Rectus capitis posterior major
Inferior oblique
Longissimus capitis
Levator scapulae
Rhomboid minor
Rhomboid major

The rhomboid minor is located just above its neighbor, the rhomboid major. The rhomboid minor courses the medial border of the scapula in line with the scapular spine to the spinous processes of C7-T1. The minor and major both lie deep to the trapezius, but are superficial to the thoracic erector spinae; therefore, firm palpation is needed to demarcate their fibers. Lesions of these tissues are present in most people with poor postural control (e.g., rounded shoulders) or with conditions of the shoulder.

Origin: C7-T1 spinous processes, lower ligamentum nuchae

Insertion: Scapula (root of the spine on the medial or vertebral border)

Action: Scapular adduction, downward rotation, and elevation

Innervation: C5 (dorsal scapular nerve)

Palpation Procedure

- Place the patient prone.
- Locate the spine of the scapula and trace over to its vertebral border. The fibers of the rhomboid minor insert on the scapula at this location.
- Stack your forefinger and middle finger and strum across the fibers of the rhomboid minor with the tips of your fingers oriented toward the shoulder of the same side.
- Note the location of any tender points or fasciculatory response at the muscle and its attachments.
- Once you have determined the most dominant tender point or fasciculation (or both), maintain light pressure with the pad(s) of the finger(s) at the location throughout the PRT treatment procedure until reassessment has occurred.

PRT Clinician Procedure

- Place the patient prone.
- Stand on the opposite side of the shoulder to be treated.
- With your far hand, grasp the cap of the shoulder and depress the shoulder down toward the opposite hip while applying scapular adduction.
- Apply scapular rotation (clockwise) with your far hand.
- Tip the vertebral border of the scapula down toward the rib cage with either your far thumb or your far hand or forearm.

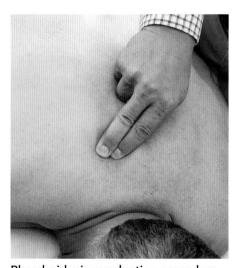

Rhomboid minor palpation procedure.

- With the palm of your near palpation hand, translate the fascia and muscular tissues up toward the rhomboid minor in line with the orientation of its fibers. The palm should be placed on the opposite side of the vertebral column, if possible.
- Corollary tissues treated: Rhomboid major, trapezius (upper and middle fibers), infraspinatus, supraspinatus

 See video 9.5 for the rhomboid minor PRT procedure.

Patient Self-Treatment Procedure

- Lie prone.
- Place a pillow under the anterior aspect of the shoulder to encourage scapular retraction or adduction.
- Place the shoulder in a slightly depressed position with the palm facing up.
- This self-treatment procedure can also be used for the rhomboid major.
- Maintain the treatment position until the fasciculatory response abates or for three to five minutes.

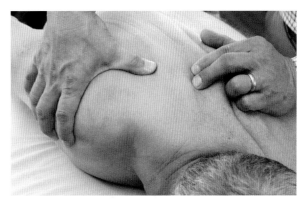

Rhomboid minor PRT clinician procedure.

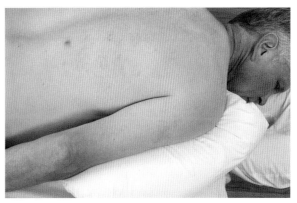

Rhomboid minor self-treatment procedure.

Rhomboid Major

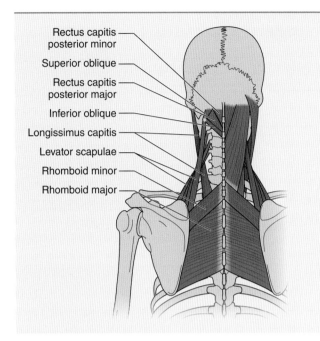

Rectus capitis posterior minor
Superior oblique
Rectus capitis posterior major
Inferior oblique
Longissimus capitis
Levator scapulae
Rhomboid minor
Rhomboid major

The rhomboid major and rhomboid minor perform similar actions at the shoulder. However, because of the major's fiber orientation and size, it produces more powerful scapular adduction. Lesions of the rhomboid major are prevalent in the majority of the population because of the postural demand on these fibers, but they are most prevalent in those who exhibit shoulder girdle weakness.

Origin: T2-T5 spinous process, supraspinous ligament

Insertion: Scapula (between the scapular root and the inferior scapular angle)

Action: Scapular adduction, downward rotation, and elevation

Innervation: C5 (dorsal scapular nerve)

Palpation Procedure

- Place the patient prone.
- Locate the spine of the scapula and trace over to its vertebral border. The upper fibers of the rhomboid major insert on the scapula at this location; the lower fibers, at the inferior angle.
- Stack your forefinger and middle finger and strum across the fibers of the rhomboid major with the tips of your fingers oriented vertically toward the head.
- Note the location of any tender points or fasciculatory response at the muscle and its attachments.
- Once you have determined the most dominant tender point or fasciculation (or both), maintain light pressure with the pad(s) of the finger(s) at the location throughout the PRT treatment procedure until reassessment has occurred.

PRT Clinician Procedure

- Place the patient prone.
- Stand on the opposite side of the shoulder to be treated.
- With your far hand, grasp the middle of the upper arm pinning it against the side of the thorax.

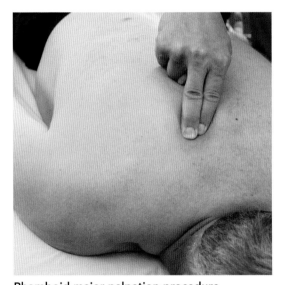

Rhomboid major palpation procedure.

- Pull the arm toward you with your far hand. Keeping the arm in contact with the thorax will retract the scapula and rotate the thorax toward the spine.
- Tip the vertebral border of the scapula down toward the rib cage with either your far thumb or your far hand or forearm.
- With the palm of your near palpation hand, translate the fascia and muscular tissues horizontally toward the rhomboid major in line with the orientation of its fibers. The palm should be on the opposite side of the vertebral column, if possible.
- Corollary tissues treated: Rhomboid minor, trapezius (middle fibers), serratus anterior, thoracic erector spinae

Patient Self-Treatment Procedure

See the rhomboid minor self-treatment procedure.

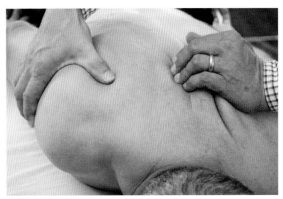

Rhomboid major PRT clinician procedure.

Levator Scapulae

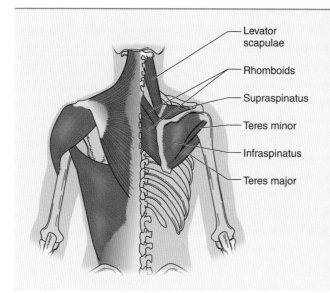

- Levator scapulae
- Rhomboids
- Supraspinatus
- Teres minor
- Infraspinatus
- Teres major

The levator scapulae extends from the superior angle of the scapula to the transverse processes of C1-C4. Its fibers are deep to the trapezius, but reveal themselves for palpation at the lateral neck, bracketed between the splenius capitis and posterior scalene. The inferior fibers, which arise from the superior angle of the scapula, can be palpated indirectly through the trapezius fibers.

Origin: C1-C4 transverse processes

Insertion: Superior angle of the scapula

Action: Scapular elevation, abduction, and downward rotation; cervical extension; lateral flexion and rotation to the same side

Innervation: C3-C4 (ventral rami); C5 (dorsal scapular nerve)

Palpation Procedure

- The patient should be prone or in a seated position.
- Locate the vertebral border of the scapula and trace it upward to the superior angle or tip of the scapula.
- Stack your forefinger and middle fingers and orient them toward the middle of the upper trapezius.
- To access the inferior fibers of the levator scapulae at the scapula, apply firm downward pressure over and through the middle trapezius fibers and strum across the fibers to feel their density.
- Note the location of any tender points or fasciculatory response along the muscle and its scapular attachment.
- Once you have determined the most dominant tender point or fasciculation (or both), maintain light pressure with the pad(s) of the finger(s) at the location throughout the PRT treatment procedure until reassessment has occurred.

PRT Clinician Procedure

- Place the patient prone.
- With your far hand, move the arm through abduction while palpating the inferior fibers of the levator scapula through the overlying trapezius fibers with the near hand. Once the most relaxed position or fasciculatory response is felt, stabilize the arm against the edge of the treatment table with your leg.
- Place the thenar aspect of your far hand at the lower lateral border of the scapula with your fingers oriented over the superior scapular angle.

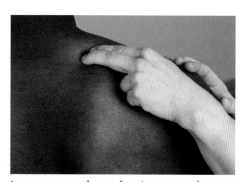

Levator scapulae palpation procedure.

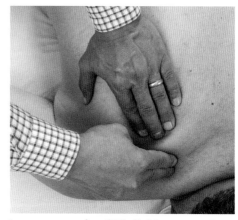

Levator scapulae PRT clinician procedure.

- With your far hand, translate the scapula upward; then apply rotation with your dominant hand.
- Tilt the superior angle of the scapula downward with the fingers of your far hand.
- Corollary tissues treated: Trapezius (upper fibers), rhomboid minor

Shoulder Impingement Syndrome

Shoulder impingement syndrome, also known as subacromial impingement syndrome, results from the impingement of tissues between the humeral head and the acromial arch, resulting in narrowing of the subacromial space (Koester, George, and Kuhn 2005). Shoulder impingement can encompass a myriad of pathologies including rotator cuff tear, calcific tendinitis, long head of the biceps tendinopathy, cervical radiculopathy, and subacromial bursitis (Koester et al. 2005; Umer et al. 2012). A thorough examination is therefore critical to determine the severity and origin of the patient's shoulder pain.

Shoulder pain typically develops gradually over a period of weeks or months and manifests at the anterolateral acromion, often radiating to the lateral mid-humerus (Koester et al. 2005). Clinically, osteopathic lesions and subsequent pain and spasm at the upper trapezius, serratus anterior, infraspinatus, and middle deltoid and its tendinous insertion are typically present, possibly as a result of subacromial pain, but also potentially from fatigue of the deltoid musculature caused by rotator cuff insufficiency. Rotator cuff pathology is often present within the shoulder (Umer et al. 2012) either from trauma, overuse, and degeneration of the rotator cuff tendon (i.e., intrinsic impingement) or from an extrinsic mechanism such as degeneration of the tendon from repetitive mechanical compression by structures external to the tendon, such as a bone spur (Umer et al. 2012). Regardless of the mechanism or underlying pathologies, the subacromial space is inflamed and frequently decreased, resulting in a disturbance of the shoulder's normal arthrokinematics (Ellenbecker and Cools 2010). Therefore, a multifactorial therapy approach should be pursued.

Ellenbecker and Cools (2010) stated that before successful rehabilitation can occur, muscle balance must be normalized. PRT may prove helpful in restoring the normal arthrokinematics of the shoulder by restoring muscular balance through the release of osteopathic lesions. However, to date, there are no well-designed trials or systematic studies demonstrating that conservative or manual therapy is more effective than surgery (Ellenbecker and Cools 2010; Umer et al. 2012), and none have examined the use of PRT for treating shoulder impingement.

Treatment Points and Sequencing

1. Anterior acromioclavicular (AC) joint
2. Deltoid (middle)
3. Serratus anterior
4. Infraspinatus
5. Upper trapezius
6. Teres minor
7. Teres major
8. Levator scapulae at the neck
9. Levator scapulae at the shoulder
10. Rhomboids

Common Signs and Symptoms

- Anterolateral acromial pain and tenderness
- Lateral mid-deltoid pain and tenderness
- Pain with overhead movements
- Pain when lying on the involved shoulder, typically at night
- Pain with ADL movements (activities of daily living such as brushing teeth and combing hair)
- Altered scapular and glenohumeral kinematics
- General loss of shoulder strength
- Weak or dysfunctional scapulothoracic musculature
- Positive Hawkins-Kennedy test and Neer's sign

Common Differential Diagnoses

- Rotator cuff tear
- Rotator cuff tendinopathy
- Long head of the biceps tendon tear
- Long head of the biceps tendinopathy
- Adhesive capsulitis
- Cervical radiculopathy
- Osteoarthritis
- Subacromial bursitis
- Subacromial osteophyte
- Infection

Clinician Therapeutic Interventions

- Perform a thorough orthopedic and biomechanical evaluation to determine whether

> continued

Shoulder Impingement Syndrome > *continued*

any underlying pathologies exist as well as to ascertain the primary areas of dysfunction.

- A radiograph is recommended for patients who present with a chronic history to ascertain osseous changes to the shoulder as well as whether a congenital abnormality at the acromion exists that could be decreasing the subacromial space (e.g., a beaked acromion).

- Request an MRI if traditional treatment and therapy fail after six weeks. If an MRI reveals a full-thickness rotator cuff tear, surgery may be warranted (Koester et al. 2005).

- If hypomobility is present at the articulating joints of the shoulder, mobilizations may help restore the normal arthrokinematics of the shoulder and scapulothoracic articulation. However, pursue the release of hypertonic tissues prior to manipulation.

- Traditional palliative modalities (e.g., heat, ice, therapeutic ultrasound, laser) may decrease the pain and improve blood flow to chronically inflamed tissues, such as the long head of the biceps tendon.

- Have the patient avoid overhead movements early in the course of rehabilitation and progress once scapulothoracic and humeral deficiencies in movement and strength have been restored.

- A taping application to the shoulder early in the course of therapy may relieve pain.

- PNF stretching after exercise or positional release may help if the patient demonstrates posterior capsule tightness.

Patient Self-Treatment Interventions

- Initially, avoid overhead movements above the shoulder during sport, work, or ADLs.

- Perform posterior capsular stretching daily, if advised.

- Perform shoulder self-releases daily (e.g., long head of the biceps tendon).

- Perform rotator cuff strengthening below the shoulder initially, progressing to overhead rotator cuff strengthening.

- Apply palliative modalities for pain and spasm (e.g., heat and ice).

Long Head of the Biceps Tendinopathy

The function, etiology, and treatment of tendon pathology of the long head of the biceps (LHB) remain controversial (Allen 2013; Galasso et al. 2012; Krupp et al. 2009). The general consensus is that the LHB tendon stabilizes the shoulder along with the rotator cuff and assists in its movement. The tendon's anchor point on the superior glenoid labrum enables the biceps brachii to assist in shoulder flexion and extremity deceleration from an overhead throwing position as well as produce elbow flexion and forearm supination (Ditsios et al. 2012). The lack of agreement swirling around LHB tendinopathy may be due in part to the multifactorial nature of tendinopathy of the LHB.

Tendinopathy at this location rarely occurs in isolation from other shoulder pathologies, such as shoulder impingement syndrome and rotator cuff tear (Ditsios et al. 2012). Ditsios and colleagues (2012) contended that LHB tendinopathy can occur from trauma or degenerative breakdown from intrinsic and extrinsic factors such as overuse, resulting in acute or chronic inflammation, partial or complete rupture of the tendon, or luxation from the bicipital groove. Because of the tendon's potential role in stabilizing and moving the shoulder, tenderness and inflammation may be present at the tendon when other stabilizing structures are insufficient, such as the rotator cuff. Allen (2013) reported on multiple studies that demonstrated a strong association (90%) between rotator cuff tear and LHB tendon disorders. Refior and Sowa (1995) posited that the pathophysiology of LHB tendinopathy may be the result of repetitive friction, traction, and excessive glenohumeral rotation that causes a superior humeral head translation and results in compression and shear of the tendon and subsequent degenerative changes (e.g., fibrosis, tendon thickening, scar adhesions). The presence of a rotator cuff tear may accelerate the pathogenesis of LHB tendinopathy because the rotator cuff cannot effectively stabilize the humeral head in the glenoid fossa, particularly during overhead movements.

Typically, conservative therapy for isolated LHB tendinopathy consists of six to eight weeks of pain management, strengthening, and restoring normal and accessory motion (Ditsios et al. 2012; Krupp et al. 2009). However, if an underlying pathology is identified, then the therapy regimen

---

Treatment Points and Sequencing

1. LHB tendon
2. Deltoid
3. Upper trapezius
4. Supraspinatus
5. Infraspinatus
6. Anterior AC joint
7. Teres minor
8. Rhomboids
9. Levator scapulae at the shoulders
10. Sternocleidomastoid
11. Supinator
12. Biceps aponeurosis

---

is modified to address specific pathology-related deficits. Inflammation of the tendon must be addressed early because it may lead to instability resulting in disruption of the shoulder's kinematics and placing further stress on the tendon and surrounding tissues (Allen 2013). Allen (2013) indicated that instability of the shoulder as a result of a subscapularis tendon tear, rotator cuff tendon and labral pathology, or subluxation of the LHB tendon may result in rupture. The two most common surgical interventions pursued when conservative treatment has failed for LHB tendinopathy is tenotomy and tenodesis (Galasso et al. 2012). Krupp and colleagues (2009) recommended manual therapy in the initial phases after surgery, particularly if capsular tightness is present. However, to date, not one mode (tenotomy, tenodesis, manual therapy, or traditional therapy) has been shown to be more effective than another for treatment of LHB tendinopathy (Ditsios et al. 2012; Galasso et al. 2012).

Common Signs and Symptoms

- Anterior shoulder pain
- Decreased shoulder range of motion
- An audible snap with overhead throwing motions
- A popping or catching sensation
- A "Popeye sign," which indicates retraction of the tendon
- Shoulder and elbow weakness
- Pain with lifting or overhead activities or at rest

> continued

- Positive LHB tendon orthopedic tests, such as Speed's test (*Note:* Most LHB tendon orthopedic tests have very low sensitivity and may be confounded by other pathologies of the shoulder.)
- Point tenderness over the LHB tendon at the bicipital groove

Common Differential Diagnoses

- Rotator cuff tear
- SLAP (superior labral tear from anterior to posterior) lesion
- Shoulder impingement syndrome
- Osteoarthritis
- Deltoid strain
- Infection
- Subacromial bursitis

Clinician Therapeutic Interventions

- Confirm through orthopedic evaluation and diagnostic imaging whether an underlying shoulder pathology is present.
- Use PRT to address the presence of osteopathic lesions at the shoulder, neck, and distal structures in the arm.
- After releasing hypertonic tissues at the shoulder, use mobilizations and PNF stretching to address capsular restrictions and restore normal and accessory movement.
- In the initial phases of rehabilitation, focus on reducing pain and spasm, restoring motion, and regaining stabilization with movement and under load.
- Use a progressive functional shoulder program incorporating open- and closed-chain exercises.
- Thermal modalities applied to the LHB tendon followed by stretching may improve the healing environment for chronic conditions.
- Transverse friction massage to the tendon may help those with chronic conditions.

Patient Self-Treatment Interventions

- Perform self-release of the LHB tendon daily.
- Initially, avoid overhead activities and aggravating ADL movements.
- Apply palliative cold and heat modalities to control pain and spasm.
- Perform myofascial self-massage of the tendon for five to eight minutes daily.
- PNF stretch the tendon and other restricted tissues.

Summary

The assessment and treatment of upper-quarter injury conditions is inherently challenging because of the influence of proximal neurological triggers and the inherent structural instability of the shoulder. Although a proximal influence is often found to affect distal structure and function, a distal influence on proximal structure and function is less commonly seen. However, the upper quarter and the core work in concert to enable upper-quarter kinetic function. Therefore, a thorough evaluation of the entire upper-quarter kinetic chain is often required to determine the root of the injury and its contributing influences.

PRT may be a preferred intervention for both acute and chronic shoulder injury for athletic and workplace injuries. As a result of its nondirect nature, PRT can safely treat adolescents (without disturbing epiphyseal growth), those with joint trauma, and those with low bone mineral density. It is an excellent therapeutic tool for treating the upper-quarter somatic dysfunction associated with acute trauma. Moreover, it may also prove to be a gold standard for treating chronic upper-extremity conditions because of its potential to address recalcitrant osteopathic lesions that have developed from weakness, fatigue, and tissue overload from repetitive movements. Given the staggering rise in upper-quarter injuries and surgical interventions among adolescent athletes and workers, the search for more effective therapeutic interventions is greatly needed.

Elbow and Forearm

The elbow, much like the knee, serves as a linkage point for the joints above and below as well as their tendinous and ligamentous attachments. Therefore, weakness or trauma proximal or distal can often manifest at this linkage point and its articulating structures. One of the most widely recognizable elbow injuries is tennis elbow, or lateral epicondylalgia (LE), formerly known as lateral epicondylitis (Ahmad et al. 2013). Tennis elbow was once thought to be the result of an inflammatory condition, but is now widely accepted as a chronic degenerative condition of the common extensor tendon or the forearm extensor tendons that attach to the lateral epicondyle (Ahmad et al. 2013; Coombes, Bisset, and Vicenzino 2010; Scott et al. 2013).

According to the consensus statement on exercise-related tendinopathies formed from the Second International Scientific Tendinopathy Symposium in 2012 (Scott et al. 2013), the metaplastic and fibrotic changes leading to tendon thickening and pain may be the result of an increased scleraxis gene expression during the later stages of healing "as the tendon attempts to restore its phenotype" (p. 1). The amount of expression depends on the amount of mechanical strain on and movement of the tendon over time. However, the pathogenesis of LE, as well as tendinopathy in general, is not yet well understood. Ahmad and colleagues (2013) proposed that LE results when the tendon is stretched beyond its tolerance. Dean and colleagues (2013) agreed that a mechanical overload of tendons often instigates tendinopathy, but they suggested that an underlying neurological mechanism may cause the continued chronic inflammatory cycle that patients often experience.

In a systematic review, Dean and colleagues found strong evidence for alterations in peripheral sensitization, potentially from upregulation of the glutaminergic system in patients experiencing tendinopathy. "Glutamate is a key metabolite and key neurotransmitter involved in the transmission of pain" (Dean et al. 2013, 3042), which, if sustained, may lead to central sensitization (Ahmad et al. 2013). Jewson and colleagues (2015) also suggested that tendon disease may involve a neurological component, but they proposed that the primary driver is an upregulation of the sympathetic nervous system, primarily at the paratendinous tissue. All studies showed larger, rounder, and irregularly shaped tenocytes, which are the building blocks of tendons. Additionally, the tenocytes possessed high levels of catecholamine production (TH-LI or THmRNA) and adrenoreceptors. These are important findings because the morphological changes to the tenocytes and their elevated levels of catecholamine may reduce blood flow to the tendon, propagating its degeneration and hypersensitivity (Jewson et al. 2015).

Meltzer and Standley's (2007) findings lend support for use of indirect osteopathic manipulative therapies such as PRT. The authors found a significant reduction in fibroblastic proliferation and interleukin secretion when a modeled indirect osteopathic therapy was applied to a vitro stain after modeled repetitive motion strain. Although the findings of this modeling study highlight the potential role of an indirect therapy on cell mechanotransduction, additional in vivo research is needed to confirm the findings. The common consensus, however, is that chronic inflammatory tendon conditions are often the result of previous injury (Hjelm, Werner, and Renstrom 2012), overuse (Ahmad et al. 2013), fatigue (Scott et al. 2013), improper sport technique or form (Scott et al. 2013), faulty work ergonomics (Da Costa and Vieira 2010), or a lack of proximal joint range of motion and stabilization (Shanley et al. 2011).

In a prospective study of risk factors for upper-extremity injury among Swedish youth girl ($n = 20$) and boy ($n = 35$) tennis players, Hjelm and colleagues (2012) found that regardless of body location, including the spine, previous injury was the greatest risk factor followed by more than six hours of play per week. Elbow tendinopathy was the most common injury, although no decrease in shoulder internal rotation was found among injured players, which has been shown to contribute to the development of elbow tendinopathy (Shanley et al. 2011). Therefore, fatigue from excessive play may have been the primary reason for elbow tendinopathy in this group. Fatigue may not only produce myofascial trigger points (MTrPs), but also lead to them (Dommerholt, Bron, and Franssen 2006). It may be plausible, then, that fatigue coupled with the development of osteopathic lesions disturbs the load-bearing matrix organization of the tendinous tissue, decreasing the tensile strength of the tissue as well as its ability to produce force.

In a pre- and posttest investigation of 12 healthy subjects with elbow tender points, Wong, Moskovitz, and Fabillar (2011) found a significant increase in isometric grip strength with the application of strain counterstrain (SCS) among the intervention group compared to the sham intervention group. The researchers applied SCS to the pronator and supinator musculature once a week over a period of two weeks with a follow-up assessment at week 3. Although the findings of Wong and colleagues are encouraging, they must be interpreted cautiously because of low subject numbers and the fact that subjects were not examined in an injured state. However, in a single-case design, Baker and colleagues (2014) also demonstrated that when PRT was applied to tendinopathy at the elbow, an increase in strength was observed as well as an increase in range of motion and a decrease in pain, and that patient satisfaction with functional performance was improved.

Although traumatic injuries do occur to the elbow and forearm, very few produce the recalci-trant pain and dysfunction associated with elbow tendinopathy (Sanders et al. 2015; Scott et al. 2013). It is now widely accepted that an "itis" at the elbow that lasts longer than a few days is not maintained by an acute inflammatory response (Coombes et al. 2010; Jewson et al. 2015), but may be the result of cellular or neurological mechanisms such as altered gene expression (Scott et al. 2013), tenocyte dysfunction (Jewson et al. 2015), elevated glutamate secretion (Dean et al. 2013), and sympathetic nervous system upregulation (Jewson et al. 2015). PRT may assist in improving the proposed cellular and neurological events associated with tendinopathy both at the tendon proper and at its paratendon by increasing its perfusion and decreasing its sensitivity. This could play a vital role in limiting the propensity for developing central sensitization and, hence, chronic inflammation.

TREATMENT
Common Anatomical Areas and Conditions for PRT

- Muscle strain
- Ligament sprain
- Osteoarthritis
- Radiculopathy
- Pronator teres syndrome

- Cubital tunnel syndrome
- Dislocation (postrelocation)
- Little Leaguer's elbow
- Golfer's elbow
- Tennis elbow

Biceps Aponeurosis

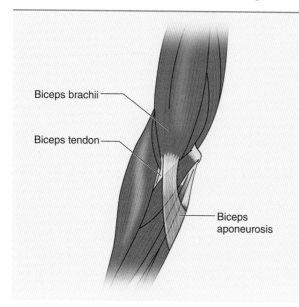

Biceps brachii

Biceps tendon

Biceps aponeurosis

At the cubital fossa of the elbow, the distal tendons of the biceps brachii conjoin to form the biceps aponeurosis, also known as the lacertus fibrosus. The aponeurosis assists in the movement of the elbow along with distal biceps tendon insertion at the radial tuberosity, but it also provides additional stability to the cubital fossa. Because the fibers of the aponeurosis blend into the deep fascia of the medial flexor tendons, lesions at the aponeurosis are often present in patients with medial elbow tendinitis, also known as golfer's elbow.

Palpation Procedure

- Place the patient supine with the elbow in a relaxed flexed position.
- Ask the patient to perform resistive supination, which will reveal the margins of the biceps aponeurosis.
- Once the aponeurosis is located, strum across its fibers with your forefinger and middle finger.
- In a well-defined patient, the aponeurosis can be traced as far as the medial epicondyle.
- Note the location of any tender points or fasciculatory response along the tissue.
- Once you have determined the most dominant tender point or fasciculation (or both), maintain light pressure with the pad(s) of the finger(s) at the location throughout the PRT treatment procedure until reassessment has occurred.

PRT Clinician Procedure

- Place the patient in a supine position with the elbow in a flexed and relaxed position.
- With your far hand, grasp the patient's hand with your palm over its dorsal aspect.
- Using the far hand, flex and extend the elbow to determine the maximal position of comfort or the fasciculatory response, or both.
- Apply supination and pronation with your far hand.
- Apply compression and distraction with your far hand.
- Apply finger flexion with your far hand for fine-tuning.

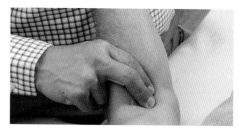

Biceps aponeurosis palpation procedure.

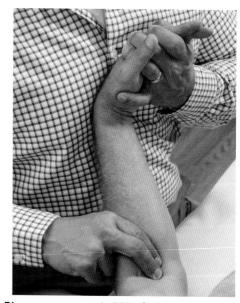

Biceps aponeurosis PRT clinician procedure.

- Corollary tissues treated: Pronator teres, medial flexors, medial epicondyle, brachioradialis, biceps brachii

Brachioradialis

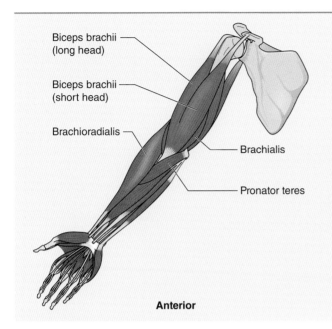

Biceps brachii (long head)

Biceps brachii (short head)

Brachioradialis

Brachialis

Pronator teres

Anterior

The brachioradialis is the most superficial muscle on the radial aspect of the forearm, and its muscle belly is readily visible with resistive hammerlike elbow movements. Proximally, the brachioradialis is often fused with the brachialis; distally, its tendon inserts just proximal to the styloid process of the radius. Even though innervation is derived from an extensor nerve, the muscle produces elbow flexion.

Origin: Proximal two thirds of the humerus

Insertion: Radius (proximal to the styloid process)

Action: Elbow flexion; assists forearm supination and pronation

Innervation: C5-C6 (radial nerve)

Palpation Procedure

- Place the patient supine or in a seated position with the forearm in a neutral position, or the thumb pointing upward.
- To visualize the brachioradialis, ask the patient to perform resistive elbow flexion with the thumb pointed upward.
- Strum across the muscle belly of the brachioradialis just below the joint line of the elbow. The belly can also be pinced.
- Trace the brachioradialis to its tendinous attachments inferior and posterior as far as possible.
- Note the location of any tender points or fasciculatory response along the muscle and its attachments.
- Once you have determined the most dominant tender point or fasciculation (or both), maintain light pressure with the pad(s) of the finger(s) at the location throughout the PRT treatment procedure until reassessment has occurred.

PRT Clinician Procedure

- Place the patient supine with the elbow at 90°.
- Place your far hand through the patient's.
- With your far hand, flex and extend the patient's elbow.
- Apply marked radial deviation of the wrist with your far hand; then apply internal and external forearm rotation.
- Apply marked compression toward the elbow at the wrist with your far hand.
- Corollary tissues treated: Extensor carpi radialis, brachialis

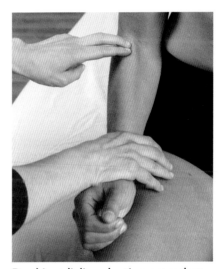

Brachioradialis palpation procedure.

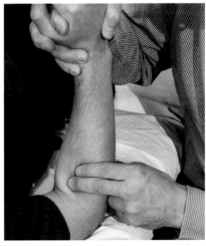

Brachioradialis PRT clinician procedure.

241

Flexors of the Wrist and Fingers

The five muscles that comprise the flexors of the wrist and fingers originate from the medial elbow. The superficial layer contains the flexor carpi radialis, ulnaris, and palmaris longus. The middle and deep layers contain the flexor digitorum superficialis and flexor digitorum profundus, respectively. The digitorum muscles are not directly accessible for palpation, but their contractions can be felt. Nevertheless, treatment of the other flexors should produce a release of these deeper tissues as well.

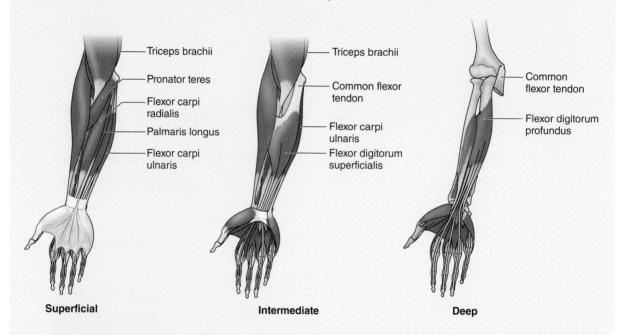

Triceps brachii
Pronator teres
Flexor carpi radialis
Palmaris longus
Flexor carpi ulnaris

Triceps brachii
Common flexor tendon
Flexor carpi ulnaris
Flexor digitorum superficialis

Common flexor tendon
Flexor digitorum profundus

Superficial   **Intermediate**   **Deep**

Flexor Carpi Radialis

Origin:	Humerus (medial epicondyle by the common flexor tendon)
Insertion:	Second and third metacarpals (base and palmar surfaces)
Action:	Wrist flexion, radial deviation, elbow flexion (weak)
Innervation:	C6-C7 (median nerve)

Flexor Carpi Ulnaris

Origin:	Humerus (medial epicondyle via the common flexor tendon), ulna (posterior upper two thirds)
Insertion:	Fifth metacarpal, pisiform
Action:	Wrist extension, ulnar deviation, elbow flexion (weak)
Innervation:	C7-C8 (ulnar nerve)

Palmaris Longus

Origin:	Humerus (medial epicondyle via the common flexor tendon)
Insertion:	Flexor retinaculum, palmar aponeurosis, intermuscular septa
Action:	Thumb abduction, tense palmar fascia and wrist flexion (weak), elbow flexion (weak)
Innervation:	C7-C8 (median nerve)

Flexor Digitorum Superficialis

Origin:	Humerus (medial epicondyle via the common flexor tendon), ulnar collateral ligament of the elbow, coronoid process, intramuscular septa
Insertion:	Second through fifth digits (sides of the middle phalanges)
Action:	Second through fifth Proximal interphalangeal (PIP) and Metacarpal phalangeal (MP) flexion; assists wrist flexion
Innervation:	C8-T1 (median nerve)

Flexor Digitorum Profundus

Origin: Ulna (upper three quarters of the anterior and medial surface and coronoid process), interosseous membrane

Insertion: Second through fifth distal phalanges, palmar surface and base

Action: Second through fifth distal interphalangeal (DIP) flexion, MP and PIP flexion; assists wrist flexion

Innervation: Second and third digits: C8-T1 (median nerve)

Fourth and fifth digits: C8-T1 (ulnar nerve)

Palpation Procedure

The superficial muscle bellies of the flexors that act on the wrist and fingers and possibly the elbow are often difficult to discern under palpation when starting at the elbow. However, working distally from the tendons at the wrist, you can trace muscle bellies proximally to the common flexor tendon at the medial elbow.

- To visually locate the wrist flexor tendons, ask the patient to flex the wrist with ulnar (wrist adduction) and radial (wrist abduction) deviation.

- Place the wrist in a neutral position and the elbow in a relaxed flexed position.

- Strum the tendon of the flexor carpi radialis (FCR) upward (most lateral tendon at the wrist) to its muscle belly and onward to the common flexor tendon.

- To determine whether the patient possesses a palmaris longus (it is absent in some people), ask the patient to move the thumb and ring finger toward one another while flexing the wrist. Its tendon will be just medial to the FCR. Repeat the palpation procedure for the FCR.

- The flexor carpi ulnaris (FCU) tendon at the wrist can be visually located by having the patient flex the wrist while performing ulnar deviation. The tendon can also be strummed upward to its muscle belly, which is located just a finger width anterolateral to the ulnar shaft as it courses toward the common flexor tendon.

- The insertion sites of the wrist flexor tendons should also be palpated.

- The density of the flexor digitorum muscles can be felt under contraction at the medial side of

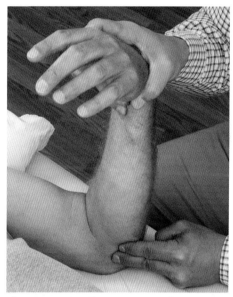

Flexor group palpation procedure.

the ulnar shaft. Place the elbow and wrist in 90° of flexion, and ask the patient to squeeze the pinky and thumb together while flexing the wrist to feel the contraction of these deep flexors.

- Note the location of any tender points or fasciculatory response at these muscles or their tendons and attachment sites.

- Once you have determined the most dominant tender point or fasciculation (or both), maintain light pressure with the pad(s) of the finger(s) at the location throughout the PRT treatment procedure until reassessment has occurred.

> continued

Flexors of the Wrist and Fingers *> continued*

PRT Clinician Procedure

- Place the patient supine with the elbow in slight flexion (approximately 20°).
- Rest the dorsum of the wrist against your torso.
- With your far hand, apply marked wrist and finger flexion.
- Apply deviation (ulnar or radial) with your far hand to target specific musculature (e.g., radial = FCR).
- Individual finger flexion can be accentuated to target specific muscles (e.g., the fifth digit for the flexor carpi ulnaris).
- Using the far hand, apply rotation coupled with wrist compression or distraction.
- Corollary tissues treated: Medial epicondyle, pronator teres, flexor group tendons at the wrist

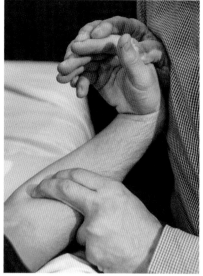

Flexor group PRT clinician procedure.

Supinator

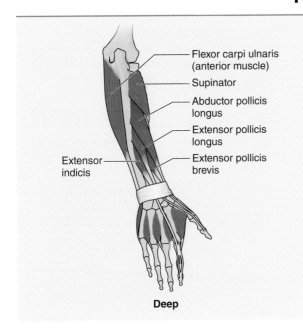

Flexor carpi ulnaris (anterior muscle)

Supinator

Abductor pollicis longus

Extensor pollicis longus

Extensor pollicis brevis

Extensor indicis

Deep

The supinator is a broad muscle located deep on the lateral side of the elbow. As the name dictates, it supinates the forearm. Its fibers originate from the lateral epicondyle and traverse to wrap around the head of the radius. Because of its deep location, indirect palpation of this muscle is used.

Origin: Lateral epicondyle of the humerus, radial collateral ligament, annular ligament, dorsal surface of the ulna

Insertion: Radius (proximal third)

Action: Forearm supination

Innervation: C6-C7 (radial nerve)

Palpation Procedure

- Place the patient supine with the elbow at 90°.
- Place your hand in the patient's as if shaking hands. Locate the humeral lateral epicondyle and the proximal anterior shaft of the radius. The supinator lies between these two landmarks underneath the extensor fibers.
- Apply firm pressure through the extensor fibers while asking the patient to supinate against your resistance while the elbow is at 90°. The deep contraction medial to the brachioradialis will be felt with this maneuver.
- Note the location of any tender points or fasciculatory response at this muscle during treatment. Rule out any tender points that may exist at the extensors prior to assessment and treatment because of the supinator's deep location.
- Determine the most dominant tender point or fasciculation (or both) and maintain light pressure with the pad(s) of the finger(s) throughout the treatment until reassessment has occurred.

PRT Clinician Procedure

- Place the patient supine with the arm off the treatment table.
- Place the patient's proximal arm on your thigh with the elbow extending beyond your thigh.
- Using your far hand, apply mild extension to the elbow at the distal wrist.
- Apply marked supination with your far hand.

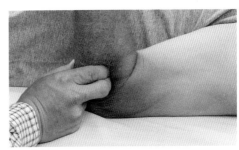

Supinator palpation procedure.

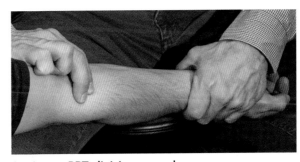

Supinator PRT clinician procedure.

- Apply a valgus force to the elbow with your far hand, using your near hand's thenar mass for stabilization.
- With your far hand, apply axial compression and distraction at the wrist to fine-tune.
- Corollary tissues treated: Forearm extensors, lateral epicondyle

Pronator Teres

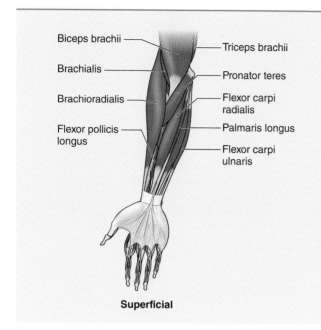

Biceps brachii
Brachialis
Brachioradialis
Flexor pollicis longus

Triceps brachii
Pronator teres
Flexor carpi radialis
Palmaris longus
Flexor carpi ulnaris

Superficial

The pronator teres is located on the anterior aspect of the forearm, coursing medially from the medial epicondyle across the cubital fossa to the middle of the radial shaft. The primary function of the muscle is to produce forearm pronation. Lesions of the pronator teres may produce nerve compression at the proximal portion of the median nerve and the anterior interosseous nerve, producing pronator teres syndrome.

Origin: Humeral (shaft proximal to the medial epicondyle), common flexor tendon, coronoid process

Insertion: Radius (middle of the lateral surface of the radial shaft)

Action: Elbow pronation; assists elbow flexion

Innervation: C6-C7 (median nerve)

Palpation Procedure

- Place the patient supine with the elbow in a flexed and relaxed position.
- Locate the medial epicondyle and the biceps aponeurosis. The pronator teres courses between these two landmarks.
- Slide medially off the bicep aponeurosis onto the proximal fibers of the pronator teres.
- Orient your forefinger and middle finger across the oblique fibers of the pronator teres and strum them until they blend into the medial flexor fibers and disappear under the brachioradialis.
- Note the location of any tender points or fasciculatory response at this muscle.
- Once you have determined the most dominant tender point or fasciculation (or both), maintain light pressure with the pad(s) of the finger(s) at the location throughout the PRT treatment procedure until reassessment has occurred.

PRT Clinician Procedure

- Place the patient supine with the involved arm at the side.
- With your far hand, grasp through the patient's hand with the palmar aspect of your hand over the dorsal aspect of the patient's.
- Using your far hand, apply marked wrist flexion and pronation while moving the dorsal aspect of the wrist toward the torso and maintaining wrist flexion.

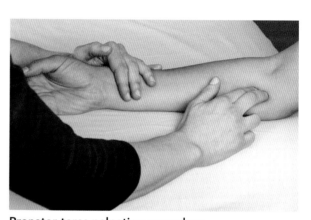

Pronator teres palpation procedure.

- Using your far hand, apply light axial compression toward the elbow.
- Fine-tune the position by applying radial and ulnar deviation with the far hand.
- Corollary tissues treated: Elbow flexors, pronator quadratus, biceps brachii, brachioradialis

▶ **See video 10.1 for the pronator teres PRT procedure.**

Patient Self-Treatment Procedure

- Lie supine with your involved arm at your side.
- Attempt to palpate the pronator teres with your other hand to determine the position of comfort or a fasciculatory response, or both, while moving into position.
- Move your arm upward in a maximally pronated position with the dorsal aspect of your wrist along your torso producing marked wrist flexion.
- Maintain the treatment position until the fasciculatory response abates or for three to five minutes.

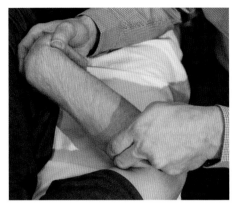

Pronator teres PRT clinician procedure.

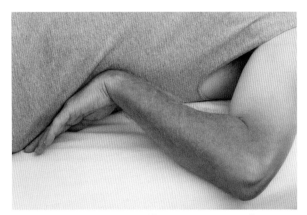

Pronator teres patient self-treatment procedure.

Medial Epicondyle and Common Flexor Tendon

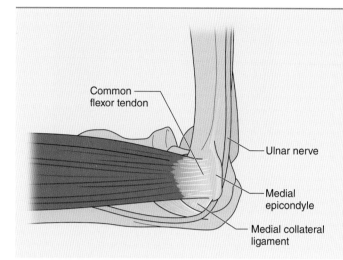

The medial epicondyle is a common site of irritation because it is a universal site of origin for all of the finger flexors and forearm pronators. Additionally, the common flexor tendon stabilizes the medial elbow against valgus and rotational forces. Therefore, the medial epicondyle and its common flexor tendon can become stressed when the joint opens during overhead throwing or a golf swing. Irritation at this site is also common among rock climbers who train primarily on indoor climbing walls.

Palpation Procedure

- Place the patient in a supine position with the elbow flexed and relaxed.
- Gently grasp the elbow across its anterior cubital fossa with your thumb and fingers over the humeral condyles.
- Gently roll over the medial condyle with either your fingers or thumb to feel its borders and its most prominent point, the medial epicondyle.
- Slide your finger or thumb distally off the medial epicondyle and strum across the common flexor tendon, moving distally. Note the distinct, but small depressions in the tendon as palpation progresses toward the flexor muscle bellies, which are the individual flexor tendons arising to fuse into the common flexor tendon.
- Note the location of any tender points or fasciculatory response at the bone and its common tendon.
- Once you have determined the most dominant tender point or fasciculation (or both), maintain light pressure with the pad(s) of the finger(s) at the location throughout the PRT treatment procedure until reassessment has occurred.

PRT Clinician Procedure

- Place the patient supine with the elbow flexed to approximately 90°.
- With your far hand, grasp the patient's hand with your thumb in the palmar aspect and your fingers over the dorsum of the patient's hand.
- Apply wrist and finger flexion with your far hand while applying compression toward the elbow. (*Note:* Apply compression over the distal radioulnar joint to avoid wrist discomfort.)

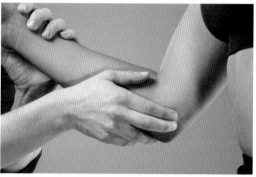

Medial epicondyle and common flexor tendon palpation procedure.

- Apply ulnar deviation and forearm rotation with your far hand.
- Apply individual finger flexion with the fingers of your far hand for fine-tuning.
- Corollary tissues treated: Flexor group, pronator teres, supinator, biceps aponeurosis

Patient Self-Treatment Procedure

- Adopt a comfortable and relaxed position with the elbow on a firm surface in a 90° flexed position.
- Use your noninvolved hand to explore the tissues for tenderness or a fasciculatory response, or both.
- Position the elbow at approximately 90° while palpating the most tender or dominant point at the medial elbow. Apply wrist flexion and ulnar deviation while simultaneously applying forearm rotation.
- Once you have found the position of comfort or fasciculatory response (or both), apply downward compression with the noninvolved hand to the top of the involved hand toward the elbow. If tenderness or a fasciculatory response is still present upon reassessment, repeat the procedure.
- Maintain the treatment position until the fasciculatory response abates or for three to five minutes.

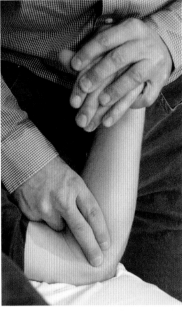

Medial epicondyle and common flexor tendon PRT clinician procedure.

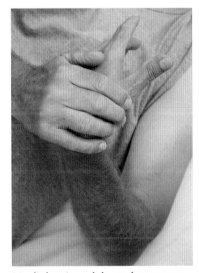

Medial epicondyle and common flexor tendon patient self-treatment procedure.

Triceps Brachii

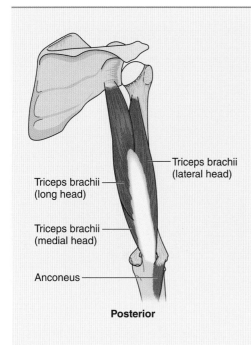

Triceps brachii
(lateral head)

Triceps brachii
(long head)

Triceps brachii
(medial head)

Anconeus

Posterior

The triceps is the only muscle on the posterior arm in the extensor compartment. The triceps is composed of three heads (long, lateral, and medial) that share a common tendon insertion on the olecranon. The triceps brachii produces elbow extension and shoulder extension and adduction. The origin of the long head at the infraglenoid tubercle of the scapula enables the triceps to produce shoulder extension and adduction. The lateral and long heads are the most accessible and visible on the dorsal arm, but the inferior fibers of the medial head can also be accessed at the medial and lateral borders of the common triceps tendon just above the olecranon.

Origin:	Long head: Scapula (infraglenoid tuberosity)
	Lateral head: Humerus (proximal posterior surface)
	Medial head: Humerus (distal posterior surface)
Insertion:	All heads: Ulna (olecranon process)
Action:	All heads: Elbow extension
	Long head: Assists shoulder extension and adduction
Innervation:	C6-C8 (radial nerve)

Palpation Procedure

- Place the patient prone with the arm at approximately 90°.
- Locate the olecranon process.
- Strum across the triceps tendon working upward to the muscular fibers of the long and lateral heads.
- Strum across the fibers of the long and lateral heads using the humerus below as a base against which to apply palpation pressure. As the proximal aspect of the long head is gained, it will dip under the posterior deltoid as its tendon slips between the teres minor and teres major on its way to its origin at the infraglenoid tuberosity. To palpate the tendon, press firmly through the posterior deltoid and strum across its fibers.
- The fibers of the medial head can be palpated by strumming up and down medial and lateral to the distal tendon with the thumb and forefinger.
- Note the location of any tender points or fasciculatory response at the muscle, its tendon, and its attachments.
- Once you have determined the most dominant tender point or fasciculation (or both), maintain light pressure with the pad(s) of the finger(s) at the location throughout the PRT treatment procedure until reassessment has occurred.

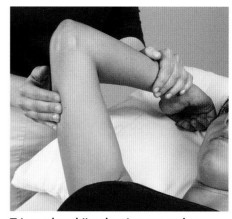

Triceps brachii palpation procedure.

PRT Clinician Procedure

- Place the patient supine with the upper arm supported by your thigh and the elbow off your thigh.
- Place the arm into approximately 30 to 50° of abduction and extension.
- With your far hand at or above the wrist, apply elbow hyperextension.
- Apply humeral rotation with your far hand according to the area being treated (internal for the medial and long heads of the triceps and external for the lateral and medial heads).
- Apply humeral compression or distraction with your far hand.
- Corollary tissues treated: Posterior deltoid, anconeus, olecranon

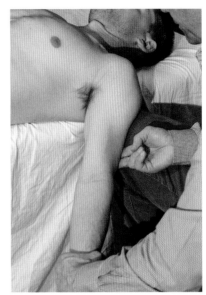

Triceps brachii PRT clinician procedure.

Olecranon

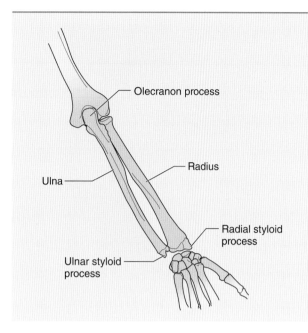

The olecranon is found at the proximal end of the ulna. The hooklike shape of the olecranon is simply the pointy part of the posterior elbow, its anterior or internal surface articulating with the trochlea of the humerus and its posterior or external surface serving as a major attachment site for the triceps brachii muscle. Lesions at the olecranon often result from either forceful hyperextension of the elbow or excessive and repetitive pulling on the bone from the triceps.

Palpation Procedure

- With the patient supine or seated, support the patient's forearm and elbow in a relaxed position.
- Palpate over the posterior aspect of the elbow while moving the elbow through flexion and extension to discern the border of the olecranon.
- Just above the olecranon, the triceps tendon can be found. Strum across the tendon, moving distally to its insertion site on the olecranon.
- Note the location of any tender points or fasciculatory response at the bone and the tendon attachment of the triceps.
- Once you have determined the most dominant tender point or fasciculation (or both), maintain light pressure with the pad(s) of the finger(s) at the location throughout the PRT treatment procedure until reassessment has occurred.

PRT Clinician Procedure

- Place the patient supine with the upper arm on your thigh and the elbow joint off your thigh.
- Place the involved upper extremity into approximately 30° of extension and abduction.
- Apply hyperextension of the elbow at or above the patient's wrist with your far hand.
- Rotate the wrist or forearm with your far hand.
- With your far hand, apply compression or distraction at the wrist for fine-tuning.
- Corollary tissue treated: Triceps brachii

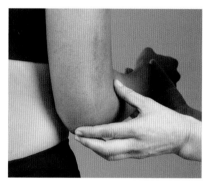

Olecranon palpation procedure.

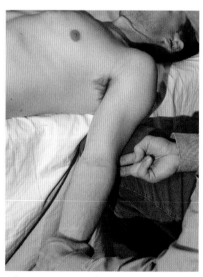

Olecranon PRT clinician procedure.

Anconeus

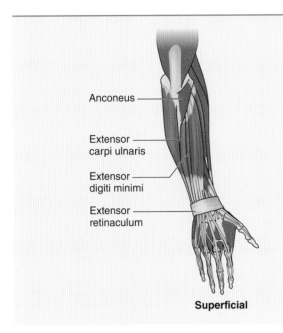

Anconeus

Extensor
carpi ulnaris

Extensor
digiti minimi

Extensor
retinaculum

Superficial

An often-forgotten elbow extensor, the triangular anconeus lies on the posterior surface of the elbow just lateral to the olecranon. The anconeus assists the triceps in extending the elbow. Lesions at the anconeus are often present with lateral and medial elbow tendinopathy.

Origin:	Humerus (lateral epicondyle)
Insertion:	Ulna (olecranon and posterior quarter of the upper ulnar shaft)
Action:	Elbow extension
Innervation:	C6-C8 (radial nerve)

Palpation Procedure

- Place the patient either prone or supine with the elbow extended.
- Locate the lateral epicondyle of the humerus and olecranon.
- Orient the palpation fingers or thumb obliquely across the fibers of the anconeus between these two landmarks. Strum across the fibers working distally toward the shaft of the ulna.
- Note the location of any tender points or fasciculatory response at the muscle, its tendon, and its attachments.
- Once you have determined the most dominant tender point or fasciculation (or both), maintain light pressure with the pad(s) of the finger(s) at the location throughout the PRT treatment procedure until reassessment has occurred.

PRT Clinician Procedure.

- Place the patient supine with the elbow off the edge of the treatment table.
- Take the patient's hand with your far hand as if shaking hands, and wrap your thumb around the hypothenar aspect of the patient's hand.
- With your far hand, apply hyperextension of the elbow with marked wrist extension.
- Using your far hand, apply rotation to the forearm.
- Apply compression or distraction to the joint of the elbow with your far hand.
- Corollary tissues treated: Triceps, posterior deltoid

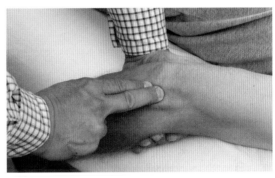

Anconeus palpation procedure.

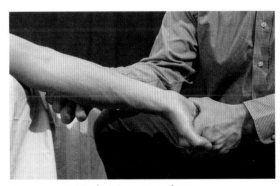

Anconeus PRT clinician procedure.

Extensors of the Wrist and Fingers

Four primary muscles produce wrist and finger extension. The extensor carpi radialis longus, extensor carpi radialis brevis, extensor carpi ulnaris, and extensor digitorum are bracketed by the brachioradialis and ulnar shaft at the posterolateral forearm. Although the extensor digiti minimi is often indicated as an extensor of the wrist and fingers as well, the minimi is typically viewed as an extension of the extensor digitorum. Like the muscles of the medial flexor group, which form a common tendon attachment at the medial epicondyle, the muscles of the extensor group also converge into a common tendon attachment at the lateral epicondyle.

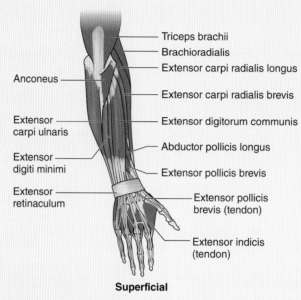

Superficial

Extensor Carpi Radialis Longus

Origin: Humerus (distal third of the lateral supracondylar ridge), common extensor tendon

Insertion: Second metacarpal (dorsal base on the radial side)

Action: Wrist extension and radial deviation; assists elbow flexion

Innervation: C6-C7 (radial nerve)

Extensor Carpi Radialis Brevis

Origin: Humerus (lateral epicondyle via the common extensor tendon), radial collateral ligament

Insertion: Third metacarpal (dorsal base on the radial side)

Action: Wrist extension and radial deviation (weak)

Innervation: C7-C8 (radial nerve)

Extensor Carpi Ulnaris

Origin: Humerus (lateral epicondyle via the common extensor tendon), ulna (posterior aponeurosis)

Insertion: Fifth metacarpal (based on the ulnar side)

Action: Wrist extension, ulnar deviation

Innervation: C7-C8 (radial nerve)

Extensor Digitorum

Origin: Humerus (lateral epicondyle via the common extensor tendon)

Insertion: Second through fifth digits (digital expansion over the proximal and middle phalanges with lateral slips to the distal phalanges)

Action: Second through fifth MP, PIP, and DIP extension; assists with wrist extension

Innervation: C7-C8 (radial nerve)

Palpation Procedure

- Place the patient in either a seated or supine position with the elbow flexed at 90° and the forearm in a neutral position, thumb pointing up.
- Grasp the brachioradialis like a hamburger and pull it up away from the radius. Directly inferior to the brachioradialis lie the extensor carpi radialis longus and brevis.
- Keeping your fingers perpendicular to the fibers of the extensor carpi radialis longus and brevis, move onto their muscle fibers (not distinguishable from one another) and continue strumming distally to their tendinous aspects. (*Note:* To determine whether you are on the brachioradialis or the extensor carpi radialis brevis and longus, instruct the patient to extend the wrist under palpation. The brachioradialis does not contract with wrist extension, but the others do.
- Drop down or move medially onto the fibers of the extensor digitorum. A distinct valley or demarcation exists between the extensor digitorum and extensor carpi radialis longus and brevis. To differentiate between them, instruct the patient to tap the fingers as though playing a piano. The digitorum fibers will produce a robust contraction.
- Move onto the ridge of the ulna. The extensor carpi ulnaris lies against the shaft of the ulna. Capture the medial border of the extensor carpi ulnaris by moving off its fibers onto the ulna and then strum over the fibers by pulling up or away from the ulnar ridge with firm pressure.
- Also explore the extensor group's distal insertion sites.
- Note the location of any tender points or fasciculatory response at the muscles, their tendons, and their attachments.
- Once you have determined the most dominant tender point or fasciculation (or both), maintain light pressure with the pad(s) of the finger(s) at the location throughout the PRT treatment procedure until reassessment has occurred.

PRT Clinician Procedure

- The patient is supine with the forearm resting on your thigh.
- Place your far palm on the patient's palm and apply marked wrist and finger extension.
- Apply wrist deviation using your far hand and either radial or ulnar deviation depending on the targeted muscle (radial deviation for the

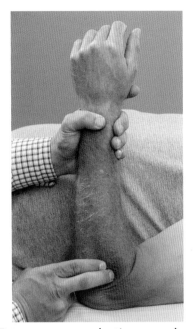

Extensor group palpation procedure.

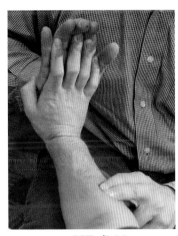

Extensor group PRT clinician procedure.

extensor carpi radialis and ulnar deviation for the extensor carpi ulnaris).
- Finger extension is accentuated according to the targeted muscles (e.g., second through fifth fingers for the extensor digitorum, second and third fingers for the extensor carpi radialis, and fifth finger digit extension for the extensor carpi ulnaris).
- Apply rotation with your far hand.
- Apply compression with your far hand for fine-tuning.
- Corollary tissues treated: Common extensor tendon, extensor group tendons at the wrist, supinator

Lateral Epicondyle and Common Extensor Tendon

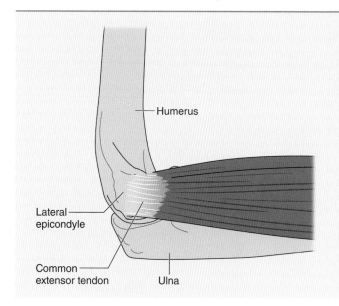

Although complaints of elbow pain on the lateral side are typically more common than those on the medial side, lateral and medial elbow pain often present together because of the synergist and antagonist relationships they perform. Much like the common flexor tendon at the medial elbow, the extensors of the fingers and supinators of the wrist also attach to the lateral epicondyle via a common extensor tendon. The extensors at the lateral elbow cocontract with the flexors, and their common tendon and its site of origin can also become stressed during overhead throwing, racket sports, climbing, or any activity that calls unduly on the extensors, such as excessive use of a screwdriver.

Palpation Procedure

- Place the patient in a supine or seated position with the elbow flexed and relaxed.
- Gently grasp the elbow across its anterior cubital fossa with your thumb and fingers over the humeral condyles.
- Gently roll over the lateral condyle with either your fingers or thumb to feel its borders and its most prominent point, the lateral epicondyle.
- Slide your finger or thumb distally off the lateral epicondyle and strum across the common extensor tendon, moving distally. Note the distinct, but small depressions in the tendon as palpation progresses toward the extensor muscle bellies, which are the individual extensor tendons arising to fuse into the common extensor tendon.
- Note the location of any tender points or fasciculatory response at the bone and its common tendon.
- Once you have determined the most dominant tender point or fasciculation (or both), maintain light pressure with the pad(s) of the finger(s) at the location throughout the PRT treatment procedure until reassessment has occurred.

PRT Clinician Procedure

- Place the patient supine with the elbow flexed to approximately 90°.
- With your far hand, grasp the patient's hand with your fingers in the palmar aspect and your thumb over the dorsum of the patient's hand.

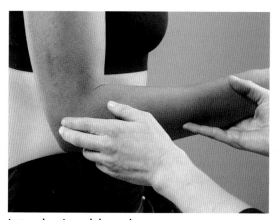

Lateral epicondyle and common extensor tendon palpation procedure.

- Apply wrist and finger extension with your far hand while applying compression toward the elbow. (*Note:* Apply compression over the distal radioulnar joint to avoid wrist discomfort.)
- Apply radial deviation and forearm rotation with your far hand.
- Apply individual finger extension with the fingers of your far hand for fine-tuning.
- Corollary tissues treated: Extensor group, pronator teres, supinator, distal biceps tendon

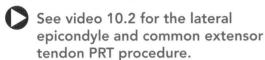 See video 10.2 for the lateral epicondyle and common extensor tendon PRT procedure.

Patient Self-Treatment Procedure

- Adopt a comfortable and relaxed position with the elbow on a firm surface in a 90° flexed position.
- Use your noninvolved hand to explore the tissues for tenderness or a fasciculatory response, or both.
- While palpating the most tender point at the lateral elbow, actively position the elbow in approximately 90° of flexion, while moving the wrist through extension, radial deviation, and forearm rotation.
- Once the position of comfort or fasciculatory response (or both) is found, apply downward compression with the noninvolved hand. If tenderness or a fasciculatory response is still present upon reassessment, repeat the procedure.
- Maintain the treatment position until the fasciculatory response abates or for three to five minutes.

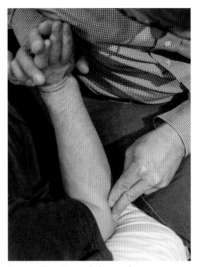

Lateral epicondyle and common extensor tendon PRT clinician procedure.

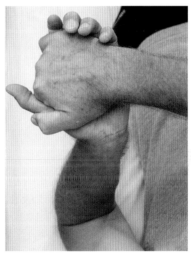

Lateral epicondyle and common extensor tendon patient self-treatment procedure.

Tennis Elbow

Tennis elbow is a tendinopathy of the common extensor tendon that originates from the lateral epicondyle of the humerus (Orchard and Kountouris 2011). The condition is no longer considered an acute inflammatory condition (it was previously termed lateral epicondylitis), but rather, a degenerative tendinopathy linked to tissue overload (Shiri and Viikari-Juntura 2011). Before the advent of lightweight tennis rackets and the two-handed backhand, the condition was commonly seen in tennis players.

Today, the condition appears to manifest in those who undertake strenuous repetitive activity that overloads the capacity of the tendon (Shiri and Viikari-Juntura 2011). Shiri and Viikari-Juntura (2011) reported in their investigation of occupational risk factors for tennis elbow that the prevalence is between 1 and 4% in the general population and between 0.8 and 29.3% in the working population. The condition is more likely to develop with age, the greatest prevalence is in those between 40 and 60 years of age, and the condition is more prevalent in women than in men (Shiri and Viikari-Juntura 2011). The increase in prevalence seen in the working population has been attributed to high force demands, repetitive movements, hand and arm vibrations, and awkward postures (Shiri and Viikari-Juntura 2011). However, a relationship of these risks factors to the development of the disorder has not yet been substantiated in the literature; nor have workplace and ergonomic modifications been shown to prevent upper-quarter injury (Andersen et al. 2011). Additionally, there is limited evidence to show that any one therapeutic or surgical intervention is superior to a wait-and-see policy or traditional eccentric therapy (Orchard and Kountouris 2011; Shiri and Viikari-Juntura 2011).

A study of the impact of growth factor injection for therapy-resistant tennis elbow (Creaney et al. 2012), autologous blood injection (ABI), and platelet-rich plasma (PRP) injection demonstrated similar efficacy of improvement at follow-up six months postinjection: 66% for the PRP group ($n = 80$) and 72% for the ABI group ($n = 70$). However, to date, growth factor injection has not been shown to be more effective than traditional treatment or a wait-and-see approach (Creaney et al. 2012).

Treatment Points and Sequencing

1. Lateral epicondyle and common extensor tendon
2. Extensors of the wrist and fingers (extensor group)
3. Medial epicondyle and common flexor tendon
4. Flexors of the wrist and fingers (flexor group)
5. Brachioradialis
6. Pronator teres
7. Anconeus
8. Triceps
9. Wrist extensors and flexors
10. Long head of the biceps tendon
11. Rotator cuff musculature
12. Upper trapezius

The good news is that in 80% of cases, the condition resolves on its own within a year without any intervention (Shiri and Viikari-Juntura 2011). However, athletes and workers are often pressed to resolve the issue more quickly. Cortisone injection, although providing significant immediate pain relief, has shown negative intermediate and long-term outcomes over exercise and stretching (Olaussen et al. 2013). Moreover, continued elbow load on the job during therapy has been shown to produce poor outcomes (Shiri and Viikari-Juntura 2011), possibly as a result of persistent weakness, overload, and fatigue of the tendon and muscular tissues. This provides an additional challenge for the therapist working with a patient who needs to remain active on the job or in a sport.

One study to date has examined the use of PRT to address tendinopathy at the elbow. In a single-case design, Baker and colleagues (2014) found significant improvement in pain, range of motion, and patient satisfaction after treatment of reactive bicipital aponeurosis in a 21-year-old competitive swimmer. The patient was treated once a day with PRT over a period of four days, and follow-up reassessment occurred at one month posttreatment. The patient did not have tennis elbow, but bicipital aponeurosis may have a similar pathogenesis. In this case, the patient continued to be physically active during treatment, which may point to PRT being an effective modality for tendinopathy for patients who must continue to perform in sport or at work. This study and that of Wong and colleagues (2011) demonstrated a marked improvement in elbow strength in a healthy population after tender point treatment. This suggests that acute reduction of pain and improvement of strength may be critical outcomes to attain early in the rehabilitation process to limit fatigue and the further development of osteopathic lesions, thereby accelerating recovery time for active people.

Common Signs and Symptoms

- Gradual onset of pain at the lateral elbow that may migrate proximally or distally
- Pain with resistive extension of the wrist and fingers and forearm supination
- Normal elbow range of motion
- Reduced grip strength and function

Common Differential Diagnoses

- Cervical radiculopathy
- Little Leaguer's elbow
- Medial epicondylitis
- Radial nerve entrapment
- Biceps tendinopathy
- Common extensor tendon longitudinal tear

Clinician Therapeutic Interventions

- Conduct a thorough orthopedic evaluation to rule out common differential diagnoses. Clinically, an association has been seen with rotator cuff weakness or pathology and the presence of tennis elbow and golfer's elbow. If proximal weakness or dysfunction exists, additional load will be placed on the elbow.
- Use PRT prior to joint mobilizations, massage, and tissue stretching.
- Consider thermal modalities such as ultrasound to the reactive tendon and tissues.
- Consider mobilizations if deficits in range of motion are present.
- Use a progressive eccentric-based therapy program, loading the tendon gradually over time.
- Consider a core strengthening regimen for patients who perform repetitive overhead activities.
- If therapy is unsuccessful, consider requesting diagnostic imaging to rule out other underlying pathologies.
- Use of cortisone for reactive tendinopathy may improve short-term outcomes, but to date it has not been shown to positively affect long-term outcomes (Orchard and Kountouris 2011).

Patient Self-Treatment Interventions

- Perform self-release on the affected tissues daily.
- Apply self-massage or myofascial stretch daily to the tendon.
- Apply palliative modalities to reduce pain and spasm.
- Avoid activities that aggravate the elbow.
- Perform PNF stretching of the tissues daily after physical activity or therapy.

Pronator Teres Syndrome

Pronator teres syndrome (PTS) involves the entrapment of the median nerve as it passes between the two heads of the pronator teres (Quan 2013). However, because of the potential for the median nerve to become entrapped at the carpal tunnel and also at the antecubital fossa of the elbow, diagnosis may prove challenging. Lee and colleagues (2014) reported that although isolated PTS is rare, it may be combined with other median neuropathies, clouding diagnosis. Moreover, because the anterior interosseous nerve (AIN) passes through the pronator teres muscle, hypertonicity of the pronator may also affect the AIN. However, the AIN is strictly a motor nerve; therefore, differential diagnosis can be confirmed with electromyographic study (Ulrich, Piatkowski, and Pallua 2011). Lee and colleagues (2014) pointed out that "entrapment of the AIN produces strictly motor weakness in the flexor pollicis longus and the radial half of the flexor digitorum profundus" (p. 3). They suggested that the crux of PTS diagnosis is the typical pattern of muscle denervation that presents in the pronator teres, flexor carpi radialis, pronator quadratus, abductor pollicis brevis, flexor digitorum superficialis, and digitorum profundus.

If somatic dysfunction exists at the elbow along with increased hypertonicity of the pronator teres, PRT may reduce compression of both the median and anterior interosseous nerves. Upon release of the pronator teres, patients often report an immediate relief of pain and numbness and improved motor function.

Common Signs and Symptoms

- Pain in the wrist and forearm
- Weakness of the thenar muscles
- Palmar triangle dysesthesia
- Median nerve distribution numbness with repetitive pronation or supination
- Fatigue of forearm musculature with repetitive pronation or supination
- Pain on resistive forearm pronation and extension of the elbow
- Positive Tinel's sign at the pronator teres
- Point tenderness over the pronator teres
- Thenar mass atrophy

Treatment Points and Sequencing

1. Pronator teres
2. Medial epicondyle and common flexor tendon
3. Bicipital aponeurosis
4. Flexors of the wrist and fingers (flexor group)
5. Supinator
6. Brachioradialis
7. Lateral epicondyle and common extensor tendon
8. Extensors of the wrist and fingers (extensor group)
9. Abductor pollicis brevis

Common Differential Diagnoses

- Lacertus fibrosus
- Flexor superficialis crossover syndrome
- C6-C7 radiculopathy
- Carpal tunnel syndrome
- Anterior interosseous entrapment
- Forearm compartment syndrome
- Supracondylar process syndrome

Clinician Therapeutic Interventions

- Conduct a thorough orthopedic evaluation to rule out common differential diagnoses such as anterior interosseous nerve entrapment.
- Use PRT prior to joint mobilizations, massage, and tissue stretching.
- Consider thermal modalities such as ultrasound to the reactive tissues.
- Consider mobilizations if deficits in range of motion are present.
- Use a progressive therapy program with a focus on eccentric loading of the pronator teres with a gradual progression toward repetitive pronation and supination.
- Consider a core strengthening regimen for patients who perform repetitive overhead activities.
- If therapy is unsuccessful, consider requesting diagnostic imaging to rule out other underlying pathologies.

Patient Self-Treatment Interventions

- Perform self-release on the affected tissues daily.
- Apply self-massage or myofascial stretching daily.
- Apply palliative modalities to reduce pain and spasm.
- Avoid activities that aggravate the elbow.
- Perform PNF stretching of the tissues daily after physical activity or therapy.

Summary

The challenge of working with a patient presenting with somatic dysfunction at the elbow and forearm is that it may be the result of a proximal influence at the shoulder or cervical spine, which may cloud the clinical presentation of the patient and the diagnosis (Ahmad et al. 2013). Moreover, if a tendinopathy is suspected, the patient is likely also suffering from peripheral and central sensitization (Jewson et al. 2015), which often results in recalcitrant recovery and places the patient at risk for relapse (Scott et al. 2013). Sanders and colleagues (2015) reported an 8.5% recurrence rate of lateral elbow tendinosis within two years and an overall incidence rate of 2.4 per 1,000 in 2012. It is now well understood that chronic tendinopathies at the elbow are not effectively treated with corticosteroid injections, and doing so may produce a negative long-term outcome and higher recurrence rate than exercise-based therapy alone (Coombes et al. 2010; Olaussen et al. 2013). Additionally, emerging evidence points to greater cellular and neurological influences on the maintenance of tendinopathies than once thought (Jewson et al. 2015; Scott et al. 2013). However, there is still no clear consensus on the best type of therapy or combination of therapies for tendinopathy patients.

Prevailing evidence to date has shown better long-term outcomes among tendinosis patients with an exercise-based therapy regimen versus no intervention or injection therapy (Drew et al. 2012; De Vos, Windt, and Weir 2014). Eccentric exercises have shown promise for improvement in short-term and intermediate outcomes for both lateral (Olaussen et al. 2013) and medial elbow tendinopathies (Tyler et al. 2014). However, exercise, including eccentric exercise coupled with stretching, demonstrated the greatest benefit (e.g., reduction in pain, improvement in strength and function) for tendinopathies in the long run (Olaussen et al. 2013). How eccentric exercise or stretching (once believed to alter the load-bearing tendon matrix) positively affects tendon healing remains unclear (Drew et al. 2012; Scott et al. 2013). Emerging evidence suggests that manipulative manual therapies coupled with an eccentric-based therapy protocol may have a positive effect on elbow tendinopathy (Baker et al. 2014; Bisset, Hing, and Vicenzino 2012; Wong et al. 2011). However, according to the *UK Evidence Report*, evidence supporting the use of manipulative therapy alone is weak, although it remains favorable (Clar et al. 2014).

Evidence supports the call for more integrative research studies using manual therapies such as PRT. When used for chronic elbow conditions, PRT likely interrupts peripheral and central sensitization pathways, positively affecting cellular and neurological processes and engendering a homeostatic environment in which effective therapy can occur. PRT may also improve tissue perfusion and limit sympathetic nervous system upregulation. However, a paucity of research exists to support and test these propositions at this time.

CHAPTER 11

Wrist and Hand

CHAPTER OBJECTIVES

After reading this chapter, you should be able to do the following:

❶ Appreciate the factors that may influence the development of somatic dysfunction of the wrist and hand.

❷ Locate and palpate wrist and hand structures to be treated with positional release therapy (PRT).

❸ Apply PRT techniques to treat the wrist and hand.

❹ Discuss how common injury conditions such as gamekeeper's thumb may be treated based on myofascial lesion patterns.

From an examination of the NEISS (National Electronic Injury Surveillance System) database, Ootes, Lambers, and Ring (2012) estimated in 2009 the number of upper-extremity injuries seen in U.S. emergency departments to be 3,468,996, which translates to an incidence of 1,130 per 100,000 people. The authors found that the most common area injured was the finger (38.4%), and the most frequent upper-extremity injury was fracture. Finger lacerations (221 per 100,000) brought the majority of patients to the emergency department followed by wrist fracture (72 per 100,000). Similar findings have also been found in European emergency departments. Sytema and colleagues (2010) examined 25,000 emergency department cases between 1995 and 2005 in a European level I trauma unit and found that, of the cases examined, 35% involved the upper extremity. Of these, 44% were the result of fracture, and the majority occurred in the home. Although no published studies have examined the effect of PRT on wrist and finger injury, because of the pain and dysfunction associated with them, it warrants investigation.

Moseley and colleagues (2014) observed a cohort of 1,549 wrist fracture patients. In those who had a numerical pain rating higher than 5 in the first week postfracture, 4% developed complex regional pain syndrome (CRPS) within four months. They wrote that CRPS "is characterized by disproportionate pain and disability, with disturbed autonomic and motor function, usually confined to 1 arm or leg" (p. 16). In a study of the use of strain counterstrain (SCS) for the treatment of CRPS in the ankle, Collins (2007) attributed significant pain relief and improved functional outcomes to a reduction in peripheral and central sensitization. However, whether the same outcomes would be observed in wrist fracture patients is unknown. Soft tissue injury is also observed frequently with wrist fracture (Ogawa et al. 2013), which may lead to upregulation of the somatic nervous system as a result of the associated pain and dysfunction.

Three soft tissues are commonly injured with distal radial fractures: the triangular fibrocartilage complex (TFCC), scapholunate interosseous ligament (SLIL), and lunotriquetral interosseous ligament (LTIL) (Ogawa et al. 2013). In a prospective study of 89 patients who received arthroscopic surgery for distal radial fracture, only 17.1% did not present with a soft tissue injury. Of those who did, 59% presented with TFCC injury, 54.5% with an SLIL injury, and 34.5% with an LTIL injury, regardless of the fracture type and whether the fracture was intra- or extra-articular. The authors attributed the high rate of soft tissue injuries to excessive compressive loading and shearing of the ligaments and carpals.

Although treating traumatic injury to the wrist and hand directly may be difficult in patients who are casted, PRT may be an excellent treatment modality for those in removable splints because of its indirect, nonpainful approach. The application of PRT for chronic wrist and hand injuries such as carpal tunnel syndrome (CTS), tenosynovitis, and osteoarthritis also shows promise because of its propensity to reduce tissue hypertonicity and nerve compression and improve blood flow.

Throughout the zones of the hand and wrist are multiple opportunities for nerve compression and chronic inflammation to develop. Ghasemi-rad and colleagues (2013) reported that the most common wrist and hand injury seen in U.S. physician offices is CTS. Within the carpal tunnel is a tightly packed area of tendons, their synovial sheaths, and the median nerve, all of which are bound by inelastic tissues such as the transverse carpal ligament and carpal bones. Compression of these tissues between the unyielding structures of the transverse carpal ligament and carpal bones can result in paresthesia and pain, minimally at the first three fingers, but not at the palm or dorsum of the hand (Ghasemi-rad et al. 2013). Siu and colleagues (2012) proposed that osteopathic manipulative therapy (OMT), consisting of myofascial release, joint manipulation, and muscle energy, is effective for the management of compression of the carpal tunnel. Compression in the carpal tunnel as well as in the forearm (Brown et al. 2011) may reduce ATP and tissue perfusion, resulting in muscle acidosis (Fry et al. 2013) that could cause the development of tender and trigger points in the affected and adjacent tissues (Gerwin, Dommerholt, and Shah 2004). This creates an environment in which somatic dysfunction can manifest and persist (Speicher and Draper 2006). Chronic inflammation of the tendons, if left to persist in these areas, may also produce tenosynovitis (Navalho et al. 2012) and osteoarthritis (Villafañe, Cleland, and Fernandez-De-Las-Peñas 2013).

The implications of a loss of wrist and hand function on activities of daily living, work duties, and sport performance are immense. Little of what we do in life does not involve the wrist and hand. Given the likelihood of wrist fracture leading to CRPS (Moseley et al. 2014) and soft tissue disruption (Ogawa et al. 2013), PRT may serve a significant role in limiting the associated pain, thereby reducing the potential for the development of somatic dysfunction. Additionally, PRT may also improve ATP and tissue perfusion by reducing tissue tonicity, which may improve tendon and nerve gliding in the tunnels and compartments of the wrist and forearm. This could limit the risk of developing compressive neuropathies such as CTS and exertional compartment syndrome (Brown et al. 2011).

TREATMENT
Common Anatomical Areas and Conditions for PRT

- Muscle strain
- Ligament sprain
- Osteoarthritis
- Radiculopathy
- Carpal tunnel syndrome
- De Quervain syndrome
- Dislocation (postrelocation)
- Tendinopathy

Wrist Flexor Tendons

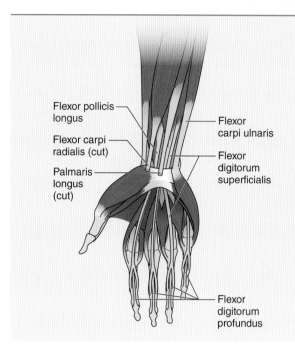

Flexor pollicis longus

Flexor carpi radialis (cut)

Palmaris longus (cut)

Flexor carpi ulnaris

Flexor digitorum superficialis

Flexor digitorum profundus

The wrist flexor tendons (flexor carpi radialis, ulnaris, palmaris longus, flexor digitorum superficialis, and flexor digitorum profundus) crossing at the wrist may exhibit osteopathic lesions. They may also become entrapped within the carpal tunnel causing pain and numbness in the hand.

Palpation Procedure

- Position the patient supine with the wrist in a relaxed flexed position.
- Start palpation at either the medial or lateral wrist.
- Strum across the wrist flexor tendons with one or two fingers, moving to the next tendon.
- Note the location of any tender points or fasciculatory response at the tendons and their attachments.
- Once the most dominant tender point or fasciculation (or both) has been determined, maintain light pressure with the pad(s) of the finger(s) at the location throughout the PRT treatment procedure until reassessment has occurred.

PRT Clinician Procedure

- Place the patient supine with the elbow flexed to approximately 70°.
- With your far hand, apply marked wrist flexion.
- Apply wrist deviation and rotation with your far hand to target specific wrist tendons (e.g., radial deviation for the flexor carpi radialis tendon).
- With your far hand, apply light compression at the wrist toward the elbow.
- Corollary tissues treated: Flexor group, common flexor tendon

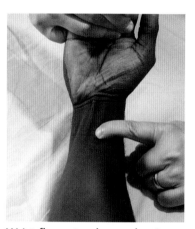

Wrist flexor tendons palpation procedure.

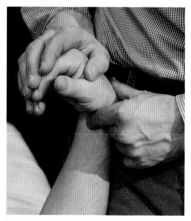

Wrist flexor tendons PRT clinician procedure.

Metacarpophalangeal Joint

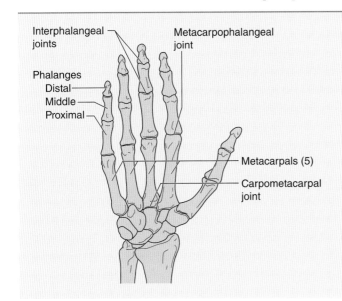

Interphalangeal joints
Metacarpophalangeal joint
Phalanges
Distal
Middle
Proximal
Metacarpals (5)
Carpometacarpal joint

The metacarpophalangeal (MCP) joints are formed by the articulation of each metacarpal and the proximal end of the associated proximal phalange. The joint is a synovial ellipsoid joint enclosed in a fibrous capsule further supported by ligaments and tendons. When the MCP joints are stabilized, their respective proximal phalanges can be translated forward, backward, and side to side and rotated about the long axis.

Palpation Procedure

- Place the patient supine with the wrist and hand in a relaxed position.
- Visually locate the MCPs, or knuckles.
- Grasp the MCP between the thumb and forefinger.
- While applying light pressure, roll over the dorsal and palmar aspects of the joint.
- Flex and extend the proximal phalange to discern the joint's articulation between the metacarpal and proximal phalange.
- Note the location of any tender points or fasciculatory response at the joint and its overlying tissues.
- Once the most dominant tender point or fasciculation (or both) has been determined, maintain light pressure with the pad(s) of the finger(s) at the location throughout the PRT treatment procedure until reassessment has occurred.

PRT Clinician Procedure

- Place the patient supine.
- With your near hand and fingers, stabilize the MCP joint and its immediate neighbors. The hand can be placed either on the table or with the elbow at 90°.
- With your far hand and fingers, apply long axis compression of the phalange toward the wrist.
- Apply phalange flexion with your far hand and fingers for palmar MCP points and extension for dorsal points.

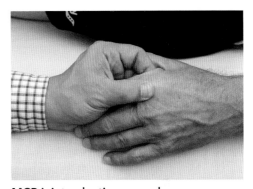

MCP joint palpation procedure.

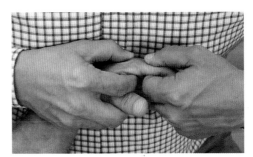

MCP joint PRT clinician procedure.

- Rotate the proximal phalange with your far hand and fingers.
- Apply extension and flexion of the metacarpal with the stabilizing fingers of your near hand.
- Corollary tissues treated: Extensor digitorum tendon, carpometacarpals

Proximal and Distal Interphalangeal Joints

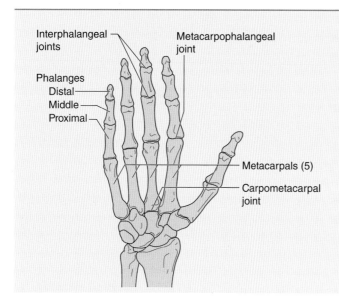

Lesions at the proximal and distal interphalangeal joints of the fingers often present with both acute and chronic injury or conditions such as a jammed finger, pulley rupture, and osteoarthritis. Each finger has two synovial hinge interphalangeal joints, proximal and distal, and the thumb has only a distal interphalangeal joint. Each joint is stabilized with collateral and palmar ligaments.

Palpation Procedure

- Place the patient's hand and wrist in a relaxed position.
- Flex the proximal joint to 90° of flexion.
- Start the palpation of the joint in its flexed position at the dorsal aspect.
- The joint line can be explored even though it is covered centrally by the extensor digitorum dorsal expansion.
- Move to the collateral ligaments and strum across them; then strum across the ventral aspect of the joint.
- To palpate the distal joint, repeat the procedure performed on the proximal joint.
- Note the location of any tender points or fasciculatory response at the joint and its overlying tissues.
- Once the most dominant tender point or fasciculation (or both) has been determined, maintain light pressure with the pad(s) of the finger(s) at the location throughout the PRT treatment procedure until reassessment has occurred.

PRT Clinician Procedure

- Place the patient's hand in a relaxed and supported position on the table or your thigh.
- Grasp both sides of the joint with the forefingers and thumbs of both hands.
- Palpate the lesion with one of your near forefingers.
- Using the fingers of both hands, apply compression to the joint.
- Extend the joint for dorsal lesions, and apply flexion for palmar lesions.

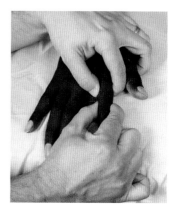

Proximal and distal interphalangeal joints palpation procedure.

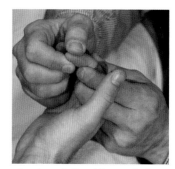

Proximal and distal interphalangeal joints PRT clinician procedure.

- Apply a valgus force for medial lesions and a varus force for lateral lesions.
- Apply rotation with either hand.
- Corollary tissues treated: MCP joints, extensor and flexor tendons or slips, digital collateral ligaments

Lumbricals of the Hand

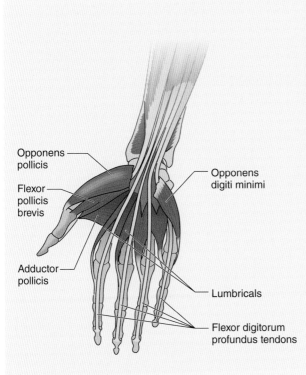

Opponens pollicis

Flexor pollicis brevis

Adductor pollicis

Opponens digiti minimi

Lumbricals

Flexor digitorum profundus tendons

The lumbricals of the hand join both the flexor and extensor tendon systems of the hand and fingers. The lumbricals arise from the flexor digitorum profundus tendon to join the extensor hood of the radial side of each middle phalange (2 through 5). Because they have a relationship with both the flexors and extensors of the fingers, the lumbricals assist with both actions at the fingers. However, they are covered by the palmar aponeurosis, occluding direct palpation of these tissues as well as the palmar interossei.

Origin: Flexor digitorum profundus tendon (second through fifth digits)

Insertion: Extensor digitorum expansion, radial side of the corresponding digit

Action: Metatarsophalangeal joint flexion (second through fifth), proximal interphalangeal (PIP) and distal interphalangeal (DIP) extension, fifth digit opposition

Innervation: First and second lumbricals: C8-T1 (median nerve)

Third and fourth lumbricals: C8-T1 (ulnar nerve)

Palpation Procedure

- Place the wrist and hand in a relaxed flexed position on the treatment table or your thigh.
- Grasp each metacarpal with your thumb and forefinger, with your thumb over the palmar side.
- Roll your thumb off the metacarpal and into the space between it and the adjacent metacarpal.
- While stabilizing the metacarpal(s) on the dorsal side with your forefinger, strum deeply between them and along their shafts.
- *Note:* Use indirect pressure to assess lesions at this location.
- Note the location of any tender points or fasciculatory response between the metacarpals and in their overlying tissues.
- Determine the most dominant tender point or fasciculation (or both) and maintain light pressure with the pad(s) of the finger(s) throughout the treatment until reassessment has occurred.

PRT Clinician Procedure

- Place the patient's hand and wrist in a supported and flexed position on your thigh or the treatment table and cup the dorsum of the hand and fingers in your far hand.
- Apply flexion as well as adduction to the metacarpals and fingers with your far hand.

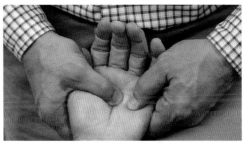

Lumbricals of the hand palpation procedure.

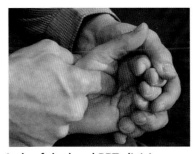

Lumbricals of the hand PRT clinician procedure.

- Adduct the metacarpals by squeezing the patient's hand together with your far hand.
- Rotate the metacarpals with your far hand for fine-tuning.
- Corollary tissues treated: Palmar interossei, palmar aponeurosis, metacarpophalangeal joints

Opponens Pollicis and Adductor Pollicis

The opponens and adductor pollicis share a common deep location within the thenar eminence of the thumb and also a similar function, which is why they are grouped for palpation and treatment. As their names indicate, these short muscles of the thumb bring it across the palm— the opponens pollicis to the fifth ray and the adductor pollicis to the second and third fingers.

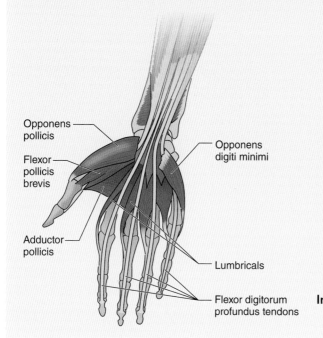

Opponens pollicis

Flexor pollicis brevis

Adductor pollicis

Opponens digiti minimi

Lumbricals

Flexor digitorum profundus tendons

Origin: Opponens pollicis: Trapezium, flexor retinaculum

Adductor pollicis: Capitate, bases of the second and third metacarpals, flexor retinaculum

Insertion: Opponens pollicis: Entire radial side of the first metacarpal

Adductor pollicis: Thumb (proximal phalange base, ulnar side), extensor retinaculum (medial aspect of the thumb)

Action: Opponens pollicis: Opposition (flexion, abduction, and medial rotation of the CMC joint)

Adductor pollicis: CMC joint adduction; assists with MCP adduction and flexion

Innervation: C8-T1 (ulnar nerve, and also median nerve for opponens pollicis)

Palpation Procedure

- Place the patient's wrist and hand in a relaxed position.
- Locate the base of the first metacarpal and place your thumb over this location with your fingers on the dorsal wrist for stabilization.
- Strum firmly over the base of the first metacarpal and through the superficial and intermediate thenar muscles to apply indirect palpatory pressure to the opponens pollicis.
- The inferior fibers of the adductor pollicis can be felt at the web space between the thumb and forefinger. To identify these fingers, have the patient oppose the thumb and forefinger and then apply firm strumming to the adductor pollicis.
- Note the location of any tender points or fasciculatory response at the muscles and their attachments.
- Once the most dominant tender point or fasciculation (or both) has been determined, maintain light pressure with the pad(s) of the finger(s) at the location throughout the PRT treatment procedure until reassessment has occurred.

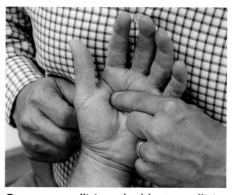

Opponens pollicis and adductor pollicis palpation procedure.

PRT Clinician Procedure

- Place the patient's wrist and hand in a supported position on your chest, thigh, or the table.
- With your far hand, apply marked first metacarpal adduction toward the medial wrist for the opponens and toward the third ray for the adductor pollicis.
- With the far hand, apply flexion and rotation to the first metacarpal for the opponens and adductor. Also apply third finger and metacarpal flexion toward the thumb for the adductor pollicis with either hand.
- Corollary tissues treated: Palmar interossei, lumbricals, abductor pollicis brevis, flexor pollicis brevis

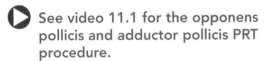 **See video 11.1 for the opponens pollicis and adductor pollicis PRT procedure.**

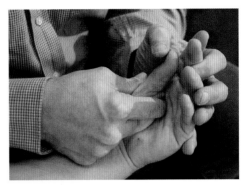

Opponens pollicis and adductor pollicis PRT clinician procedure.

Abductor Pollicis Brevis and Flexor Pollicis Brevis

The abductor and flexor pollicis brevis are the superficial and intermediate muscles that form the thenar eminence of the thumb along with their deeper neighbors, the opponens pollicis and adductor pollicis. As their names denote, they abduct and flex the thumb. The individual bellies of these muscles are difficult to differentiate from one another; therefore, they are palpated and treated as a group.

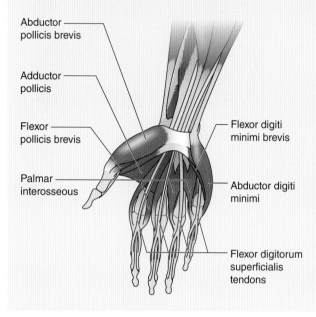

Abductor pollicis brevis
Adductor pollicis
Flexor pollicis brevis
Palmar interosseous
Flexor digiti minimi brevis
Abductor digiti minimi
Flexor digitorum superficialis tendons

Origin: Abductor pollicis brevis: Flexor retinaculum, scaphoid, trapezium, abductor pollicis longus tendon

Flexor pollicis brevis: Flexor retinaculum and trapezium (superficial head) and trapezoid; capitate and palmar ligaments (deep head)

Insertion: Abductor pollicis brevis: Proximal radial base of the first phalange

Flexor pollicis brevis: Proximal ulnar base of the first phalange

Action: Carpometacarpal (CMC) and MCP joint abduction, thumb opposition

Innervation: Abductor pollicis brevis: C8-T1 (median nerve)

Flexor pollicis brevis: C8-T1 (superficial head: median nerve; deep head: ulnar nerve)

Palpation Procedure

- Place the patient's hand in a relaxed position.
- Grasp the thenar eminence with your thumb and forefinger, and place the thumb on the dorsal metacarpal for stabilization.
- Start at the MCP joint of the thumb and strum toward it, capturing both the abductor and flexor pollicis brevis; use the metacarpal as a base against which to apply palpatory pressure.
- Continue the palpation down the thumb toward the wrist.
- Note the location of any tender points or fasciculatory response at the muscles and their attachments.
- Determine the most dominant tender point or fasciculation (or both) and maintain light pressure with the pad(s) of the finger(s) throughout the treatment until reassessment has occurred.

PRT Clinician Procedure

- Place the patient's hand and wrist on your chest, thigh, or the treatment table.
- With your far hand, apply marked thumb flexion.
- Apply adduction to the first metacarpal with your far hand.
- Apply long axis compression to the first metacarpal with the thumb of your far hand.
- Rotate the thumb with your far hand to fine-tune.

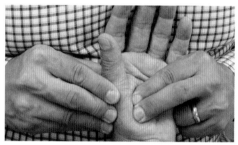

Abductor pollicis brevis and flexor pollicis brevis palpation procedure.

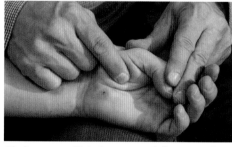

Abductor pollicis brevis and flexor pollicis brevis PRT clinician procedure.

- Corollary tissues treated: Opponens pollicis, adductor pollicis

 See video 11.2 for the abductor pollicis brevis and flexor pollicis brevis PRT procedure.

Dorsal Interossei of the Hand

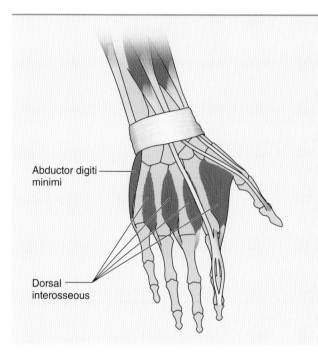

Abductor digiti minimi

Dorsal interosseous

The dorsal interossei of the hand are accessible to palpation between the metacarpals. The four bipennate dorsal interossei muscles arise from the sides of each of the metacarpals. Their primary function is finger abduction.

Origin: Sides of the first through fourth metacarpals

Insertion: Dorsal extensor expansion, base of the associated proximal phalanges

Action: Finger abduction; assist with flexion of the MCP joints and extension of the interphalangeal (IP) joints, as well as thumb abduction

Innervation: C8-T1 (ulnar nerve)

Palpation Procedure

- Place the patient's wrist and hand in a relaxed position.
- Grasp the patient's hand with your thumb on the palmar hand for stabilization and your forefinger between the metacarpals.
- Stroke up and down each side of the metacarpals and the overlying interossei.
- Note the location of any tender points or fasciculatory response along the metacarpals and their interossei.
- Once the most dominant tender point or fasciculation (or both) has been determined, maintain light pressure with the pad(s) of the finger(s) at the location throughout the PRT treatment procedure until reassessment has occurred.

PRT Clinician Procedure

- Place the patient's hand and wrist in a supported position on your thigh or the treatment table.
- While stabilizing the hand against your thigh or the table with your near hand, use one of the fingers for palpation while also extending the phalange with your far hand.
- Using your far hand, abduct and adduct the opposing phalanges together for the area being treated.
- Apply rotation to the phalanges with your far hand and fingers.
- Corollary tissues treated: Wrist extensor tendons, metatarsophalangeal joints, CMC joints, extensor digitorum

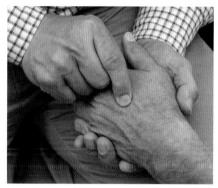

Dorsal interossei of the hand palpation procedure.

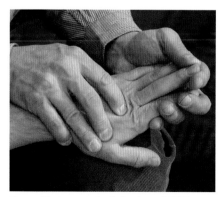

Dorsal interossei of the hand PRT clinician procedure.

Wrist Extensor Tendons

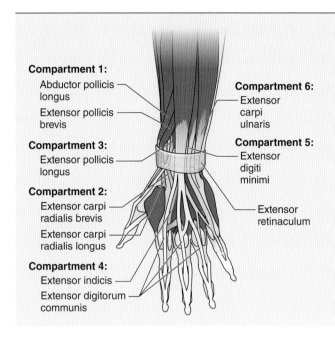

Compartment 1:
Abductor pollicis longus
Extensor pollicis brevis

Compartment 3:
Extensor pollicis longus

Compartment 2:
Extensor carpi radialis brevis
Extensor carpi radialis longus

Compartment 4:
Extensor indicis
Extensor digitorum communis

Compartment 6:
Extensor carpi ulnaris

Compartment 5:
Extensor digiti minimi

Extensor retinaculum

The wrist extensor tendons (extensor carpi radialis longus and brevis, extensor carpi ulnaris, and extensor digitorum) crossing at the wrist may also exhibit osteopathic lesions. Lesions of the extensor tendons are often the result of repetitive eccentric wrist flexion or an acute injury such as falling on an outstretched arm.

Palpation Procedure

- Position the patient supine with the wrist in a relaxed position.
- Start palpation at about 1 cm (just under 1/2 in.) medial to the radial styloid. The two tendons crossing the wrist at this location are the extensor carpi radialis longus and brevis. The lateral tendon is the longus, which can be followed to the base of the second metacarpal. The medial brevis tendon can be traced to its distal insertion on the third metacarpal. Moving medially across the wrist, the extensor digitorum tendon can be found almost at the center of the wrist, medial to the extensor pollicis longus tendon. The extensor carpi ulnaris can be found just lateral to the styloid process of the ulna.
- Strum across the wrist extensor tendons with one or two fingers, moving to the next tendon.
- Note the location of any tender points or fasciculatory response at the tendons and their attachments.
- Determine the most dominant tender point or fasciculation (or both) and maintain light pressure with the pad(s) of the finger(s) throughout the treatment until reassessment has occurred.

PRT Clinician Procedure

- Place the patient supine with the elbow flexed to approximately 90°.
- With your far hand on the patient's palm, apply marked wrist extension.
- Apply wrist deviation and rotation with your far hand to target specific wrist tendons (e.g., radial deviation for the extensor carpi radialis).

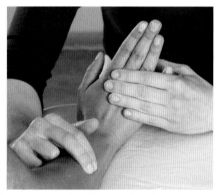

Wrist extensor tendons palpation procedure.

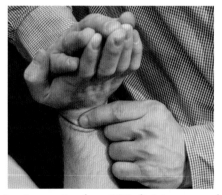

Wrist extensor tendons PRT clinician procedure.

- Using your far hand, apply light compression at the wrist toward the elbow.
- Corollary tissues treated: Extensor group, common extensor tendon

Extensor Pollicis Longus and Brevis Tendons

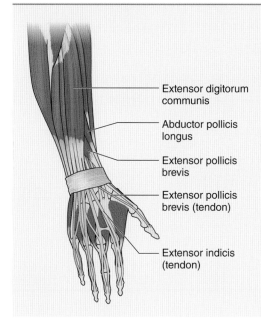

Extensor digitorum communis

Abductor pollicis longus

Extensor pollicis brevis

Extensor pollicis brevis (tendon)

Extensor indicis (tendon)

The tendons of the extensor pollicis longus and brevis form the borders of the anatomic snuff box at the posterior thumb. The scaphoid bone, or navicular, is located within the snuff box and can be a site of tenderness when a fracture is present. Because the extensor pollicis longus and brevis tendons course upward to the middle of the posterior forearm, deep to the forearm extensors, these tendons are not accessible to palpation. Lesions of these tendons are often present with conditions such as osteoarthritis of the CMC joint of the thumb and de Quervain syndrome.

Origin: Extensor pollicis longus: Ulna (middle of the posterior shaft)

Extensor pollicis brevis: Radius (posterior shaft)

Insertion: Thumb (base of the proximal dorsal phalange)

Action: Extension of the interphalangeal joints of the thumb including the CMC and MP joints; assist with radial deviation of the wrist

Innervation: C8-T1 (median nerve)

Palpation Procedure

- Place the patient's hand in a neutral, supported position with the thumb pointing up.
- To visually identify both tendons, ask the patient to pull the thumb upward and back to reveal the border of the anatomic snuff box.
- Starting at the MP joint of the thumb, strum over each of the tendons (the brevis is most medial when the hand is in a neutral position and is the smaller of the two) to the wrist joint.
- Note the location of any tender points or fasciculatory response at the tendons and their attachments.
- Once the most dominant tender point or fasciculation (or both) has been determined, maintain light pressure with the pad(s) of the finger(s) at the location throughout the PRT treatment procedure until reassessment has occurred.

PRT Clinician Procedure

- Place the patient's wrist and hand in a neutral, supported position.
- Apply marked thumb extension with your far hand or fingers.
- Apply compression of the thumb toward the wrist with your far hand.
- Using your far hand and fingers, apply rotation to the thumb.
- Fine-tune the treatment by applying abduction and adduction to the thumb with your far hand.
- Corollary tissues treated: Abductor pollicis longus, extensor carpi radialis tendon at the wrist

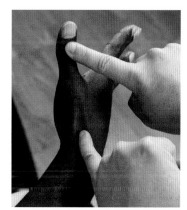

Extensor pollicis longus and brevis tendons palpation procedure.

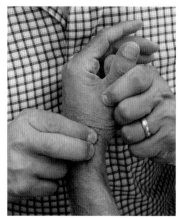

Extensor pollicis longus and brevis tendons PRT clinician procedure.

De Quervain Syndrome

De Quervain syndrome, or disease, results from a thickening of the synovial sheath of the extensor pollicis brevis (EPB) and abductor pollicis longus (APL) tendons, which decreases the space within the first dorsal compartment in which they function (Shaefer and Speier 2012). The etiology of the condition is not well understood, but Sharan and Ajeesh (2012) found a 7.41% incidence in an adult sample who reported excessive text messaging. Shaefer and Speier (2012) observed that the condition was prevalent among instrumental athletes (musicians). Patel, Kashyap, Tadisina, and Gonzalez (2013) reported on studies that indicate that the tendon sheaths demonstrate thickening and fibrotic nodules, but an absence of an inflammatory process. Therefore, the reported success (62 to 93%) of cortisone injection (Patel et al. 2013) is confounding because no inflammation is present. Traditional treatment of de Quervain syndrome involves cortisone injections, anti-inflammatory medications, splinting, and physical medicine and rehabilitation (PMR). Surgical decompression of the first dorsal compartment is typically reserved for when conservative therapy has failed.

Given the risks involved with surgery and cortisone injections, clinicians would do well to explore the use of PRT as a nonpainful alternative for decompressing the EPB and APL tendons at the first dorsal compartment. Release of these tendons and their muscles may reduce thickening and fascial restriction at the compartment and reduce chronic inflammation, if present.

Common Signs and Symptoms

- Pain at the anatomical snuff box and the radial side of the wrist that may radiate into the forearm
- Thumb motion that is painful with decreased motion
- Point tenderness over the CMC joint and overlying tendons at the dorsal thumb and radial wrist
- Decreased pinch and grip strength
- Pain with gripping and active and passive ulnar deviation
- Positive Finkelstein's test

Treatment Points and Sequencing

1. Extensor pollicis longus and brevis tendons
2. CMC joint of the thumb
3. Lateral epicondyle and common extensor tendon
4. Brachioradialis
5. Extensors of the wrist and fingers (extensor group)
6. Pronator teres
7. Medial epicondyle and common flexor tendon

Common Differential Diagnoses

- Scaphoid fracture of the wrist
- Abductor pollicis and extensor pollicis tendon tear
- Intersection syndrome
- Osteoarthritis of the thumb and CMC joint
- Wartenberg's syndrome

Clinician Therapeutic Interventions

- In addition to evaluating the wrist and hand, assess proximal upper-extremity tissues for weakness and osteopathic lesions that may also be affecting the function of the wrist and hand (e.g., the elbow and shoulder).
- Determine aggravating movements to eliminate or modify them in the early phases of rehabilitation.
- Apply PRT to the tendons and affected tissues to normalize tissue tonicity and reduce pain and spasm.
- Following PRT, apply thermal modalities (e.g., ultrasound, laser, diathermy) to increase blood flow and extensibility of the tendons and joint.
- Consider mobilizations of the CMC joint, wrist, and elbow to restore normal arthrokinematics and encourage joint nourishment.
- When the tissues are warm, apply myofascial release, massage, or other therapeutic techniques to encourage collagen reorganization.

- Apply instrumented soft tissue mobilization in a nonpainful manner to encourage collagen reorganization and the reduction of myofascial restriction.
- The use of KT Tape or splinting early in rehabilitation may provide relief, particularly during sleep.

Patient Self-Treatment Interventions

- Attempt to self-release tissues daily (e.g., pronator teres).

- Apply heat to the affected tissues (20 to 30 minutes).
- Self-massage the affected tendons daily (five to eight minutes).
- After exercise or rehabilitation, stretch the affected tissues daily in a nonpainful manner.
- Apply ice if an acute flare-up occurs.

Gamekeeper's Thumb

Acute or chronic injury of the ulnar collateral ligament (UCL) of the thumb is a common injury seen with athletic activity; it is often called gamekeeper's or skier's thumb (Patel et al. 2010). Campbell (1955) was the first to describe the injury after finding a high incidence of UCL injury in Scottish gamekeepers who used their hands to break the necks of rabbits. However, the injury can also result from falling on an outstretched arm, a ball hitting the end of the thumb, or the thumb getting caught in the drop of a ski pole; the mechanism of injury dictates the term used (Mahajan and Rhemrev 2013). A partial or full rupture of the ligament occurs when the thumb's MCP joint receives either a repetitive or traumatic valgus force resulting in excessive abduction and hyperextension.

The MCP joint of the thumb receives its primary static support from the UCL of the thumb, which has two parts, the proper collateral ligament (PCL) and the accessory collateral ligament (ACL). The shape of the joint along with the dorsal capsule and volar plate also provide static stability to the MCP joint (Mahajan and Rhemrev 2013). Dynamically, the muscles of the thumb provide stability, particularly the adductor pollicis (Mahajan and Rhemrev 2013). When the dynamic stabilizers fail, the static stabilizers are often injured. The nature of the evaluation and treatment to be performed are based on whether the PCL or the ACL ligament is injured.

Caution must be exercised when assessing the severity of gamekeeper's thumb. Because a ligamentous laxity test may disrupt the ligament or bony avulsion fragments further, radiographs should be taken prior to ligamentous testing to rule out fracture or partial tendon avulsion. An MRI follow-up helps to ascertain the extent of UCL disruption (Koplay et al. 2014). If ligamentous laxity without a firm end point is found in full extension, then both ligaments are injured indicating a complete tear. When a complete tear is suspected, a Stener lesion is likely present (Koplay et al. 2014). A Stener lesion occurs when the distal end of the UCL is caught between the adductor aponeurosis and the bone (Mahajan and Rhemrev 2013). A small bump may be felt at the ulnar side of the joint. Because the ligament–bone interface is blocked by the aponeurosis, it has been proposed that the UCL will not heal and,

Treatment Points and Sequencing
1. UCL of the thumb
2. Adductor pollicis
3. Opponens pollicis
4. Abductor or flexor pollicis, or both
5. Dorsal interossei
6. Extensor pollicis longus
7. Lateral epicondyle and common extensor tendon

therefore, requires surgical intervention (Koplay et al. 2014; Mahajan and Rhemrev 2013).

It is generally agreed that patients with complete tears should pursue surgery and those with incomplete tears should receive immobilization for four to six weeks followed by hand therapy (Patel et al. 2010). Werner and colleagues (2014) reported favorable long-term outcomes for 17 U.S. collegiate football players who underwent anchor repair of the UCL; however, they did not use a comparison group. To date, no evidence exists suggesting that a surgical or nonsurgical route is optimal for treating a complete UCL rupture.

PRT can be used for both acute and chronic partial and complete UCL tears because it does not involve a valgus stress to the joint. In fact, it does just the opposite: it closes the joint to relax the MCP capsule, UCL, and associated tissues. Therefore, PRT is an excellent intervention in the acute stage of injury because of its ability to reduce pain and associated somatic dysfunction. PRT can also address chronic osteopathic lesions that reside in static and dynamic tissues without disrupting the UCL ligament. However, imaging should still be done to assess the severity of the injury to determine whether surgery is required. Additionally, if the patient is not casted, PRT can be performed on the affected tissues by removing the splint, if used.

Common Signs and Symptoms

- History of trauma or repeated strain to the MCP joint
- Pain and swelling at the MCP joint
- Point tenderness over the MCP joint
- Pincer grip weakness

- Pain and functional difficulty with routine ADL tasks (activities of daily living such as grasping objects, opening jars, and turning keys and door knobs)
- Ecchymosis at the UCL with acute injury
- Small nodular mass at the MCP joint

Common Differential Diagnoses

- Osteoarthritis of the MCP joint
- Stener lesion
- Phalangeal fracture
- MCP joint dislocation

Clinician Therapeutic Interventions

- Primary to ligamentous testing, order radiographs to rule out the presence of facture and ligamentous avulsion. An MRI is helpful for determining the extent of the tear. However, because pain may limit ligamentous findings, laxity testing may be done with an anesthetic by a physician.
- Treat pain and spasm as soon as possible with PRT; then stabilize the joint with either a splint or cast to avoid reaggravation.
- Continue PRT during the immobilization phase as long as the manipulations do not cause pain.

- Once the immobilization phase is over, the patient should undergo therapy for the hand and possibly the forearm and elbow to improve dynamic and static stabilization of the UCL at the thumb.
- Use traditional modalities (e.g., laser, ultrasound) to facilitate an optimal healing environment of the UCL of the thumb.
- Consider grade I and II joint mobilizations for partial UCL tears; apply them throughout the rehabilitation process to help control pain and spasm and limit abnormal scar formation.

Patient Self-Treatment Interventions

- If not casted, wear a splint throughout the day, particularly when sleeping, to avoid reaggravation.
- Use palliative modalities to control pain, swelling, and spasm.
- Daily self-massage may provide relief.
- Compression tape may help to control soft tissue swelling at the joint.
- Perform daily mobilization exercise as directed by the attending therapist or physician.

Summary

Injuries to the wrist and hand pose a significant financial and health care burden, particularly when left untreated. A Danish population-based study revealed that hand and wrist injuries cost the most of any type of injury annually ($740 million in U.S. dollars); the greatest cost is to productivity rather than health care (De Putter et al. 2012). Using ultrasound imaging of 35 patients with recent inflammatory arthritis of the wrist, Navalho and colleagues (2012) found that the majority showed tenosynovitis of the extensor carpi ulnaris and at the flexor tendon of the second finger as well as radiocarpal joint synovitis. This was significantly associated with the development of early rheumatory arthritis (ERA) at a one-year follow-up. Although a similar association has not been made for de Quervain syndrome (Shaefer and Speier 2012), the chronic inflammation that may develop and persist at the thumb and wrist coupled with implications for an impact on the carpometacarpal (CMC) joint may suggests a threat of the development of ERA.

The ability of PRT to address the etiology of tenosynovitis or osteoarthritis of the wrist and fingers is unknown. However, releasing hypertonic tissues in the wrist and hand may improve tissue perfusion, increase ATP production, and limit the propensity for the development of peripheral and central sensitization. It may also address complex regional pain syndrome (CRPS), an extremely painful disorder known to be associated with one of the most common wrist injuries, the fracture (Moseley et al. 2014).

CHAPTER 12

Cranium

Regis Turocy, DHCE, MPT, PRT-c

CHAPTER OBJECTIVES

After reading this chapter, you should be able to do the following:

1. Locate the structures of the craniofacial system.

2. Appreciate that the craniofacial system is like any other part of the body and can be a source of direct or referred pain, or both.

3. Palpate key anatomical reference points on the cranium.

4. Locate and palpate craniofacial structures to be treated with positional release therapy (PRT).

5. Treat tender points on craniofacial structures with PRT.

The evaluation and treatment of the cranium has been controversial since the 1939 publication of William G. Sutherland's book *The Cranial Bowl.* His initial writings were an attempt to incite professional interest in cranio-membranous-articular mobility and the involvement of the cranium in somatic dysfunction. Dr. Sutherland's premise was that the bones of the cranium and face have mobility: "There is mobility throughout the articulations of the craniofacial bones which is a primary requisite to the consideration of cranial membranous articular strains or lesions as etiologic factors found frequently in association with head maladies" (Sutherland 1939, 23). This was a radical idea that contradicted what was written in the American and British anatomy texts of that time. Since then, numerous other parallel and derivative approaches to treating the cranium have been proposed, including craniopathy (Chaitow 1999), sacro-occipital techniques (DeJarnett 1975, 1978), and craniosacral therapy (Upledger and Vredevoogd 1983). These writings have added to the confusion and debate regarding the theories that underpin the methodologies involved in treating the cranium.

Although numerous practitioners are attracted to the dramatic results claimed by those who use these methodologies, skepticism about the science of cranial therapy remains (Becker 1977). Dr. Lawrence Jones, who developed the strain counterstrain (SCS) approach for treating somatic dysfunction, believes that the cranium is like any other part of the body and can present with tender points from either direct or indirect trauma to its structures or related structures (Jones et al. 1995). His treatment approach is based on sound neurophysiological principles, and it is the basis for the evaluation and treatment of the cranium within the neurophysiological framework of PRT, as discussed in chapter 2. Using common tender point locations is an evaluative and diagnostic tool in the treatment of craniofacial somatic dysfunction.

Many common craniofacial conditions are interrelated, suggesting that dysfunction in one area may cause symptomology in another area. Nociceptive input in one area can produce secondary reflex muscle contractions and, if prolonged, can contribute to the development of myofascial trigger points in associated areas (Simons, Travell, and Simons 1999). For example, there is a close association between the trigeminal neurons and those of C1 and C2 (Bogduk 1998). Sustaining a forward head posture can facilitate the muscles of mastication as well as produce atypical facial pain. Not only will tender points be found in the region of the upper cervical spine, but the masseter, temporalis, and pterygoids could also exhibit tender points (Simons et al. 1999). Another example is chest breathers whose abnormal breathing patterns produce excessive stress in the supra- and infrahyoid regions. Prolonged stress in these areas can alter mandibular function creating reflex muscle spasm in the muscles of mastication and atypical facial pain (Simons et al. 1999). Because of their interrelatedness, the evaluation of the head, neck, and masticatory and stomatognathic systems (speech, swallowing, eating) can be daunting.

It is beyond the scope of this chapter to provide an all-inclusive and effective treatment approach for using PRT for all of the abnormal conditions that can produce craniofacial pain. However, common cranial conditions that can be treated readily with PRT are presented. Rocabado and Iglarsh's text *Musculoskeletal Approach to Maxillofacial Pain* (1991) provides a more thorough review of craniofacial dysfunction and treatment.

A plethora of pathology can produce craniofacial pain, but one of the most common is myofascial in origin (Simons et al. 1999). Myofascial pain can influence the intracranial pain pathways and their interconnections, especially the trigeminocervical pathways (Dutton 2004) involving the atlanto-occipital joint (Dreyfuss, Michaelson, and Fletcher 1994), atlanto-axial joint (Ehni 1984), C2 spinal nerve (Bovin, Berg, and Dale 1992), and temporomandibular joint (TMJ). One of the most common complaints of involvement of these associated areas is benign headache. Pain distribution from these interrelated pathways can be to the frontal region, orbit, vertex (C1), temporal and suboccipital regions (C1 and C2), occiput, mastoid, and frontal regions (C3) (Dutton 2004). These benign headaches can be classified as tension-type headaches, occipital headaches, or cervicogenic-type headaches (Dutton 2004).

Dutton (2004) provided additional considerations when assessing headache. Following are signs and symptoms requiring neurological assessment:

- Headaches that are sudden, severe, and diffuse

- Headaches that awaken one from sleep
- Headaches associated with projectile vomiting, but not nausea
- Unilateral pulsating pain in synchrony with the heartbeat
- Headaches that worsen with activity or exertion
- Headaches that begin or worsen with recumbency
- Focal tenderness over the temporal artery in someone over age 60
- Sudden, intense, sharp pain of short duration that is either spontaneous or triggered by a mild stimulus
- Severe pain around sinuses or teeth
- Headaches associated with other symptoms
- Cognitive impairment
- Visual disturbances
- Numbness or altered sensation
- Loss of strength or coordination
- Loss or alteration of smell, taste, or hearing
- Fever or associated systemic illness
- Difficulty swallowing
- Loss or impairment of voice or chronic cough

As a general rule, most health care providers receive only a cursory exposure to the cranium and its structures. This chapter does not provide an exhaustive anatomical description of the craniofacial complex. However, therapists pursuing the treatment of the cranium as part of their therapeutic armamentarium should have knowledge of the cranial structures. Numerous American and British anatomical texts that address the external and internal cranial structures are available. Following are a few anatomical points to facilitate the treatment of cranial structures with PRT.

The human cranium is made up of 8 cranial bones and 14 facial bones (figure 12.1). These bones help protect the organs involved in motor control, equilibrium, cognition, emotion, vision, hearing, taste, and smell. They also provide for the attachment of muscles that move the head, control facial expression, and facilitate mastication, which are some of the strongest muscles in the body (figure 12.2).

The following pages present therapeutic techniques for the craniofacial structures. Tender points on select osseous landmarks are provided to facilitate treatment as previously identified by D'Ambrogio and Roth (1997) and Jones and colleagues (1996). When applicable, muscle origin, insertion, action, and innervation are presented to assist in determining the origin of the osteopathic lesion (Biel 1989; Warwick and Williams 1973).

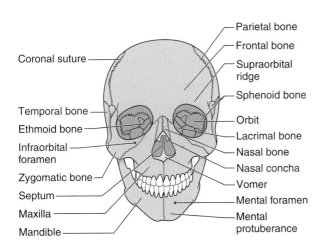
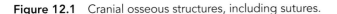
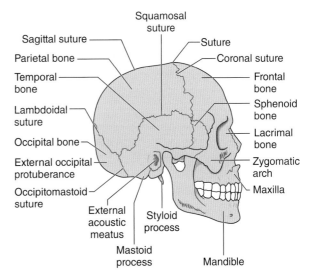

Figure 12.1 Cranial osseous structures, including sutures.

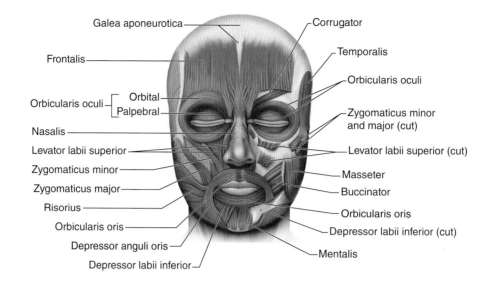

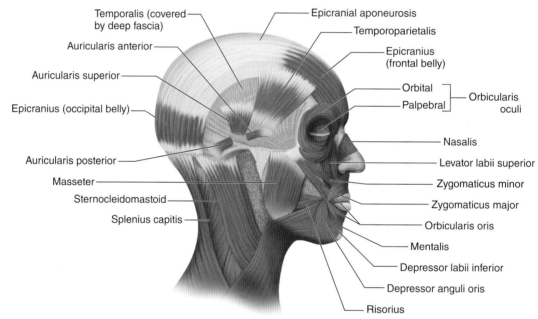

Figure 12.2 Muscles of the cranium.

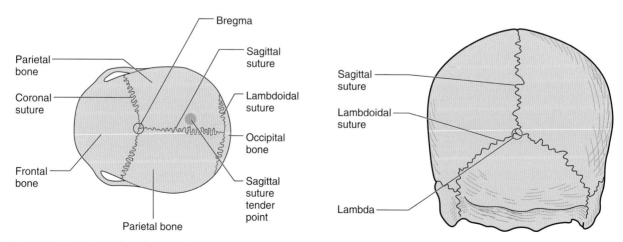

Figure 12.3 Sagittal and coronal sutures.

Figure 12.4 Posterior sutures.

General Procedures for Cranial Sutures

Greenman (2003) provided a palpation exercise to identify the sutures in a living subject (figure 12.1). Practitioners should perform this exercise numerous times on multiple patients until they are confident of their ability to palpate these landmarks of the skull.

1. Palpate the depression at the top of the nose and between the orbits. This is the junction of the two nasal bones and the frontal bone called the nasion.

2. Proceed laterally over the upper margin of the orbit and follow laterally and inferiorly and feel the frontal zygomatic suture.

3. Continue inferiorly along the lateral aspect of the orbit and begin to move medially to feel the zygomaticomaxillary suture.

4. Continue medially along the inferior aspect of the orbit, moving to the superior aspect to palpate the suture of the maxillonasal junction and the maxillofrontal suture.

5. Return to the nasion and move upward between the two supraorbital ridges of the frontal bone; the midline depression is the glabella.

6. Continue to move toward the vertex of the skull in the midline and palpate a depression approximately one third of the way posteriorly on the vertex. This depression is the junction of the sagittal and coronal sutures and the remnant of the fontanel called the bregma (figure 12.3).

7. Moving posteriorly from the bregma along the midline, the sagittal suture is palpable.

8. Starting from the bregma, palpate bilaterally along the coronal suture feeling the junction of the frontal and parietal bone on each side. At the lower end of the coronal suture, the palpating finger will move deeper; palpate the junction of the sphenoid, frontal, parietal, and temporal bones. This junction is termed the pterion. The inferior aspect of this junction is the greater wing of the sphenoid (figure 12.2).

9. From the pterion, follow the suture line posteriorly along the junction of the parietal and temporal squama. This suture courses over the top of the ear in a circular fashion and ends just posterior to the ear.

10. Moving straight posteriorly from the posterior, inferior aspect of the suture between the parietal and the temporal squama, you will come to a short suture between the parietal bone and the mastoid portion of the temporal bone. At the posterior aspect of this suture is a slight depression at the junction of the parietal bone, the mastoid portion of the temporal bone, and the occiput called the asterion (figure 12.2).

11. From the asterion on each side, course medially and superiorly along the lambdoidal suture separating the parietal from the occipital squama. The point at which these two sutures join with the sagittal suture is called the lambda (figure 12.4).

Common Anatomical Areas and Conditions for PRT

Common Cranial Conditions

- Tension headache
- Migraine
- Temporomandibular dysfunction (TMD)
- Atypical facial pain

- Whiplash syndrome
- Forward head posture
- Abnormal breathing patterns (chest breathers)
- Concussion

Potential Causes of Craniofacial Pain

- Trauma
- Headache
- Occipital neuralgia
- TMD
- Upper cervical spine somatic dysfunction
- Osteoarthritis
- Rheumatoid arthritis and related rheumatoid arthritis variants (dermatomyositis, temporal arteritis)
- Lyme disease

- Fibromyalgia
- Arteriovenous malformation
- Intracranial infection (meningitis)
- Cerebrovascular disease
- Tumor
- Encephalitis
- Systemic infections
- Multiple sclerosis

Occipitomastoid

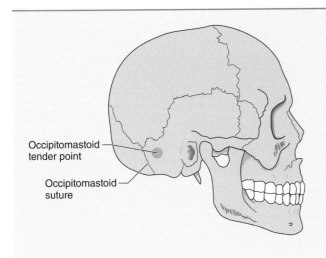

The occipitomastoid tender points can be found medial and superior to the mastoid process on the occipitomastoid suture. This area can be tender in patients with cervical spine dysfunction and concussion.

Occipitomastoid tender point

Occipitomastoid suture

Palpation Procedure

- Position the patient supine (can also be performed in seated position).
- Palpate the mastoid process and move medially (approximately two finger widths) and slightly superiorly.
- Ask the patient to exhale and apply pressure anteriorly and superiorly.
- Note the location of any tender points or fasciculatory response at the bony structure and its overlying tissue.
- Once you have determined the most dominant tender point or fasciculation (or both), maintain light pressure with the pad(s) of the finger(s) at the location throughout the PRT treatment procedure until reassessment has occurred.

PRT Clinician Procedure

- The patient is supine on the treatment table.
- Place a bolster under the patient's knees for comfort.
- Sit at the head of the table.
- For unilateral involvement, grasp the cranium with both hands with the thenar or hypothenar areas over the temporal bones and the inferior fingers on the tender tissues.
- Apply pressure medially while counterrotating the temporal bones around a transverse axis. Determine the direction of rotation based on patient comfort.
- For bilateral involvement, grasp the occiput in your near hand; your far hand should be just above the frontal bone. With your near hand, apply pressure in an anterior and caudal direc-

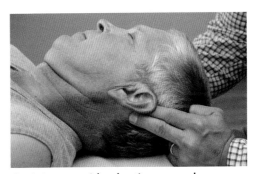

Occipitomastoid palpation procedure.

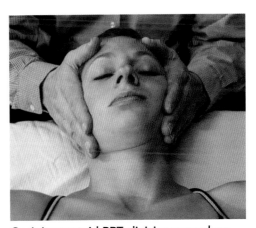

Occipitomastoid PRT clinician procedure.

tion on the occiput; with your far hand, apply pressure in a posterior and caudal direction on the frontal bone.

 See video 12.1 for the occipitomastoid PRT procedure.

Occipital

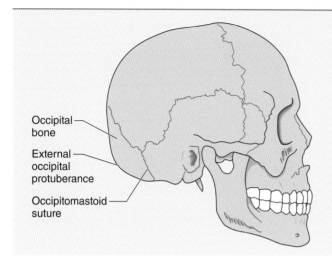

Occipital bone

External occipital protuberance

Occipitomastoid suture

Tender points are often present in the occipital region just slightly superior to the occipitomastoid tender point and approximately one to two finger widths from the posterior occipital protuberance. This area can be tender with cervical dysfunction, concussions, and headache.

Palpation Procedure

- The patient is supine or prone on the treatment table.
- Apply pressure anteriorly when you are over the region of the tender point.
- Note the location of any tender points or fasciculatory response at the bony structure and its overlying tissue.
- Once you have determined the most dominant tender point or fasciculation (or both), maintain light pressure with the pad(s) of the finger(s) at the location throughout the PRT treatment procedure until reassessment has occurred.

PRT Clinician Procedure

- The patient is supine on the treatment table.
- Place a bolster under the patient's knees for comfort.
- Sit at the head of the table.
- Grasp the occiput with the near hand.
- Place the far hand on the anterior aspect of the frontal bone.
- Apply an anterior-posterior (AP) pressure on the frontal bone with the far hand.
- A rolled towel can be placed under the superior shoulders to accentuate cranial extension.

Patient Self-Treatment Procedure

- Place a rolled towel under the superior shoulders and gently tuck the base of head in toward the shoulders to accentuate cranial extension.
- Palpate either side of the occiput for tenderness and the presence of a fasciculation.
- If tenderness is unilateral, flex the neck toward the tender side while monitoring for the stron-

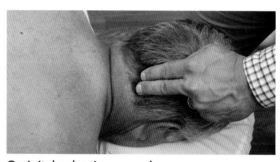

Occipital palpation procedure.

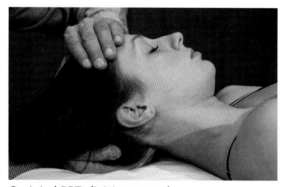

Occipital PRT clinician procedure.

gest fasciculation in the range or feeling of greatest comfort.
- When the greatest feeling of comfort or fasciculation has been found, rotate the head toward the tender point using the same approach for optimal positioning as previously done for cervical flexion toward the tender point.
- Maintain the self-treatment position until the fasciculation subsides or three to five minutes have elapsed, then move out of the position slowly.

Posterior Sphenobasilar

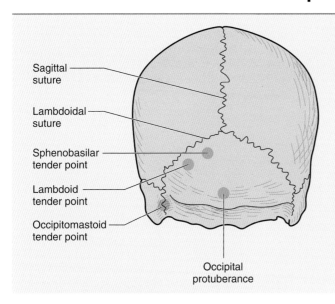

- Sagittal suture
- Lambdoidal suture
- Sphenobasilar tender point
- Lambdoid tender point
- Occipitomastoid tender point
- Occipital protuberance

Posterior sphenobasilar tender points are often located medial to the lambdoid suture approximately two finger widths superior to and two finger widths lateral to the occipital protuberance. This area can be tender with cervical dysfunction, headache, concussion, and sphenoid tenderness.

Palpation Procedure

- The patient is supine or prone on the treatment table.
- Apply pressure anteriorly when you are over the region of the tender point.
- Note the location of any tender points or fasciculatory response at the bony structure or overlying tissue.
- Once you have determined the most dominant tender point or fasciculation (or both), maintain light pressure with the pad(s) of the finger(s) at the location throughout the PRT treatment procedure until reassessment has occurred.

PRT Clinician Procedure

- The patient is supine on the treatment table.
- Place a bolster under the patient's knees for comfort.
- Sit at the head of the table.
- Grasp the occiput with the near hand and the frontal bone with the far hand. Apply a counterrotation force around an imaginary AP axis with the far hand. Determine the counterrotation direction based on patient comfort or a change in tender point tenderness.

 See video 12.2 for the posterior sphenobasilar PRT procedure.

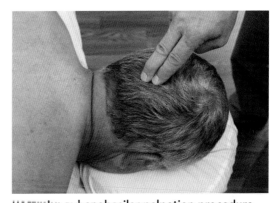

Posterior sphenobasilar palpation procedure.

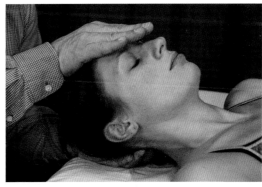

Posterior sphenobasilar PRT clinician procedure.

Stylohyoid

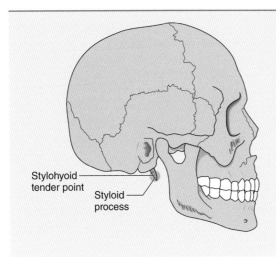

Stylohyoid — tender point
Styloid — process

Stylohyoid tender points are often found anterior and slightly medial to the mastoid process over the styloid process. This area can be tender with TMD and upper cervical spine dysfunction (whiplash syndrome).

Palpation Procedure

- The patient is supine on the treatment table.
- Place your palpating finger on the mastoid process. Then move your finger approximately one finger width anteriorly and slightly medially.
- Apply pressure medially.
- Note the location of any tender points or fasciculatory response at the bony structure or overlying tissue.
- Once you have determined the most dominant tender point or fasciculation (or both), maintain light pressure with the pad(s) of the finger(s) at the location throughout the PRT treatment procedure until reassessment has occurred

PRT Clinician Procedure

- The patient is supine on the treatment table.
- Place a bolster under the patient's knees for comfort.
- Use the index finger of your near hand to palpate the tender point. Grasp as much of the occiput as possible with your near hand and flex the upper cervical spine.
- Have the patient open the mouth slightly and then relax. Place your far hand on the opposite mandible and gently push the mandible toward the tender point.

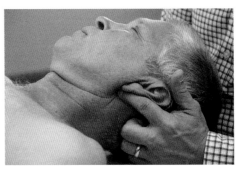

Stylohyoid palpation procedure.

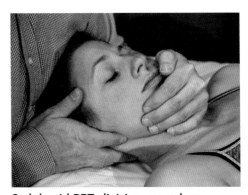

Stylohyoid PRT clinician procedure.

Maxilla

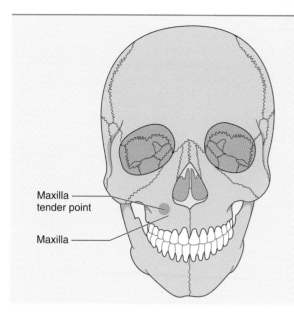

Maxilla tender point

Maxilla

Tender points at the maxilla are commonly found inferior to the infraorbital region approximately two finger widths lateral to the nose. Pressure is applied posteriorly. This point can be tender with sinus conditions, headache, blunt trauma to the eye socket, and TMD.

Palpation Procedure

- The patient is supine on the treatment table or seated.
- From the mid-infraorbital region, move your finger one finger width from the infraorbital foramen (two finger widths from the distal end of the nose).
- Note the location of any tender points or fasciculatory response at the bony structure or overlying tissue.
- Once you have determined the most dominant tender point or fasciculation (or both), maintain light pressure with the pad(s) of the finger(s) at the location throughout the PRT treatment procedure until reassessment has occurred.

PRT Clinician Procedure

- The patient is supine on the treatment table.
- Place a bolster under the patient's knees for comfort.
- Place the heels of your hands on the zygomatic portion of both maxillary bones. Apply a medial compression force bilaterally.

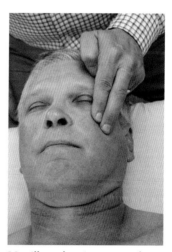

Maxilla palpation procedure.

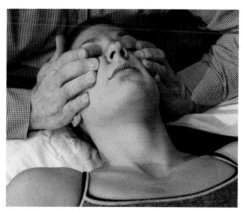

Maxilla PRT clinician procedure.

Nasal

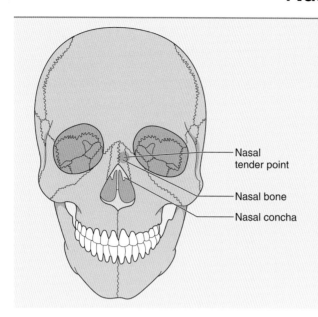

Nasal tender point

Nasal bone

Nasal concha

Tenderness at the nasal bone is often found on the anterolateral aspect of the nose (typically the bridge of the nose). This area can be tender in those with sinus problems, trauma to the nose, and nasolacrimal duct occlusion.

Palpation Procedure

- The patient is supine on the treatment table.
- From the nasion, move your palpating finger inferior one to one and a half finger widths and one finger width lateral to find the tender point on the nasal bone.
- Note the location of any tender points or fasciculatory response at the bony structure or overlying tissue.
- Once you have determined the most dominant tender point or fasciculation (or both), maintain light pressure with the pad(s) of the finger(s) at the location throughout the PRT treatment procedure until reassessment has occurred.

PRT Clinician Procedure

- The patient is supine on the treatment table.
- Place a bolster under the patient's knees for comfort.
- With the far hand, push the contralateral nasal bone medially toward the tender point.

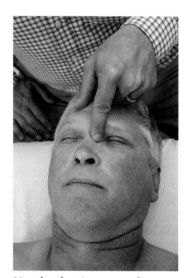

Nasal palpation procedure.

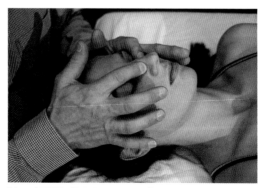

Nasal PRT clinician procedure.

Supraorbital

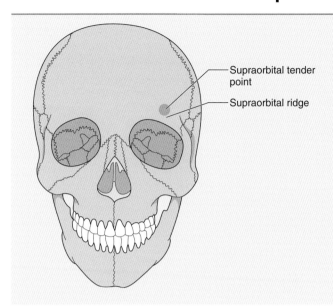

Tender points at the supraorbital ridge often manifest on the inner edge of the orbit near the supraorbital foramen. This point can be tender in those with sinus problems, headaches, visual disturbances, and concussions.

Palpation Procedure

- The patient is supine on the treatment table.
- Stabilize the cranium with the opposite hand.
- From the nasion, the tender points are often found one to one and a half finger widths laterally near the supraorbital foramen.
- Note the location of any tender points or fasciculatory response at the bony structure or overlying tissue.
- Once you have determined the most dominant tender point or fasciculation (or both), maintain light pressure with the pad(s) of the finger(s) at the location throughout the PRT treatment procedure until reassessment has occurred.

PRT Clinician Procedure

- The patient is supine on the treatment table.
- Place a bolster under the patient's knees for comfort.
- Place the far hand on the patient's frontal bone (forehead) and with the near hand pinch the nasal bones while monitoring the lesion with the fingers of the near or far hand.
- Move the hand that is resting on the frontal bone in a cephalad direction while applying traction in a caudal direction with the near hand that is pinching the nose.

 See video 12.3 for the supraorbital PRT procedure.

Patient Self-Treatment Procedure

- Palpate the lateral ridge of the eye with one or two fingers while lying down.

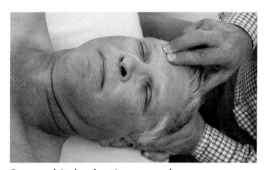

Supraorbital palpation procedure.

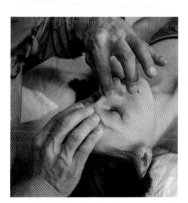

Supraorbital PRT clinician procedure.

- With the other hand, place two fingers above the brow of the eye where the tender area is located and translate the tissue downward toward the tender tissue.
- While translating the tissue above the brow of the eye downward, feel for a fasciculatory, or twitch, response from the tissue or the area where the greatest amount of tissue relaxation is felt. Hold until the fasciculation subsides or three to five minutes have elapsed.

Frontal

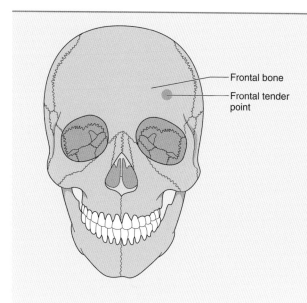

Frontal tender points are commonly located approximately two finger widths superior to the lateral portion of the orbit on the frontal bone. Pressure is applied medially. This area can be tender with headache (especially above the eye), concussion, and blunt trauma to the frontal bone.

Palpation Procedure

- The patient is supine on the treatment table.
- Stabilize the cranium with the opposite hand.
- Palpate the frontal bone approximately two finger widths above the lateral aspect of the orbit.
- Note the location of any tender points or fasciculatory response at the bony structure or overlying tissue.
- Once you have determined the most dominant tender point or fasciculation (or both), maintain light pressure with the pad(s) of the finger(s) at the location throughout the PRT treatment procedure until reassessment has occurred.

PRT Clinician Procedure

- The patient is supine on the treatment table.
- Place a bolster under the patient's knees for comfort.
- While pressing lightly on the tender point with the fingers of the near hand, place your far hand on top of the frontal bone and push the frontal bone caudally.
- The frontal bones can also be compressed bilaterally when tenderness is present bilaterally.

▶ See video 12.4 for the frontal PRT procedure.

Patient Self-Treatment Procedure

- While lying supine, place a finger over the tender area at the forehead.

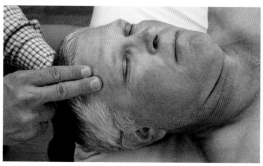

Frontal palpation procedure.

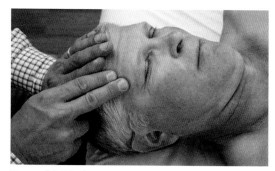

Frontal PRT clinician procedure.

- Place two fingers from the other hand above the tender tissue and translate the tissue down toward the tender area.
- While translating the tissue downward, feel for a fasciculatory, or twitch, response from the tissue or the area where the greatest amount of tissue relaxation is felt. Hold until the fasciculation subsides or three to five minutes have elapsed.

Sagittal Suture

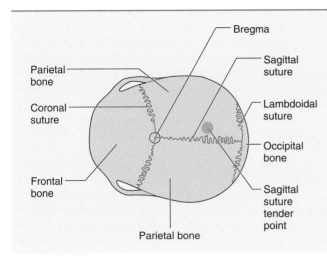

Bregma
Sagittal suture
Parietal bone
Lambdoidal suture
Coronal suture
Occipital bone
Frontal bone
Sagittal suture tender point
Parietal bone

Tender points at the sagittal suture often manifest on the top of the head and lateral to the sagittal suture on either side. This point can be tender in those with headaches or concussions.

Palpation Procedure

- The patient is supine on the treatment table.
- Palpate along either side of the sagittal suture.
- Note the location of any tender points or fasciculatory response at the bony structure or overlying tissue.
- Once you have determined the most dominant tender point or fasciculation (or both), maintain light pressure with the pad(s) of the finger(s) at the location throughout the PRT treatment procedure until reassessment has occurred.

PRT Clinician Procedure

- The patient is supine on the treatment table.
- Place a bolster under the patient's knees for comfort.
- Place your near thumb on the tender point. With the far thumb, apply a caudal pressure on the parietal bone lateral to the sagittal suture and opposite the tender point.

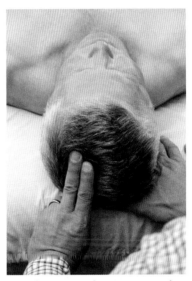

Sagittal suture palpation procedure.

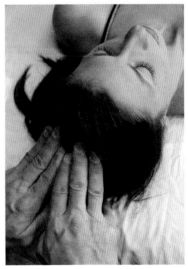

Sagittal suture PRT clinician procedure.

Sphenoid: Lateral Sphenobasilar

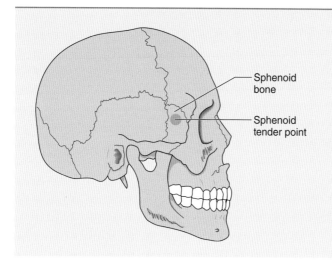

Sphenoid bone

Sphenoid tender point

Sphenoid (lateral sphenobasilar) tender points are often found approximately two to two and a half finger widths posteriorly from the lateral ridge of the orbit. A small depression can be felt in this area. This point can be tender in those with TMD, headaches, concussion symptoms such as blurred vision, and an aversion to light.

Palpation Procedure

- The patient is supine on the treatment table.
- While moving your finger posteriorly from the lateral ridge of the orbit, you will feel a slight depression in the greater wing of the sphenoid. This is usually the tender point area.
- Note the location of any tender points or fasciculatory response at the bony structure or overlying tissue.
- Once you have determined the most dominant tender point or fasciculation (or both), maintain light pressure with the pad(s) of the finger(s) at the location throughout the PRT treatment procedure until reassessment has occurred.

PRT Clinician Procedure

- The patient is supine on the treatment table.
- Place a bolster under the patient's knees for comfort.
- Using the near hand, monitor the tender point while placing the heel of the same hand over the frontal bone and zygoma for counterpressure, then apply a lateral pressure on the opposite greater wing of the sphenoid with the far hand toward the tender point.

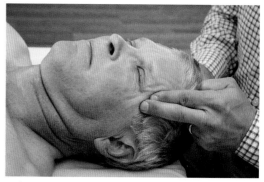

Sphenoid (lateral sphenobasilar) palpation procedure.

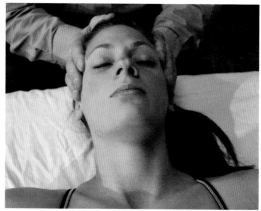

Sphenoid (lateral sphenobasilar) PRT clinician procedure.

Temporalis

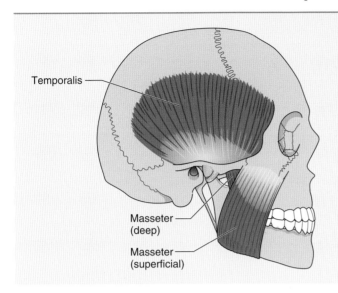

The temporalis muscle is located on the temporal aspect of the cranium; its extensive origin attaches to the frontal, temporal, and parietal bones. Its fibers converge in a thick mass that extends under the zygomatic arch to connect to the coronoid process. This muscle can be involved with TMD, headaches, and stomatognathic dysfunction.

Origin:	Temporal fossa and fascia
Insertion:	Coronoid process of the mandible
Action:	Elevates and retracts the mandible
Innervation:	Temporal branch of the mandibular nerve

Palpation Procedure

- The patient is supine on the treatment table.
- Place your fingers approximately one and a half finger widths superior to the zygomatic arch and palpate the fibers from anterior to posterior. Tenderness may be present in the anterior, middle, or posterior fibers, or a combination of all three.
- Note the location of any tender points or fasciculatory response at the bony structure or overlying tissue.
- Once you have determined the most tender point or fasciculation (or both), maintain light pressure with the pad(s) of the finger(s) at the location throughout the PRT treatment procedure until reassessment has occurred.

PRT Clinician Procedure

- Sit at the head on the side opposite that of the tender point. With the near finger, monitor the tender point while the rest of the hand grasps the frontal bone. Place the heel of the far hand under the zygomatic arch.
- With the near hand on the frontal bone, apply a force around an AP axis toward the tender point on the zygomatic arch while applying a cephalad force with the heel of the far hand (anterior fiber involvement).
- For middle and posterior involvement, grasp the parietal bone with the near hand that is monitoring the tender point. Place the heel of the far hand under the zygomatic arch. With the near hand that is monitoring the tender point,

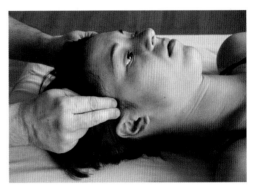

Temporalis palpation procedure.

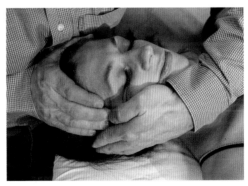

Temporalis PRT clinician procedure.

exert a force along an AP axis toward the tender point. Apply a force in a cephalad direction with the heel of the far hand.

 See video 12.5 for the temporalis PRT procedure.

Masseter

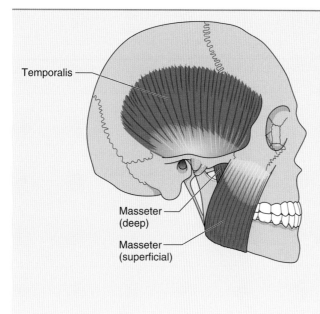

Temporalis

Masseter (deep)

Masseter (superficial)

The masseter muscle is the strongest muscle in the body in proportion to its size. The two masseters acting together can exert forces greater than 150 pounds (68 kg). The masseter is located on the side of the mandible and extends from the zygomatic arch to the angle of the mandible. It is composed of two bellies: a superficial belly that can be accessed from the face, and a deep belly that can be palpated from inside the mouth. This muscle can be involved in TMD, stomatognathic dysfunction, whiplash syndrome, atypical facial pain, and headaches.

Origin:	Zygomatic arch
Insertion:	Angle and ramus of the mandible
Action:	Elevates the mandible; is the primary chewing muscle and is also used in speech and swallowing
Innervation:	Mandibular nerve via the masseteric nerve

Palpation Procedure

- The patient is supine on the treatment table.
- Sit at the head of the table. Palpate an area between the zygomatic arch and the angle of the mandible. The tender point is usually halfway between the structures. This is the superficial belly of the masseter.
- The deep belly can be palpated from inside the mouth between the zygomatic arch and the angle of the mandible.
- *Caution:* Be very careful when placing your fingers in a patient's mouth. If there is any concern that the patient could reflexively close the mouth, you may want to avoid this procedure. The masseter can exert enough force to bite off a finger.
- Note the location of any tender points or fasciculatory response at the bony structure or overlying tissue.
- Once you have determined the most dominant tender point or fasciculation (or both), maintain light pressure with the pad(s) of the finger(s) at the location throughout the PRT treatment procedure until reassessment has occurred.

PRT Clinician Procedure

- The patient is supine on the treatment table.
- Place a bolster under the patient's knees for comfort.
- Stabilize the patient's head against your chest and, using your near hand, monitor the tender point with your fingertips.

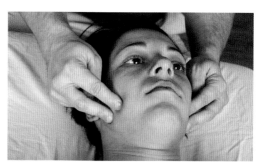

Masseter palpation procedure.

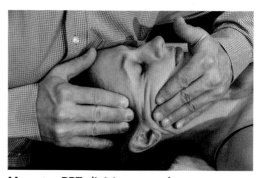

Masseter PRT clinician procedure.

- With the near hand, grasp the mandible, and with the mandible relaxed, move it toward the tender point while applying a light closure force toward the tender point.

 See video 12.6 for the masseter PRT procedure.

Medial Pterygoid

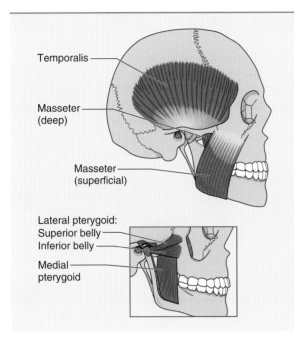

The medial pterygoid muscle assists the masseter and temporalis in elevating the mandible. It also protracts the mandible. This muscle can be involved in TMD, stomatognathic dysfunction, and whiplash syndrome.

Origin: Medial surface of the lateral pterygoid plate of the sphenoid bone, tuberosity of the maxilla

Insertion: Medial surface of the ramus of the mandible

Action: Elevates the mandible; protracts the mandible; when acting unilaterally, can deviate the mandible to the opposite side

Innervation: Mandibular nerve

Palpation Procedure

- The patient is supine on the treatment table.
- The tender point is just slightly superior to the angle of the mandible on the medial surface of the ascending ramus.
- Note the location of any tender points or fasciculatory response at the bony structure or overlying tissue.
- Once you have determined the most tender point or fasciculation (or both), maintain light pressure with the pad(s) of the finger(s) at the location throughout the PRT treatment procedure until reassessment has occurred.

PRT Clinician Procedure

- The patient is supine on the treatment table.
- Place a bolster under the patient's knees for comfort.
- Position yourself at the patient's head.
- While monitoring the tender point with the fingers of the near hand grasping the mandible, place the far hand over the cranium with the fingers above the TMJ for stabilization.
- Translate the far fingers downward toward the tender point while using the near hand to move the mandible toward the tender point.

 See video 12.7 for the medial pterygoid PRT procedure.

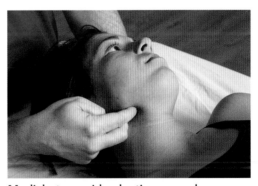

Medial pterygoid palpation procedure.

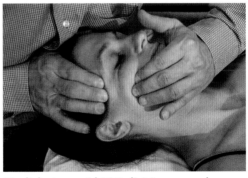

Medial pterygoid PRT clinician procedure.

Lateral Pterygoid

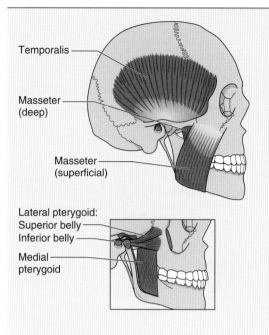

Temporalis

Masseter (deep)

Masseter (superficial)

Lateral pterygoid:
Superior belly
Inferior belly

Medial pterygoid

The lateral pterygoid muscle has horizontal fibers that run from the sphenoid bone to the joint capsule and articular disc of the TMJ. The lateral pterygoid works in coordination with the medial pterygoid and the masseter to protrude the mandible. When acting unilaterally, it can produce mandibular deviation to the same side. The lateral pterygoid also guides the disc during its anterior excursion on opening the mouth and posterior movement on closing the mouth (eccentric contraction of the superior fibers). This muscle can be involved in TMD (especially of the articular disc), stomatognathic dysfunction, headaches, whiplash syndrome, and tinnitus (a close association exists among the anatomy of the lateral pterygoid, articular disc of the TMJ, and middle ear).

Origin: Infratemporal surface and crest of the greater wing of the sphenoid (superior head); lateral surface of the lateral pterygoid plate of the sphenoid (inferior head)

Insertion: Articular disc and capsule of the TMJ

Action: Protracts the mandible; moves the capsule and articular disc anteriorly and posteriorly; when contracting unilaterally, deviates the mandible to the opposite side

Innervation: Mandibular nerve

Palpation Procedure

- The patient is supine on the treatment table.
- The muscle can be palpated extraorally a finger width anterior to the articular process of the mandible and one finger width inferior to the zygomatic arch.
- With a gloved hand, palpate this muscle by placing your index finger in the superior posterior cheek pouch on the lateral aspect of the lateral pterygoid plate. Make sure the patient will not react by suddenly closing the mouth on your finger.
- Determine the most dominant tender point or fasciculation (or both) and maintain light pressure with the pad(s) of the finger(s) throughout the treatment until reassessment has occurred.

PRT Clinician Procedure

- The patient is supine on the treatment table.
- Position yourself at the head of the patient. Place a bolster under the patient's knees for comfort.
- Extraorally: While monitoring the external tender point with the fingers of the near hand, grasp the mandible (jaw) with the far hand and, with the mandible slightly open and relaxed, move it toward the tender point.
- Intraorally: Monitor the tender point with the fingers of the near hand and, with the far hand,

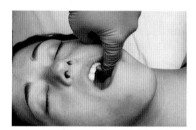

Lateral pterygoid palpation procedure.

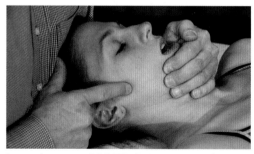

Lateral pterygoid PRT clinician procedure.

support the head and move it into a slightly flexed position, rotating and side bending the head away from the tender point. Observe the caution mentioned earlier.

 See video 12.8 for the lateral pterygoid PRT procedure.

Digastric

The digastric muscle has two bellies; the posterior belly is more readily palpable. Lesions of the digastric are often found in patients with chronic headache, TMD, and neck pain because of its multiple functions and location.

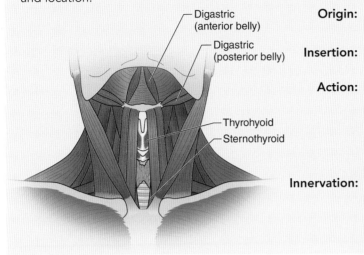

Origin:	Posterior: Temporal bone (mastoid notch)
	Anterior: Mandible (digastric fossa)
Insertion:	Intermediate tendon coursing to the hyoid bone via a fibrous sling
Action:	Depresses the mandible (TMJ); retracts the mandible (TMJ); elevates the hyoid bone during swallowing; retracts the hyoid (posterior); protracts the hyoid (anterior); assists with capital flexion (weak synergist)
Innervation:	Posterior: Facial (VII) nerve (digastric branch)
	Anterior: Trigeminal (V) nerve (mylohyoid branch)

Palpation Procedure

- Place the patient supine. Position yourself behind the patient.
- To locate the posterior belly of the digastric, find the mastoid process and the angle of the mandible. The posterior belly of the digastric runs in line with these two landmarks.
- Using your index finger, roll your fingers between these two landmarks to locate the pencil-width posterior digastric.
- To accentuate the muscle's density under palpation, ask the patient to open the jaw against your light resistance.
- To locate the anterior digastric, place your index finger just under the front of the mandible's inferior ridge just off center at its tip, and ask the patient to open the jaw against light resistance to feel this wirelike muscle contract.
- Determine the most dominant tender point or fasciculation (or both) and maintain light pressure with the pad(s) of the finger(s) throughout the treatment until reassessment has occurred.

PRT Clinician Procedure

- Place the patient supine. Place your far hand under the cranium with the fingers pointing toward the involved side.
- Place the index finger of your near hand over the posterior belly of the digastric with the thumb and the thenar mass over the TMJ.
- With your far hand, apply cranial flexion, then apply cranial lateral flexion toward the lesion.

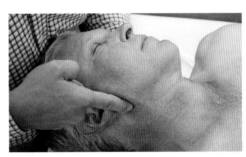

Digastric palpation procedure.

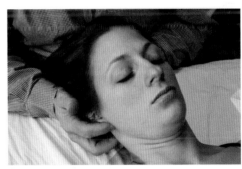

Digastric PRT clinician procedure.

- Translate the underlying tissue down toward the digastric with your near thumb and thenar mass.
- Rotate the underlying tissue toward the lesion with your far hand.
- Corollary tissues treated: Suprahyoids, sternocleidomastoid, levator scapulae, rectus capitis anterior and lateralis

 See video 12.9 for the digastric PRT procedure.

Suprahyoids

The suprahyoids comprise the geniohyoid, mylohyoid, and stylohyoid. The suprahyoids as a group assist with masticating, swallowing, and speaking. Even though they are not distinguishable separately, they are palpable as a group between the inferior tip of the mandible to the hyoid bone.

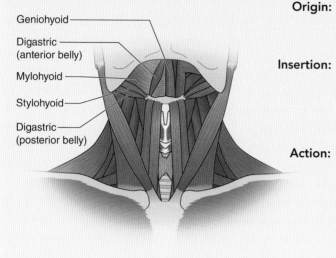

Geniohyoid
Digastric (anterior belly)
Mylohyoid
Stylohyoid
Digastric (posterior belly)

Origin: Geniohyoid: Mandible

Mylohyoid: Mandible

Stylohyoid: Temporal bone, styloid process

Insertion: Geniohyoid: Hyoid bone (anterior surface)

Mylohyoid: Hyoid bone (superior surface), mylohyoid raphe

Stylohyoid: Hyoid bone (junction between its body and greater horn)

Action: Geniohyoid: Elevates and protracts the hyoid bone; depresses the mandible; assists with capital flexion (weak)

Mylohyoid: Elevates the hyoid and tongue during swallowing; depresses the mandible (hyoid fixed), assists with capital flexion (weak)

Stylohyoid: Elevates and retracts the hyoid during swallowing; assists with mandible depression; assists with mastication and speech; assists with capital flexion (weak)

Innervation: Geniohyoid: C1 spinal nerve via hypoglossal (XII) nerve

Mylohyoid: Trigeminal (V) nerve

Stylohyoid: Facial (VII) nerve

Palpation Procedure

- Place the patient supine and position yourself at the head of the table.
- Position the pads of one or two fingers under the angle of the mandible.
- Instruct the patient to push the tongue to the roof of the mouth to feel the contraction of the suprahyoids.
- Trace the muscles to the hyoid bone.
- You can also feel the contraction of the suprahyoids during swallowing and resistive depression of the mandible.
- Note the location of any tender points or fasciculatory response along the tissue.
- Once you have determined the most dominant tender point or fasciculation (or both), maintain light pressure with the pad(s) of the finger(s) at the location throughout the PRT treatment procedure until reassessment has occurred.

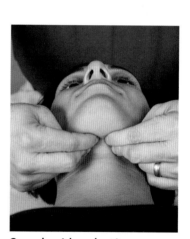

Suprahyoids palpation procedure.

PRT Clinician Procedure

- Place the patient supine and position yourself at the head of the table.
- Place the far hand at the posterior cranium and use it to move the cervical spine and cranium into flexion while palpating the tender point with the fingers of the near hand.
- With the near hand, grasp the inferior angle of the mandible and move the jaw up and down to find the optimal open position.
- Once you have found the jaw opening position, translate the jaw toward the tender point.
- Use the pinky finger to translate the mandible toward the tender point to move the hyoid bone gently toward the tender point as well.
- With the near hand apply slight backward translation of the mandible during positioning for fine-tuning.
- Corollary tissues treated: Platysma, digastric (anterior belly)

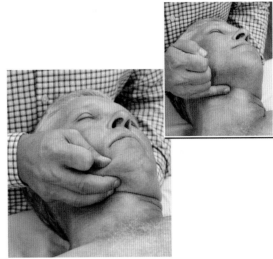

Suprahyoids PRT clinician procedure.

Infrahyoids

Four muscles comprise the infrahyoids (which are superficial to the trachea): the sternothyroid, thyrohyoid, sternohyoid, and omohyoid. Although they are not individually distinguishable, the sternohyoid and sternothyroid are accessible to palpation lateral to the trachea. The other two are deep and not readily accessible to palpation. As a group, they depress the hyoid bone and thyroid cartilage. These muscles can be involved with TMD, stomatognathic dysfunction, whiplash syndrome, and postural dysfunction (forward head).

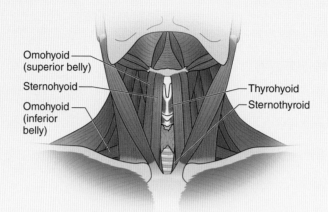

Omohyoid (superior belly)
Sternohyoid
Omohyoid (inferior belly)
Thyrohyoid
Sternothyroid

Origin: Sternothyroid: Sternum (posterior surface), cartilage of the first rib

Thyrohyoid: Thyroid cartilage

Sternohyoid: Clavicle (posterior surface), sternum (posterior surface), sternoclavicular ligament

Omohyoid, inferior belly: Scapula (subscapular notch), superior transverse ligament

Omohyoid, superior belly: Omohyoid intermediate tendon

Insertion: Sternothyroid: Thyroid cartilage

Thyrohyoid: Hyoid bone (greater horn inferior border)

Sternohyoid: Hyoid bone (lower body)

Omohyoid, inferior belly: Omohyoid intermediate tendon

Omohyoid, superior belly: Hyoid bone (lower body)

Action: Sternothyroid: Depression of the larynx after swallowing or speaking; depression of the mandible, hyoid, and tongue after elevation; cervical flexion (weak)

Thyrohyoid: Depression of the hyoid bone; elevation of the larynx and thyroid cartilage; cervical flexion

Sternohyoid: Depression of the hyoid bone after swallowing; cervical flexion (weak)

Omohyoid: Depression of the hyoid bone after elevation; cervical flexion

Innervation: Sternothyroid: C1-C3

Thyrohyoid: Hypoglossal (XII) nerve and C1

Sternohyoid: Hypoglossal (XII) nerve and C1-C3

Omohyoid: Hypoglossal (XII) nerve via C1-C3

Palpation Procedure

- Place the patient supine, and place yourself at the head of the table.
- Use gentle pressure during palpation to avoid aggravating the thyroid gland.
- Place the pads of one or two fingers just below and lateral to the thyroid cartilage (Adam's apple).
- Translate the palpation fingers medial to lateral over the bellies of the infrahyoids.
- The infrahyoids can be palpated in a superior and inferior direction along the lateral border of the trachea.
- Note the location of any tender points or fasciculatory response along the tissue.
- Once you have determined the most dominant tender point or fasciculation (or both), maintain light pressure with the pad(s) of the finger(s) at the location throughout the PRT treatment procedure until reassessment has occurred.

PRT Clinician Procedure

- Place the patient supine, and position yourself at the head of the table.
- While monitoring the tender point with the fingers of the near hand, use the far hand at the base of the posterior cranium to apply cervical flexion and then cranial flexion.
- Apply cervical rotation toward the tender point using the far hand.
- Typically, more cervical flexion is needed for more inferior tender points.
- Corollary tissues treated: Platysma, digastric, longus colli, longus capitis

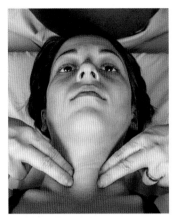

Infrahyoids palpation procedure.

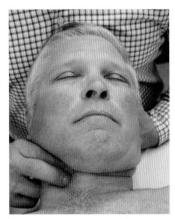

Infrahyoids PRT clinician procedure.

Headache

According to the Headache Classification Committee of the International Headache Society (1998), a cervicogenic headache is defined as one that meets the following criteria: pain that is localized to the neck and occipital regions and may project to the forehead, orbital region, temples, vertex of the cranium, and ears; pain precipitated or aggravated by specific neck movements or sustained neck postures; resistance to or limitation of active or passive physiological movements and accessory movements; and abnormal tenderness over neck musculature. These headaches tend to be unilateral with palpable tenderness along the articular pillars of C1 and C2 on the affected side. There is often a dull to moderate aching pain that begins in the neck or suboccipital region and spreads to include the greater part of the cranium. It is not unusual for patients with these headaches to develop pain that is referred to the cranium, TMJ, and face. For clarification and because of their symptomatic similarities, tension headaches and occipital headaches are included in the category of benign cervicogenic headaches.

Tension-Type Headaches
Tension-type headache is the term designated by the International Headache Society (1988) to replace *musculoskeletal-tension headache, stress headache, muscle-tension headache, psychosomatic headache,* and *psychomyogenic headache.* The society distinguishes between episodic and chronic varieties and divides those into two groups: those that are associated with disorders of the pericranial muscles and those that are not. These types of headaches constitute up to 70% of headaches reported by patients. They occur more in women than in men and have a large stress component (Cohen and McArthur 1981; Friedman and Nelson 1996). Primary complaints are a bilateral ache in the frontal and temporal areas of the cranium, an ache or pain behind the eye, and spasm or hypertonus of the cervical muscles (Nicholson and Gaston 2001).

Occipital Headache
An occipital headache is thought by many clinicians to be a result of cervical dysfunction. The underlying mechanism is often structural and includes cervical hypomobility, hypermobility, joint subluxation, degenerative joint disease (DJD), and poor sustained postures (Fredrickson,

Hovdal, and Sjaastad 1987; Hunter and Mayfield 1949; Wilson 1991). A close relationship to the trigeminocervical neurological complex is often found, resulting in cervical muscle disorders, atypical facial pain, and TMD (Abrahams, Richmond, and Rose 1975; Kerr and Olafsson 1961). This suggests the need to perform a clarifying examination to the TMJ and associated structures.

Headaches are difficult to define because of their variable distribution and symptoms. Diagnosis is usually one of exclusion. Dutton (2004) provided a simple diagnostic algorithm to assist clinicians in determining whether the symptoms are cervicogenic.

- Exclude possible intracranial causes during the history and physical exam. If intracranial pathology is suspected, an urgent workup is required.

- Exclude headaches associated with viral or other infective illness.

- Exclude a drug-induced headache (alcohol, drugs).

- Consider an exercise-related (or sex-related) headache.

- Differentiate among vascular, tension, cervicogenic, and other causes of headache.

Common Signs and Symptoms
- Suboccipital headache radiation to the frontal region or behind the eye, or both

- Headache (chronic or intermittent)

Treatment Points and Sequencing
1. Suboccipitals
2. Splenius capitis
3. Cervical interspinalis
4. Digastric
5. Occipital
6. Occipitomastoid
7. Frontal
8. Supraorbital
9. Temporalis
10. Upper trapezius
11. Sternocleidomastoid
12. Scalenes
13. Suprahyoids and infrahyoids

- Spasm or hypertonus of the cervical muscles
- Spasm or increased tension of the upper trapezius
- Decreased cervical range of motion

Common Differential Diagnoses

- Upper cervical spine somatic dysfunction
- TMD
- DJD
- Osteoarthritis
- Intracranial infection (meningitis)

Clinician Therapeutic Interventions

- Perform a thorough systems screening examination.
- Perform a detailed examination of the upper cervical spine and cervical-occipital region.
- Assess upper-quarter posture.
- Use modalities to decrease pain, inflammation, and muscle spasm, and to increase soft tissue extensibility.
- Perform soft tissue techniques for the upper cervical spine, suboccipital region, and associated areas of the upper quarter (upper trapezius, scalenes, sternocleidomastoid).
- Use joint mobilization techniques.
- Reestablish nonpainful range of motion.
- Reestablish the length–tension relationships of the upper quarter.

- Perform posture correction and education.
- Strengthen the upper quarter, especially the scapular stabilizers and rotator cuff musculature.

Patient Self-Treatment Interventions

- Self-mobilizations should be performed daily (can be taught using a towel, strap, or belt).
- Dorsal glides of the cranium (chin tucks) should also be done daily.
- The patient should perform the following active cervical mobilization on a daily basis if tolerable: Reach behind the head with both hands and interlock the fingers around the C1-C2 region. Then, perform a head-nodding motion with slight lateral flexion and rotation to the opposite side of where the pain resides.
- Resistive band exercises should be done to strengthen the scapular stabilizers and rotator cuff.
- Myofascial trigger point release can be done daily or several times a day for two to three minutes per session as long as it does not cause more than mild discomfort. The patient should place two tennis balls in a sock and tie the ends together and then lie on a firm surface with the tennis balls under the suboccipital region.
- The patient should perform self-releases for the cervical area daily.

Temporomandibular Dysfunction (TMD)

Temporomandibular dysfunction (TMD) refers to a group of clinical musculoskeletal (somatic) problems that involve the TMJ and the muscles of the mastication and stomatognathic systems (speech and swallowing). Because of the proximity of the craniofacial and cervical regions, symptoms of the upper cervical spine and craniofacial areas can occur simultaneously, or one area can produce symptoms in another. This can be caused by the trigeminocervical complex, which consists of neural interconnections between the trigeminal, facial, glossopharyngeal, and vagus nerves and those of the upper four cervical spinal nerves (Castenada 1991). For example, poor posture can be the cause of suboccipital compression, which could produce atypical facial pain (Chaitow 1999), pain in the cranium, dizziness, or nystagmus (Dutton 2004). Or, spasm of the lateral pterygoid muscle could affect the tensor tympani resulting in tinnitus, or ringing in the ears (Ochi, Ohashi, and Kinoshita 2002; Warwick and Williams 1973).

The most common condition, which comprises 90 to 95% of all cases of TMD, is a complex scenario with multiple upper-quarter and facial complaints and a variety of mandibular impairments all without identified structural causes (Stohler 1995). Females seek clinical intervention for TMD four times more often than do males (Dworkin et al. 1990; Salonen and Hellden 1990). One expression of the overrepresentation is the psychosocial nature of the dysfunction (Rocabado and Iglarsh 1991). Because of the complex nature of TMD, it is best approached as a biopsychosocial disorder. Although described as one syndrome in 1934 by Costen in Kraus (1994), current research suggests that TMD is a cluster of related dysfunctions involving the masticatory system, the stomatognathic system, and the cervical spine (Bell 1985; Dimitroulis 1998; Kraus 1994). McNeill (1991), Gelb and colleagues (1977), and Dutton (2004) described the following three primary etiological factors involved in TMD:

1. Predisposing factors: Structural, neurological, hormonal, and metabolic

2. Precipitating factors

   a. Overt, extrinsic trauma to the head, neck, or jaw

   b. Repeated low-grade trauma such as nail biting and gum chewing

Treatment Points and Sequencing

1. Masseter
2. Pterygoids
3. Temporalis
4. Digastric
5. Suprahyoids and infrahyoids
6. Omohyoid
7. Scalenes
8. Sternocleidomastoid
9. Pectoralis major and minor
10. Lateral sphenobasilar
11. Frontal
12. Stylohyoid
13. Occipital

   c. Repeated low-grade intrinsic trauma such as teeth clenching or grinding (bruxism)

   d. Stress that passes an individual threshold

3. Perpetuating factors that aid in the continuation of symptoms such as cervical pathology and systemic disease

Because considerable overlap exists in the clinical presentation of TMD, the diagnostic challenge to clinicians is considerable. An accurate diagnosis is the key to successful treatment. Therefore, clinicians presented with TMD symptoms must be familiar with the many underlying conditions that can give rise to pain in the cranium, facial region, throat, and neck. The information in this section outlines some of the major signs and symptoms and differential diagnostic categories that must be considered when evaluating complaints of TMD (Kraus 1994).

Common Signs and Symptoms

- Pain centered in front of the tragus of the ear and projecting to the ear, temple region, and cheeks and along the mandible
- Headache
- Atypical facial pain
- Orofacial pain
- Earache
- Tinnitus
- Neck pain
- Tightness in the jaw muscles
- Abnormal parafunctional activity (oral habits)

- Associated factors
  - Malocclusion
  - Muscle dyskinesis
  - Trauma
  - Recent dental work or examination (iatrogenic)

Common Differential Diagnoses

- Headache types
  - Migraine
  - Cluster
- Headaches associated with the following:
  - Head trauma
  - Vascular disorders
  - Nonvascular intracranial disorder
  - Substance withdrawal
  - Noncephalic infection
  - Metabolic disorder
- Headache associated with disorders of the following:
  - Cranium
  - Neck
  - Eyes, ears, nose, sinuses, teeth, mouth
- Cranial neuralgias, nerve trunk pain
- Arthritides
  - Osteoarthritis
  - Osteroarthrosis
  - Polyarthritides
- Inflammatory conditions
  - Synovitis
  - Capsulitis
  - Neoplasms
- Psychosocial issues

Clinician Therapeutic Interventions

- Explain to the patient the cause and nature of the disorder.
- Perform a thorough history and systems review.
- Once serious pathology has been ruled out, perform a functional examination of the TMJ and related structures.
- Perform an upper-quarter examination that includes the upper cervical spine and a posture assessment.
- In chronic behavioral presentations, a psychological examination may be warranted.

- Apply modalities to decrease pain and inflammation.
- Reestablish the normal resting position of the TMJ (lips together, teeth slightly apart) and nasal breathing.
- Evaluate the swallowing technique. There should be no tongue thrust or head movement.
- Teach the patient using Rocabado and Iglarsh's (1991) 6x6 exercise protocol, which was developed to restore upper-quarter posture, TMJ mobility, and muscle length, and to help in the self-management of symptoms.
- As a general rule, a multimodal therapeutic approach is the most effective for TMD (e.g., various modalities, manual therapy, pharmacotherapy, occlusal splint therapy, and counseling).

Patient Self-Treatment Interventions

- Limit mandibular function by avoiding large mouth opening (cut food into smaller, bite-size pieces) and avoid excessive yawning (when a yawn is about to happen, place the tongue on the roof of the mouth).
- Limit mandibular stress by chewing soft foods.
- Modify excessive habitual parafunctional activity.
- Practice upper-quarter posture modification.
- Identify and address stressors.
- Home exercise program
  - Strengthen the cervicothoracic stabilizers.
  - Strengthen the scapular stabilizers.
  - Perform mandibular mouth-opening exercises daily within a pain-free range to increase soft tissue elongation (place the tip of the tongue on the roof of the mouth while performing).
  - If there is abnormal mandibular deviation with jaw opening, use the toothpick exercise: Place toothpicks between the upper and lower incisors, and while sitting in front of a mirror, open and close the mouth, keeping the toothpicks in alignment.
  - Perform stretching exercises daily for the upper cervical spine (dorsal glide), scalenes, sternocleidomastoid, and pectoralis musculature.

Postconcussion Syndrome

A concussion is a traumatically induced disturbance in brain function that may or may not involve the loss of consciousness (Reddy 2011). Injury to the brain is mainly considered a neurometabolic dysfunction, which occurs as a result of imparted linear and rotational forces to the brain within the cranial vault (Herring et al. 2011). Concussion statistics are becoming alarming. It has been estimated that each year in the United States there are 1.7 to 3.8 million sport-related concussions and 275,000 hospitalizations and 52,000 deaths related to concussions (Selassie et al. 2013). Fortunately, 80% of concussion symptoms resolve within 6 to 12 weeks after injury (Reddy 2011). However, a percentage of patients, termed the "miserable minority" (Reddy 2011), have symptoms that last for months or years causing significant impairment in social and occupational functioning. These people are often classified as having postconcussion syndrome. Besides the presence of a headache, people with postconcussion syndrome typically present with clustered symptoms that typically fall into three categories (Gladstone 2009):

- Somatic: Dizziness, tinnitus, photophobia, phonophobia, blurred vision, diminished sense of smell, fatigability

- Cognitive: Impaired attention, concentration, speed of processing, and memory

- Psychological: Depression, anxiety, irritability, apathy, and insomnia

Postconcussion syndrome patients may have just a headache or a combination of all of the clustered symptoms. Treatment to date for an acute concussion has consisted of rest (physical and cognitive), pharmacological intervention, and neurocognitive rehabilitation.

Recently, studies in the literature have focused on other treatment options such as vestibular rehabilitation (Alsalaheen et al. 2010; Weightman et al. 2010), visual training (Greenwald, Kapoor, and Singh 2012; Weightman et al. 2010), cardiorespiratory training (Griesbach, Houda, and Gomez-Pinella 2009; Kozlowski et al. 2013; Willer and Leddy 2006), and treatment of the cervical spine (Weightman et al. 2010) with promising results. Of particular interest are the cervical spine structures that are closely linked to structures that cause many of the symptoms of concussion and postconcussion syndrome.

Treatment Points and Sequencing

1. Sphenoid (lateral sphenobasilar)
2. Posterior sphenobasilar
3. Occipital
4. Temporalis
5. Frontal
6. Supraorbital
7. Occipitomastoid
8. Maxilla
9. Masseter
10. Pterygoids
11. Suboccipitals
12. Longus capitis and longus colli
13. Cervical interspinalis
14. Splenius capitis
15. Levator scapulae at the neck
16. Levator scapulae at the shoulder
17. Upper trapezius
18. Scalenes
19. Sternocleidomastoid

Cervicogenic headache frequently coexists with complaints of dizziness, tinnitus, nausea, imbalance, hearing problems, and eye and ear pain. Baron, Cherian, and Tepper (2011) and Biondi (2005) identified the greater occipital nerve as the source of these symptoms. Referral patterns for the three occipital nerve roots (C1-C3) and their convergence on the nucleus caudalis of the trigeminal tract, along with their joint complexes, have been identified as possible sources of head pain and myofascial trigger points in the head and neck (Simons et al. 1999). The receptors in the cervical spine also have many connections to the vestibular and visual apparatus. Dysfunction of the cervical spine receptors can alter afferent input, subsequently changing the integration of timing and sensorimotor control (Stirimpakos 2011; Treleaven 2008).

Another area of interest that requires attention is the sphenobasilar synchondrosis and the important neurological structures that overlay this anatomical structure. Involvement of the sphenobasilar synchondrosis has been controversial since the publication of Dr. William Sutherland's classic work *The Cranial Bowl* (1939). Some anatomists and clinicians firmly believe that this synchondrosis does not move after age 25 (Chaitow 1999). Upledger and Vredevoogd (1983) and Chaitow (1999) wrote that sphenobasilar dysfunction in somatic illness may be a result of external forces from muscles, soft tissues, and dural membrane tension (Chaitow 1999).

It is not my intent to focus on the movement debate in this section; however, important neurological structures that lie over the sphenobasilar-occipital complex and the caudal side of the brain may be affected with concussion, such as the cranial nerves, especially the oculomotor and optic chiasm (Moore 1985; Warwick and Williams 1973). Practitioners who believe that the sphenobasilar complex can be involved in head trauma report treating the following symptoms: headaches; eye–motor difficulties; head, neck, and back pain; TMJ pain; endocrine disturbances; reading and focus difficulties; anxiety; and depression (Koren 2006). It is interesting to note that these symptoms are similar to those experienced by patients who are treated for acute concussion and postconcussion syndrome.

Considering the forces the brain is subjected to that result in a concussion, I propose that the abnormal movement of the brain during a concussion event imparts tension forces on the sphenobasilar complex and the neurological structures closely associated with this area. Involvement to the structures in this area not only produces symptoms similar to those of concussion and postconcussion syndrome, but also results in tender points on the cranium, in the suboccipital and spheno-occipital areas, and at the cervical spine segments C1-C3. The method of injury can also affect the upper cervical spine, whose involvement can magnify headaches and craniofacial pain. It is my contention that the tender points recorded on the cranium, suboccipital, and cervical regions must be treated for a complete resolution of symptoms in the acute or postconcussion phases of this injury. I realize that this proposed mechanism implicating the sphenobasilar complex in the development of symptoms related to acute concussion and postconcussion syndrome is devoid of research. However, the clinical experience of the authors of this text when working with postconcussive patients has shown that the treatment of tender points of the cranial, cervical, and shoulder regions with PRT provides promising clinical outcomes and expedient return to athletic and daily activities. To date, no studies have mapped out tender points on the cranium, cervical spine, and upper quarter for patients who have experienced acute concussions or developed postconcussion syndrome. Case studies would provide much-needed information to help develop PRT treatment protocols for postconcussive patients.

Common Signs and Symptoms

- Headache
- Poor memory
- Learning impairment
- Fatigue
- Emotional problems
- Dizziness
- Decreased eye–motor coordination
- Poor concentration
- Reading problems
- Insomnia
- Taking longer to think
- Obsessive-compulsive disorders
- Blurred vision
- Endocrine disorders
- Light sensitivity
- Restlessness
- Depression
- Nausea
- TMD
- Balance problems
- Decreased reaction time

Common Differential Diagnoses

- Severe traumatic brain injury
- Headache disorders
- Intracranial bleeds
- Cervical fracture
- Vertebral artery problems
- Depression
- Fibromyalgia
- Posttraumatic stress disorder

Clinician Therapeutic Interventions

- Conduct a thorough history and systems review.

> continued

Postconcussion Syndrome *> continued*

- Assess balance, eye–hand coordination, and motor control.
- Conduct a postural and upper-quarter screen.
- Evaluate the length–tension relationships of upper-quarter tissues.
- Apply modalities for pain control.
- Continue with cognitive training.
- Conduct balance, coordination, and vestibular rehabilitation.
- If needed, address posture education.
- Strengthening of cervical and scapular stabilizers may be needed if somatic dysfunction is chronic.

Patient Self-Treatment Interventions

- Practice daily postural awareness training.
- Perform dorsal glide exercises (chin tucks).
- Continue with eye–hand coordination exercises, balance activities, and vestibular rehabilitation.
- Engage in pain-free cervical and shoulder girdle strengthening and stretching exercises as prescribed (e.g., Ys , Ts, and Ws).

Forward Head Posture (FHP)

It is well known that habitual forward head postures (FHP) can place significant stress on the TMJ and associated soft tissue structures, the upper cervical spine, the upper thoracic facet joints, and the shoulder and shoulder girdle musculature (Dutton 2004; Simons et al. 1999). A sustained FHP produces altered length–tension relationships between the anterior and posterior musculature of the upper quarter. These changes alter the neurological activity of the tissues resulting in inefficient movement patterns (Dutton 2004; Janda 1994; Sharmann 2001; Simons et al. 1999). For example, in the FHP position, the lateral neck musculature (scalenes and sternocleidomastoid) shortens, the kyphosis of the cervicothoracic junction becomes exaggerated, the midcervical spine flexes, and the upper cervical spine compensates by extending. This position causes the mandible to experience opening forces that place increased stress on the muscles of mastication as well as on the supra- and infrahyoid musculature. This may have an effect on breathing and swallowing. A forward head posture promotes shoulder girdle protraction, lengthening and weakness of the scapular stabilizers and tightness of the pectoralis major and minor, subclavius, and upper trapezius. This ultimately produces abnormal arthrokinematics of the shoulder. If not corrected, this abnormal posture can cause a myriad of myofascial pain syndromes and tender points in the upper quarter (Kraus 1994).

Treatment Points and Sequencing

1. Suboccipitals
2. Scalenes
3. Longus capitis and longus colli
4. Sternocleidomastoid
5. Pectoralis major and minor
6. Subclavius
7. Xiphoid process
8. Upper trapezius
9. Levator scapulae
10. Rhomboids
11. Thoracic erector spinae
12. Omohyoid
13. Digastric
14. Suprahyoids and infrahyoids
15. Cranium: Temporalis, masseter, pterygoids, coronal suture, supraorbital

Common Signs and Symptoms

- Headache (cervicogenic)
- Jaw pain or tightness (masseter)
- Temporalis pain
- Greater occipital nerve irritation (frontal headaches, retro-orbital pain)
- Upper trapezius pain or tightness
- Shoulder aches and limited range of motion
- Altered breathing patterns (chest breather)
- Altered swallowing (tongue thrust with cervical motion)
- Limited cervical range of motion
- Sitting fatigue
- Dizziness

Common Differential Diagnoses

- Acute trauma (motor vehicle accident)
- Upper cervical spine fracture (odontoid instability)
- Head trauma
- Cervical spine pathology (cervical DJD)
- TMJ acute or chronic trauma
- TMJ disc or capsular dysfunction
- Pathology of the stomatognathic system
- Vertigo (benign, central, reflex, ischemic)
- Fibromyalgia
- Occlusion problems

Clinician Therapeutic Interventions

- Perform a thorough upper-quarter history and systems review.
- Apply modalities to decrease pain and soften involved tissues.
- Perform posture correction including sitting, standing, and sleeping.
- Teach the patient how to perform dorsal glide exercises of the upper cervical segments (chin tuck).
- Teach the patient scapular strengthening and stabilizing exercises.
- If applicable, instruct the patient in PNF stretching to address tight anterior structures of the upper quarter.

Summary

Although the clinical approach to treatment of the cranium has been controversial and has been met with much skepticism, a knowledge of the more common somatic dysfunctions that can refer pain to the cranium can help clinicians clear the muddy waters. PRT can be a primary clinical treatment for the cranium or be used to augment or facilitate other treatment approaches. It is especially clinically relevant for postconcussion syndrome. PRT practitioners must perform a thorough systems reviews and screening evaluations of the upper quarter and cranium in patients with complaints of cranial pain. Even though a specific structure may be difficult to identify as the primary source of pain, treatment of the cranium with PRT is safer than direct techniques and may provide pain relief with less reliance on addictive pain medications, thereby improving function and quality of life.

👆 Scanning and Mapping Evaluation: Foot

Patient: _____ Diagnosis: _____

Note the location of tenderness to palpation (left of right side, L/R) and numerical pain rating scale (NPRS) pre- and posttreatment with the associated treatment date. Additional structures can be noted in the blank boxes, as can additional location descriptors, where applicable (e.g., proximal to the joint line).

Key: O = Origin, MB = Muscle belly, I = Insertion, PMTJ = Proximal musculotendinous junction, DMTJ = Distal musculotendinous junction

	Date:			Date:			Date:		
	O/MB/I PMTJ DMTJ	Pre NPRS L/R	Post NPRS L/R	O/MB/I PMTJ DMTJ	Pre NPRS L/R	Post NPRS L/R	O/MB/I PMTJ DMTJ	Pre NPRS L/R	Post NPRS L/R
Dorsal									
Interossei									
First and second metatarsal space									
Second and third metatarsal space									
Third and fourth metatarsal space									
Fourth and fifth metatarsal space									
Cuneiforms									
First									
Second									
Third									
Talus									
Anterior									
Medial									
Lateral									
Extensor digitorum longus tendons									
Second									
Third									
Fourth									
Fifth									
Extensor digitorum brevis									

> continued

Scanning and Mapping Evaluation: Foot > *continued*

	Date:			Date:			Date:		
	O/MB/I PMTJ DMTJ	Pre NPRS L/R	Post NPRS L/R	O/MB/I PMTJ DMTJ	Pre NPRS L/R	Post NPRS L/R	O/MB/I PMTJ DMTJ	Pre NPRS L/R	Post NPRS L/R
Plantar									
Plantar aponeurosis									
Flexor hallucis brevis									
Abductor hallucis									
Abductor digiti minimi									
Plantar interossei and lumbricals									
First and second metatarsal space									
Second and third metatarsal space									
Third and fourth metatarsal space									
Fourth and fifth metatarsal space									

Notes:

Numerical Pain Rating Scale (NPRS)

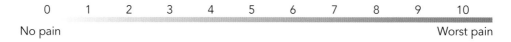

0	1	2	3	4	5	6	7	8	9	10

No pain   Worst pain

From T.E. Speicher, 2016, *Clinical guide to positional release therapy* (Champaign, IL: Human Kinetics).

👆 Scanning and Mapping Evaluation: Ankle and Lower Leg

Patient: _____   Diagnosis: _____

Note the location of tenderness to palpation (left of right side, L/R) and numerical pain rating scale (NPRS) pre- and posttreatment with the associated treatment date. Additional structures can be noted in the blank boxes, as can additional location descriptors, where applicable (e.g., proximal to the joint line).

Key: O = Origin, MB = Muscle belly, I = Insertion, PMTJ = Proximal musculotendinous junction, DMTJ = Distal musculotendinous junction

	Date:			Date:			Date:		
	O/MB/I PMTJ DMTJ	Pre NPRS L/R	Post NPRS L/R	O/MB/I PMTJ DMTJ	Pre NPRS L/R	Post NPRS L/R	O/MB/I PMTJ DMTJ	Pre NPRS L/R	Post NPRS L/R
Anterior									
Tibialis anterior muscle									
Tibialis anterior tendon									
Extensor digitorum longus muscle									
Anterior talofibular ligament									
Medial									
Tibialis posterior muscle									
Tibialis posterior tendon									
Deltoid ligament complex									
Posterior tibiotalar									
Tibiocalcaneal									
Tibionavicular									
Anterior tibiotalar									

> continued

Scanning and Mapping Evaluation: Ankle and Lower Leg *> continued*

	Date:			Date:			Date:		
	O/MB/I PMTJ DMTJ	Pre NPRS L/R	Post NPRS L/R	O/MB/I PMTJ DMTJ	Pre NPRS L/R	Post NPRS L/R	O/MB/I PMTJ DMTJ	Pre NPRS L/R	Post NPRS L/R
Posterior									
Gastrocnemius									
Achilles tendon									
Soleus									

_____

_____

Lateral									
Peroneus longus and brevis									
Calcaneofibular ligament									

_____

_____

_____

Notes:

Numerical Pain Rating Scale (NPRS)

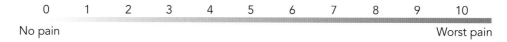

0 1 2 3 4 5 6 7 8 9 10

No pain   Worst pain

From T.E. Speicher, 2016, *Clinical guide to positional release therapy* (Champaign, IL: Human Kinetics).

👆 Scanning and Mapping Evaluation: Knee and Thigh

Patient: _____   Diagnosis: _____

Note the location of tenderness to palpation (left of right side, L/R) and numerical pain rating scale (NPRS) pre- and posttreatment with the associated treatment date. Additional structures can be noted in the blank boxes, as can additional location descriptors, where applicable (e.g., proximal to the joint line).

Key: O = Origin, MB = Muscle belly, I = Insertion, PMTJ = Proximal musculotendinous junction, DMTJ = Distal musculotendinous junction

	Date:			Date:			Date:		
	O/MB/I PMTJ DMTJ	Pre NPRS L/R	Post NPRS L/R	O/MB/I PMTJ DMTJ	Pre NPRS L/R	Post NPRS L/R	O/MB/I PMTJ DMTJ	Pre NPRS L/R	Post NPRS L/R
Anterior									
Patellar tendon									
Patella									
Quadriceps tendon									
Rectus femoris									
Medial									
Pes anserine									
Medial collateral ligament (MCL)									
Vastus medialis oblique (VMO)									
Adductor group									
Adductor magnus									
Adductor longus									
Pectineus									
Gracilis									

> continued

Scanning and Mapping Evaluation: Knee and Thigh *> continued*

	Date:			Date:			Date:		
	O/MB/I PMTJ DMTJ	Pre NPRS L/R	Post NPRS L/R	O/MB/I PMTJ DMTJ	Pre NPRS L/R	Post NPRS L/R	O/MB/I PMTJ DMTJ	Pre NPRS L/R	Post NPRS L/R
Posterior									
Popliteus									
Hamstrings									
Biceps femoris									
Semitendinosus									
Lateral									
Iliotibial band									
Lateral collateral ligament (LCL)									
Vastus lateralis									

Notes:

Numerical Pain Rating Scale (NPRS)

0   1   2   3   4   5   6   7   8   9   10

No pain   Worst pain

From T.E. Speicher, 2016, *Clinical guide to positional release therapy* (Champaign, IL: Human Kinetics).

✋ Scanning and Mapping Evaluation: Pelvis

Patient: _____ Diagnosis: _____

Note the location of tenderness to palpation (left of right side, L/R) and numerical pain rating scale (NPRS) pre- and posttreatment with the associated treatment date. Additional structures can be noted in the blank boxes, as can additional location descriptors, where applicable (e.g., proximal to the joint line).

Key: O = Origin, MB = Muscle belly, I = Insertion, PMTJ = Proximal musculotendinous junction, DMTJ = Distal musculotendinous junction

	Date:			Date:			Date:		
	O/MB/I PMTJ DMTJ	Pre NPRS L/R	Post NPRS L/R	O/MB/I PMTJ DMTJ	Pre NPRS L/R	Post NPRS L/R	O/MB/I PMTJ DMTJ	Pre NPRS L/R	Post NPRS L/R
Anterior									
Iliacus muscle									
Psoas major muscle									
Rectus abdominis muscle									
Sartorius tendon and muscle									
Rectus femoris tendon									
Tensor fasciae latae									
Superior pubis									
Inferior pubis									
Posterior									
Gluteus medius									
Gluteus maximus: superior fibers									
Gluteus maximus: inferior fibers									
Lateral rotator tendons of the hip									
Piriformis									
Quadratus femoris									
Sacrotuberous ligament									
Sacroiliac joint									

Notes:

Numerical Pain Rating Scale (NPRS)

0 1 2 3 4 5 6 7 8 9 10

No pain   Worst pain

From T.E. Speicher, 2016, *Clinical guide to positional release therapy* (Champaign, IL: Human Kinetics).

👆 Scanning and Mapping Evaluation: Spine

Patient: _____ Diagnosis: _____

Note the location of tenderness to palpation (left of right side, L/R) and numerical pain rating scale (NPRS) pre- and posttreatment with the associated treatment date. Additional structures can be noted in the blank boxes, as can additional location descriptors, where applicable (e.g., proximal to the joint line).

Key: O = Origin, MB = Muscle belly, I = Insertion, PMTJ = Proximal musculotendinous junction, DMTJ = Distal musculotendinous junction

	Date:			Date:			Date:		
	O/MB/I PMTJ DMTJ	Pre NPRS L/R	Post NPRS L/R	O/MB/I PMTJ DMTJ	Pre NPRS L/R	Post NPRS L/R	O/MB/I PMTJ DMTJ	Pre NPRS L/R	Post NPRS L/R
Anterior									
Cervical									
Sternocleidomastoid									
Anterior and middle scalenes									
Digastric									
Longus capitis and longus colli									
Suprahyoids									
Infrahyoids									
Thoracic									
Upper rectus abdominis									
Intercostals (Note level:_____)									
Xiphoid									
Sternum									
Posterior									
Cervical									
Splenius capitis									
Suboccipitals									
Levator scapulae									
Posterior scalene									
Interspinalis (Note level:_____)									

	Date:			Date:			Date:		
	O/MB/I PMTJ DMTJ	Pre NPRS L/R	Post NPRS L/R	O/MB/I PMTJ DMTJ	Pre NPRS L/R	Post NPRS L/R	O/MB/I PMTJ DMTJ	Pre NPRS L/R	Post NPRS L/R
Posterior									
Thoracic									
Intercostals (Note level:_____)									
Erector spinae (Note level: _____)									
Lumbar									
Coccyx									
Quadratus lumborum									
Lumbar erector spinae (Note level: _____)									
Lumbar interspinalis (Note level:_____)									
Lumbar multifidi									

Notes:

Numerical Pain Rating Scale (NPRS)

0   1   2   3   4   5   6   7   8   9   10

No pain   Worst pain

From T.E. Speicher, 2016, *Clinical guide to positional release therapy* (Champaign, IL: Human Kinetics).

Scanning and Mapping Evaluation: Shoulder

Patient: _____ Diagnosis: _____

Note the location of tenderness to palpation (left of right side, L/R) and numerical pain rating scale (NPRS) pre- and posttreatment with the associated treatment date. Additional structures can be noted in the blank boxes, as can additional location descriptors, where applicable (e.g., proximal to the joint line).

Key: O = Origin, MB = Muscle belly, I = Insertion, PMTJ = Proximal musculotendinous junction, DMTJ = Distal musculotendinous junction

	Date: O/MB/I PMTJ DMTJ	Pre NPRS L/R	Post NPRS L/R	Date: O/MB/I PMTJ DMTJ	Pre NPRS L/R	Post NPRS L/R	Date: O/MB/I PMTJ DMTJ	Pre NPRS L/R	Post NPRS L/R
Anterior									
Upper trapezius									
Subclavius									
Acromioclavicular joint									
Deltoid									
Anterior									
Middle									
Posterior									
Biceps brachii long head tendon									
Biceps brachii short head tendon									
Subscapularis									
Serratus anterior									
Pectoralis minor									
Pectoralis major									

	Date:			Date:			Date:		
	O/MB/I PMTJ DMTJ	Pre NPRS L/R	Post NPRS L/R	O/MB/I PMTJ DMTJ	Pre NPRS L/R	Post NPRS L/R	O/MB/I PMTJ DMTJ	Pre NPRS L/R	Post NPRS L/R
Posterior									
Supraspinatus									
Infraspinatus									
Teres minor									
Teres major									
Latissimus dorsi									
Acromioclavicular joint									
Lower trapezius									
Rhomboid minor									
Rhomboid major									
Levator scapulae									

Notes:

Numerical Pain Rating Scale (NPRS)

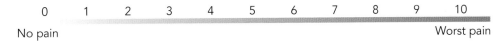

0   1   2   3   4   5   6   7   8   9   10

No pain   Worst pain

From T.E. Speicher, 2016, *Clinical guide to positional release therapy* (Champaign, IL: Human Kinetics).

Scanning and Mapping Evaluation: Elbow and Forearm

Patient: _____   Diagnosis: _____

Note the location of tenderness to palpation (left of right side, L/R) and numerical pain rating scale (NPRS) pre- and posttreatment with the associated treatment date. Additional structures can be noted in the blank boxes, as can additional location descriptors, where applicable (e.g., proximal to the joint line).

Key: O = Origin, MB = Muscle belly, I = Insertion, PMTJ = Proximal musculotendinous junction, DMTJ = Distal musculotendinous junction

	Date:			Date:			Date:		
	O/MB/I PMTJ DMTJ	Pre NPRS L/R	Post NPRS L/R	O/MB/I PMTJ DMTJ	Pre NPRS L/R	Post NPRS L/R	O/MB/I PMTJ DMTJ	Pre NPRS L/R	Post NPRS L/R
Anterior									
Biceps aponeurosis									
Brachioradialis									
Supinator									
Pronator teres									
Flexors of the wrist and fingers									
Flexor carpi radialis									
Flexor carpi ulnaris									
Palmaris longus									
Flexor digitorum									
Medial									
Medial epicondyle									
Common flexor tendon									
Posterior									
Olecranon									
Triceps brachii									
Lateral head									
Long head									
Medial head									

	Date:			Date:			Date:		
	O/MB/I PMTJ DMTJ	Pre NPRS L/R	Post NPRS L/R	O/MB/I PMTJ DMTJ	Pre NPRS L/R	Post NPRS L/R	O/MB/I PMTJ DMTJ	Pre NPRS L/R	Post NPRS L/R
Posterior									
Anconeus									
Extensors of the wrist and fingers									
Extensor carpi radialis									
Extensor carpi ulnaris									
Extensor digitorum									

Lateral									
Lateral epicondyle									
Common extensor tendon									

Notes:

Numerical Pain Rating Scale (NPRS)

0   1   2   3   4   5   6   7   8   9   10

No pain   Worst pain

From T.E. Speicher, 2016, *Clinical guide to positional release therapy* (Champaign, IL: Human Kinetics).

Scanning and Mapping Evaluation: Wrist and Hand

Patient: _____ Diagnosis: _____

Note the location of tenderness to palpation (left of right side, L/R) and numerical pain rating scale (NPRS) pre- and posttreatment with the associated treatment date. Additional structures can be noted in the blank boxes, as can additional location descriptors, where applicable (e.g., proximal to the joint line).

Key: O = Origin, MB = Muscle belly, I = Insertion, PMTJ = Proximal musculotendinous junction, DMTJ = Distal musculotendinous junction

	Date:			Date:			Date:		
	O/MB/I PMTJ DMTJ	Pre NPRS L/R	Post NPRS L/R	O/MB/I PMTJ DMTJ	Pre NPRS L/R	Post NPRS L/R	O/MB/I PMTJ DMTJ	Pre NPRS L/R	Post NPRS L/R
Anterior									
Wrist flexor tendons									
Flexor carpi radialis									
Flexor carpi ulnaris									
Palmaris longus									
Metacarpophalangeal joint									
Circle: 1st / 2nd / 3rd / 4th / 5th									
Proximal interphalangeal joint									
Circle: 1st / 2nd / 3rd / 4th / 5th									
Distal interphalangeal joint									
Circle: 2nd / 3rd / 4th / 5th									
Lumbricals									
Second and third metacarpal space									
Third and fourth metacarpal space									
Fourth and fifth metacarpal space									
Abductor and flexor pollicis brevis									
Opponens pollicis									
Adductor pollicis									

_____
_____
_____

	Date:			Date:			Date:		
	O/MB/I PMTJ DMTJ	Pre NPRS L/R	Post NPRS L/R	O/MB/I PMTJ DMTJ	Pre NPRS L/R	Post NPRS L/R	O/MB/I PMTJ DMTJ	Pre NPRS L/R	Post NPRS L/R
Posterior									
Dorsal interossei									
Second and third metacarpal space									
Third and fourth metacarpal space									
Fourth and fifth metacarpal space									
Wrist extensor tendons									
Extensor carpi ulnaris									
Extensor carpi radialis									
Extensor digitorum tendons									
Circle: 2nd / 3rd / 4th / 5th									
Extensor pollicis longus tendon									
Extensor pollicis brevis tendon									
Metacarpophalangeal joint									
Circle: 1st / 2nd / 3rd / 4th / 5th									
Proximal interphalangeal joint									
Circle: 1st / 2nd / 3rd / 4th / 5th									
Distal interphalangeal joint									
Circle: 2nd / 3rd / 4th / 5th									

Notes:

Numerical Pain Rating Scale (NPRS)

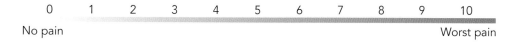

0   1   2   3   4   5   6   7   8   9   10

No pain   Worst pain

From T.E. Speicher, 2016, *Clinical guide to positional release therapy* (Champaign, IL: Human Kinetics).

✋ Scanning and Mapping Evaluation: Cranium

Patient: _____ Diagnosis: _____

Note the location of tenderness to palpation (left of right side, L/R) and numerical pain rating scale (NPRS) pre- and posttreatment with the associated treatment date. Additional structures can be noted in the blank boxes, as can additional location descriptors, where applicable (e.g., proximal to the joint line).

Key: O = Origin, MB = Muscle belly, I = Insertion, PMTJ = Proximal musculotendinous junction, DMTJ = Distal musculotendinous junction

	Date:			Date:			Date:		
	O/MB/I PMTJ DMTJ	Pre NPRS L/R	Post NPRS L/R	O/MB/I PMTJ DMTJ	Pre NPRS L/R	Post NPRS L/R	O/MB/I PMTJ DMTJ	Pre NPRS L/R	Post NPRS L/R
Osseous structures									
Occipitomastoid									
Occipital									
Posterior sphenobasilar									
Stylohyoid									
Maxilla									
Nasal									
Supraorbital									
Frontal									
Sagittal suture									
Sphenoid (lateral sphenobasilar)									

_____

_____

Muscular structures									
Temporalis									
Masseter									
Medial pterygoid									
Lateral pterygoid									
Digastric									
Suprahyoids									
Infrahyoids									

_____

_____

_____

	Date:			Date:			Date:		
	O/MB/I PMTJ DMTJ	Pre NPRS L/R	Post NPRS L/R	O/MB/I PMTJ DMTJ	Pre NPRS L/R	Post NPRS L/R	O/MB/I PMTJ DMTJ	Pre NPRS L/R	Post NPRS L/R
Associated tissues									
Upper trapezius									
Sternocleidomastoid									
Scalenes (anterior and middle)									
Splenius capitis									
Cervical interspinalis									
Levator scapulae									
Rhomboids									
Suboccipitals									

Notes:

Numerical Pain Rating Scale (NPRS)

| 0 | 1 | 2 | 3 | 4 | 5 | 6 | 7 | 8 | 9 | 10 |

No pain   Worst pain

From T.E. Speicher, 2016, *Clinical guide to positional release therapy* (Champaign, IL: Human Kinetics).

REFERENCES

Preface

D'Ambrogio, K.J., and Roth, G.B. 1997. *Positional release therapy: Assessment & treatment of musculoskeletal dysfunction.* St. Louis: Mosby.

Jones, L.H. 1964. Spontaneous release by positioning. *The D.O.* (Jan): 109–116.

Speicher, T.E., and Draper, D.O. 2006. Top 10 positional-release therapy techniques to break the chain of pain. Part 1. *Athletic Therapy Today* 11 (5): 60–62.

Chapter 1

Aguilera, F., Martín, D.P., Masanet, R.A., Botella, A.C., Soler, L.B., and Morell, F.B. 2009. Immediate effect of ultrasound and ischemic compression techniques for the treatment of trapezius latent myofascial trigger points in healthy subjects: A randomized controlled study. *Journal of Manipulative and Physiological Therapeutics* 32 (7): 515–520.

Brandt, B., and Jones, L.H. 1976. Some methods of applying counterstrain. *Journal of the American Osteopathic Association* 75 (9): 786–789.

Busch, V., Magerl, W., Kern, U., Haas, J., Hajak, G., and Eichhammer, P. 2012. The effect of deep and slow breathing on pain perception, autonomic activity, and mood processing: An experimental study. *Pain Medicine* 13 (2): 215–228.

Chaitow, L. 2002. *Positional release techniques.* London: Elsevier Health Sciences.

D'Ambrogio, K.J., and Roth, G.B. 1997. *Positional release therapy: Assessment & treatment of musculoskeletal dysfunction.* St. Louis: Mosby.

Deig, D. 2001. *Positional release technique.* Woburn, MA: Butterworth Heinemann.

Delaney, G.A., and McKee, A.C. 1993. Inter-and intra-rater reliability of the pressure threshold meter in measurement of myofascial trigger point sensitivity. *American Journal of Physical Medicine & Rehabilitation* 72 (3): 136–139.

Dommerholt, J., Bron, C., and Franssen, J. 2006. Myofascial trigger points: An evidence-informed review. *Journal of Manual & Manipulative Therapy* 14 (4): 203–221.

Gemmell, H., Miller, P., and Nordstrom, H. 2008. Immediate effect of ischaemic compression and trigger point pressure release on neck pain and upper trapezius trigger points: A randomised controlled trial. *Clinical Chiropractic* 11 (1): 30–36.

Gerwin, R.D., Dommerholt, J., 2002. Treatment of myofascial pain syndromes. In: Weiner, R. (Ed.), Pain Management; A Practical Guide for Clinicians. CRC Press, Boca Raton.

Hong, C. 1994. Lidocaine injection versus dry needling to myofascial trigger point: The importance of the local twitch response. *American Journal of Physical Medicine & Rehabilitation* 73 (4): 256–263.

Hong, C., Torigoe, Y., and Yu, J. 1995. The localized twitch responses in responsive taut bands of rabbit skeletal muscle fibers are related to the reflexes at spinal cord level. *Journal of Musculoskeletal Pain* 3 (1): 15–33.

Hong, C. 2000. Myofascial trigger points: Pathophysiology and correlation with acupuncture points. *Acupuncture in Medicine* 18 (1): 41–47.

Hoover, H.V. 1949. Fundamentals of technic. *AAO Yearbook,* 94.

Howell, J.N., Cabell, K.S., Chila, A.G., and Eland, D.C. 2006. Stretch reflex and Hoffmann reflex responses to osteopathic manipulative treatment in subjects with Achilles tendinitis. *Journal of the American Osteopathic Association* 106 (9): 537–545.

Jensen, K., Andersen, H.O., Olesen, J., and Lindblom, U. 1986. Pressure-pain threshold in human temporal region: Evaluation of a new pressure algometer. *Pain* 25 (3): 313–323.

Johnson, S.M., and Kurtz, M.E. 2003. Osteopathic manipulative treatment techniques preferred by contemporary osteopathic physicians. *Journal of the American Osteopathic Association* 103 (5): 219–224.Jones, L.H. 1964. Spontaneous release by positioning. *The D.O.* (Jan): 109–116.

Jones, L.H. 1973. Foot treatment without hand trauma. *Journal of the American Osteopathic Association* 72 (5): 481–489.

Jones, L.H., Kusunose, R.S., and Goering, E.K. 1995. *Jones strain-counterstrain.* Boise, ID: Jones Strain-CounterStrain, Inc.

Korr, I.M. 1975. Proprioceptors and somatic dysfunction. *Journal of the American Osteopathic Association* 74 (7): 638–650.

Loveless, J., Speicher, T.,E. Evaluation of the relationship between pressure sensitivity, numerical rating score and visual analog scale assessment of upper trapezius trigger points. Paper presented at: Rocky Mountain Athletic Trainers' Association Annual Symposium; 2012; Meza, AZ.

Melzack, R., Stillwell, D.M., and Fox, E.J. 1977. Trigger points and acupuncture points for pain: Correlations and implications. *Pain* 3 (1): 3–23.

Myers, H.L., Devine, W.H., Fossum, C., Glover, J., Kuchera, M., Kusunose, R.S., and Buskirk. R.V. 2006. *Clinical application of counterstrain.* Tucson, AZ: Osteopathic Press.

Peters, T., MacDonald, R., and Leach, C.M.J. 2012. Counterstrain treatment in the treatment of restless leg syndrome: A pilot single-blind randomized controlled trial: The CARL trial. *International Musculoskeletal Medicine* 34 (4): 136-140.

Simons, D.G., and Travell, J. 1981. Myofascial trigger points: A possible explanation. *Pain* 10 (1): 106.

Speicher, T.E., and Draper, D.O. 2006. *Positional release therapy techniques.* Paper presented at the Rocky Mountain Athletic Trainers' Association Annual Symposium, Salt Lake City, UT.

Speicher, T.E., and Draper, D.O. 2006a. Top 10 positional-release therapy techniques to break the chain of pain. Part 1. *Athletic Therapy Today* 11 (5): 60–62.

Speicher, T.E., and Draper, D.O. 2006b. Top 10 positional-release therapy techniques to break the chain of pain. Part 2. *Athletic Therapy Today* 11 (6): 56–88.

Speicher, T.E., and Kehrhahn, M. 2009. Analogical reasoning: A process for fostering learning transfer from the classroom to clinical practice. *International Forum of Teaching and Studies* 5 (2): 52–58.

Still, A.T. 1902. *The philosophy and mechanical principles of osteopathy.* Hudson-Kimberly: Kansas City.

Takala, E.P. 1990. Pressure pain threshold on upper trapezius and levator scapulae muscles: Repeatability and relation to subjective symptoms in a working population. *Scandinavian Journal of Rehabilitation Medicine* 22 (2): 63.

Travell, J. 1949. Basis for the multiple uses of local block of somatic trigger areas: Procaine infiltration and ethyl chloride spray. *Mississippi Valley Medical Journal* 71 (1): 13.

Williamson, A., and Hoggart, B. 2005. Pain: A review of three commonly used pain rating scales. *Journal of Clinical Nursing* 14 (7): 798–804.

Wong, C.K. 2012. Strain counterstrain: Current concepts and clinical evidence. *Manual Therapy* 17 (1): 2–8.

Wong, C.K., and Schauer-Alvarez, C. 2004. Effect of strain counterstrain on pain and strength in hip musculature. *Journal of Manual & Manipulative Therapy* 12 (4): 215–223.

Woolbright, J.L. 1991. An alternative method of teaching strain/counterstrain manipulation. *Journal of the American Osteopathic Association* 91 (4): 370–373.

Wynne, M.M., Burns, J.M., Eland, D.C., Conatser, R.R., and Howell, J.N. 2006. Effect of counterstrain on stretch reflexes, Hoffmann reflexes, and clinical outcomes in subjects with plantar fasciitis. *Journal of the American Osteopathic Association* 106 (9): 547–556.

Chapter 2

Appelberg, B., Hulliger, M., Johansson, H., and Sojka, P. 1983. Actions on gamma-motoneurones elicited by electrical stimulation of group III muscle afferent fibres in the hind limb of the cat. *The Journal of Physiology* 335 (February): 275–292.

Bailey, M., and Dick, L. 1992. Nociceptive considerations in treating with counterstrain. *The Journal of the American Osteopathic Association* 92 (3): 334, 337–341.

Bear, M.F., Connors, B.W., and Paradiso, M.A. 2007. *Neuroscience.* Vol. 2. Boston: Lippincott Williams & Wilkins.

Byrne, J.H. (Ed.). 1997. *Neuroscience online: An electronic textbook for the neurosciences.* http://nba.uth.tmc.edu/neuroscience.

Capra, N.F., Hisley, C.K., and Masri, R.M. 2007. The influence of pain on masseter spindle afferent discharge. *Archives of Oral Biology* 52 (4): 387–390.

Dommerholt, J., Bron, C., and Franssen, J. 2006. Myofascial trigger points: An evidence-informed review. *Journal of Manual and Manipulative Therapy* 14 (4): 203–221.

Dolezal, V., and Tucek, S. 1992. Effects of tetrodotoxin, Ca2+ absence, d-tubocurarine and vesamicol on spontaneous acetylcholine release from rat muscle. *The Journal of Physiology* 458 (1): 1–9.

Gerwin, R.D., Dommerholt, J., and Shah, J.P. 2004. An expansion of Simons' integrated hypothesis of trigger point formation. *Current Pain and Headache Reports* 8 (6): 468–475.

Herbert, R.D., and Gabriel, M. 2002. Effects of stretching before and after exercising on muscle soreness and risk of injury: Systematic review. *British Medical Journal (Clinical Research Ed.)* 325 (7362): 468.

Hocking, M.J.L. 2013. Exploring the central modulation hypothesis: Do ancient memory mechanisms underlie the pathophysiology of trigger points? *Current Pain and Headache Reports* 17 (7): 347.

Hong, C.Z., and Yu, J. 1998. Spontaneous electrical activity of rabbit trigger spot after transection of spinal cord and peripheral nerve. *Journal of Musculoskeletal Pain* 6 (4): 45–58.

Houdusse, A., Love, M.L., Dominguez, R., Grabarek, Z., and Cohen, C. 1997. Structures of four Ca2+-bound troponin C at 2.0 AA resolution: Further insights into the Ca2+-switch in the calmodulin superfamily. *Structure* 5 (12): 1695–1711.

Howell, J.N., Cabell, K.S., Chila, A.G., and Eland D.C. 2006. Stretch reflex and Hoffmann reflex responses to osteopathic manipulative treatment in subjects with Achilles tendinitis. *Journal of the American Osteopathic Association* 106 (9): 537–545.

Hubbard, D.R., and Berkoff, G.M. 1993. Myofascial trigger points show spontaneous needle EMG activity. *Spine* 18 (13): 1803–1807.

Johansson, H., and Sojka, P. 1991. Pathophysiological mechanisms involved in genesis and spread of muscular tension in occupational muscle pain and in chronic musculoskeletal pain syndromes: A hypothesis. *Medical Hypotheses* 35 (3): 196–203.

Jones, L.H. 1973. Foot treatment without hand trauma. *Journal of the American Osteopathic Association* 72 (5): 481–490.

Kandel, E.R., Schwartz, J.H., and Jessell, T.M. 2000. *Principles of neural science.* New York: McGraw-Hill.

Korr, I. M. 1947. The neural basis of the osteopathic lesion. *The Journal of the American Osteopathic Association* 47 (4): 191–98.

Knight, K.L., and Draper, D.O. 2012. *Therapeutic modalities: The art and science*. Boston: Lippincott Williams & Wilkins.

Korr, I.M. 1975. Proprioceptors and somatic dysfunction. *Journal of the American Osteopathic Association* 74 (7): 638–638.

Kostopoulos, D., Nelson Jr., A.J., Ingber, R.S., and Larkin, R.W. 2008. Reduction of spontaneous electrical activity and pain perception of trigger points in the upper trapezius muscle through trigger point compression and passive stretching. *Journal of Musculoskeletal Pain* 16 (4): 266–278.

Kovyazina, I.,V., Nikolsky, E.,E., Rashid, A., Giniatullin, A., Adámek, S., and Vyskočil, F. 2003. Dependence of miniature endplate current on kinetic parameters of acetylcholine receptors activation: a model study. *Neurochemical Research* 28 (3-4): 443–48.

Larsson, R.,P., Öberg A., and Larsson, S. 1999. Changes of trapezius muscle blood flow and electromyography in chronic neck pain due to trapezius myalgia. *Pain* 79 (1): 45–50.

Maekawa, K., Clark, G.T., and Kuboki, T. 2002. Intramuscular hypoperfusion, adrenergic receptors, and chronic muscle pain. *The Journal of Pain* 3 (4): 251–260.

Matthews, P.C. 1981. Muscle spindles: Their messages and their fusimotor supply. *Comprehensive Physiology*. http://onlinelibrary.wiley.com/doi/10.1002/cphy.cp010206/full.

McKillop, D.F., and Geeves, M.A. 1993. Regulation of the interaction between actin and myosin subfragment 1: Evidence for three states of the thin filament. *Biophysical Journal* 65 (2): 693–701.

McPartland, J.,M. 2004. Travell trigger points-molecular and osteopathic perspectives. *Journal of the American Osteopathic Association* 104: 244–50.

McPartland, J.M., and Simons, D.G. 2006. Myofascial trigger points: Translating molecular theory into manual therapy. *Journal of Manual and Manipulative Therapy* 14 (4): 232–239.

Moore, M. 2007. Golgi tendon organs neuroscience update with relevance to stretching and proprioception in dancers. *Journal of Dance Medicine and Science* 11 (3): 85–92.

O'Halloran, D.J., and Bloom, S.R. 1991. Calcitonin gene related peptide. *British Medical Journal (Clinical Research Ed.)* 302 (6779): 739–740.

Proske, U., and Morgan, D.L. 2001. Muscle damage from eccentric exercise: Mechanism, mechanical signs, adaptation and clinical applications. *The Journal of Physiology* 537 (2): 333–345.

Reinöhl, J., Hoheisel, U., Unger, T., and Mense, S. 2003. Adenosine triphosphate as a stimulant for nociceptive and non-nociceptive muscle group IV receptors in the rat. *Neuroscience Letters* 338 (1): 25–28.

Rosas-Ballina, M., Olofsson, P.S., Ochani, M., Valdés-Ferrer, S.I., Levine, Y.A., Reardon, C., Tusche, M.W., Pavlov, V.A., Andersson, U., Chavan, S., et al. 2011. Acetylcholine-synthesizing T cells relay neural signals in a vagus nerve circuit. *Science* 334 (6052): 98–101.

Shah, J.P., Phillips, T., Danoff, J.V., and Gerber, L.H. 2003. A novel microanalytical technique for assaying soft tissue demonstrates significant quantitative biochemical differences in 3 clinically distinct groups: Normal, latent, and active. *Archives of Physical Medicine and Rehabilitation* 84 (9): E4.

Simons, D.G., Travell, J.G., and Simons, L.S. 1999. *Travell and Simons' myofascial pain and dysfunction: Upper half of body*. Vol. 1. Baltimore: Lippincott Williams & Wilkins.

Sluka, K.A., Kalra, A., and Moore, S.A. 2001. Unilateral intramuscular injections of acidic saline produce a bilateral, long-lasting hyperalgesia. *Muscle & Nerve* 24 (1): 37–46.

Sluka, K.A., Price, M.P., Breese, N.M., Stucky, C.L., Wemmie, J.A., and Welsh, M.J. 2003. Chronic hyperalgesia induced by repeated acid injections in muscle is abolished by the loss of ASIC3, but not ASIC1. *Pain* 106 (3): 229–239.

Speicher, T.E., and Draper, D.O. 2006. *Positional release therapy techniques*. Paper presented at the Rocky Mountain Athletic Trainers' Association Annual Symposium, Salt Lake City, UT.

Stauber, W.T., Clarkson, P.M., Fritz, V.K., and Evans, W.J. 1990. Extracellular matrix disruption and pain after eccentric muscle action. *Journal of Applied Physiology* 69 (3): 868–874.

Thunberg, J., Ljubisavljevic, M., Djupsjöbacka, M., and Johansson, H. 2002. Effects on the fusimotor-muscle spindle system induced by intramuscular injections of hypertonic saline. *Experimental Brain Research* 142 (3): 319–326.

Vandenboom, R. 2004. The myofibrillar complex and fatigue: A review. *Canadian Journal of Applied Physiology* 29 (3): 330–56.

Wessler, I. 1996. Acetylcholine release at motor endplates and autonomic neuroeffector junctions: A comparison. *Pharmacological Research* 33 (2): 81–94.

Wong, K.C., and Schauer-Alvarez, C. 2004. Effect of strain counterstrain on pain and strength in hip musculature. *Journal of Manual and Manipulative Therapy* 12 (4): 215–223.

Wynne, M.M., Burns, J.M., Eland, D.C., Conatser, R.R., and Howell, J.N. 2006. Effect of counterstrain on stretch reflexes, Hoffmann reflexes, and clinical outcomes in subjects with plantar fasciitis. *Journal of the American Osteopathic Association* 106 (9): 547–556.

Chapter 3

American Cancer Society. 2014. What are the key statistics about breast cancer? Accessed October 12, 2004. www.cancer.org/cancer/breastcancer/detailedguide/breast-cancer-key-statistics.

American Diabetes Association. 2014. Statistics about diabetes. Accessed November 23, 2014. www.diabetes.org/diabetes-basics/statistics.

American Obesity Treatment Association. 2004. Related conditions to obesity. Accessed November 23, 2004. www.americanobesity.org/relatedConditions.htm.

Andrews, L.R., Cofield, R.H., and O'Driscoll, S.W. 2000. Shoulder arthroplasty in patients with prior mastectomy for breast cancer. *Journal of Shoulder and Elbow Surgery* 9 (5): 386–388.

Bates, T., and Grunwaldt, E. 1958. Myofascial pain in childhood. *The Journal of Pediatrics* 53 (2): 198–209.

Blackburn, E.H. 1991. Structure and function of telomeres. *Nature* 350 (6319): 569–573.

Blagojevic, M.C., Jinks, J.A., and Jordan, K.P. 2010. Risk factors for onset of osteoarthritis of the knee in older adults: A systematic review and meta-analysis. *Osteoarthritis and Cartilage* 18 (1): 24–33.

Boissonnault, J.S., Klestinski, J.U., and Pearcy, K. 2012. The role of exercise in the management of pelvic girdle and low back pain in pregnancy: A systematic review of the literature. *Journal of Women's Health Physical Therapy* 36 (2): 69–77.

Campisi, J., Andersen, J.K., Kapahi, P., and Melov, S. 2011. Cellular senescence: A link between cancer and age-related degenerative disease? *Seminars in Cancer Biology* 21 (6): 354–359.

Chai, N.C., Scher, A.I., Moghekar, A., Bond, D.S., and Peterlin, B.L. 2014. Obesity and headache: Part I—A systematic review of the epidemiology of obesity and headache. *Headache: The Journal of Head and Face Pain* 54 (2): 219–234.

Clemente-Fuentes, R.J.W., Pickett, H., and Carney, M. 2013. How can pregnant women safely relieve low-back pain? *The Journal of Family Practice* 62 (5): 260, 268.

Colberg, S.R., Sigal, R.J., Fernhall, B., Regensteiner, J.G., Blissmer, B. J., Rubin, R.R., and et al. 2010. Exercise and Type 2 Diabetes: The American College of Sports Medicine and the American Diabetes Association: joint position statement. *Diabetes Care* 33 (12): 147–167.

Cooper, C., Dennison, E., Edwards, M., and Litwic, A. 2013. Epidemiology of osteoarthritis. *Medicographia* 35 (2): 145–151.

Dawes, L.J., Duncan, G., and Wormstone, I.M. 2013. Age-related differences in signaling efficiency of human lens cells underpin differential wound healing response rates following cataract surgery. *Investigative Ophthalmology & Visual Science* 54 (1): 333–342.

De Souza, M.J., Nattiv, A., Joy, E., Misra, M., Williams, N.,I., Mallinson, R.,J., Gibbs, J.,C., et al. 2014. 2014 Female athlete triad coalition consensus statement on treatment and return to play of the female athlete triad: 1st international conference held in San Francisco, California, May 2012 and 2nd international conference held in Indianapolis, Indiana, May 2013. *British Journal of Sports Medicine* 48 (4): 1–20.

Easton, D.F., Ford, D., and Bishop, D.T. 1995. Breast and ovarian cancer incidence in BRCA1-mutation carriers. Breast cancer linkage consortium. *American Journal of Human Genetics* 56 (1): 265.

Ebaugh, D., Spinelli, B., and Schmitz, K.H. 2011. Shoulder impairments and their association with symptomatic rotator cuff disease in breast cancer survivors. *Medical Hypotheses* 77 (4): 481–487.

Ee, C.C., Manheimer, E., Pirotta, M.V., and White, A.R. 2008. Acupuncture for pelvic and back pain in pregnancy: A systematic review. *American Journal of Obstetrics and Gynecology* 198 (3): 254–259.

Ellulu, M., Abed, Y., Rahmat, A., Ranneh, Y., and Ali, F. 2014. Epidemiology of obesity in developing countries: Challenges and prevention. *Global Epidemic Obesity* 2 (1): 2.

Finckh, A., and Turesson, C. 2014. The impact of obesity on the development and progression of rheumatoid arthritis. *Annals of the Rheumatic Diseases* 73 (11): 1911–1913.

Fourie, W.J., and Robb, K.A. 2009. Physiotherapy management of axillary web syndrome following breast cancer treatment: Discussing the use of soft tissue techniques. *Physiotherapy* 95 (4): 314–320.

Fridén, J., and Lieber, R.L. 1998. Segmental muscle fiber lesions after repetitive eccentric contractions. *Cell and Tissue Research* 293 (1): 165–171.

Gerwin, R.D. 2005. A review of myofascial pain and fibromyalgia: Factors that promote their persistence. *Acupuncture in Medicine* 23 (3): 121–134.

Gerwin, R.D, Dommerholt, J., and Shah, J.P. 2004. An expansion of Simons' integrated hypothesis of trigger point formation. *Current Pain and Headache Reports* 8 (6): 468–475.

Gouin, J., and Kiecolt-Glaser, J.K. 2011. The impact of psychological stress on wound healing: Methods and mechanisms. *Immunology and Allergy Clinics of North America* 31 (1): 81–93.

Gowers, W.R. 1904. A lecture on lumbago: Its lessons and analogues: Delivered at the National Hospital for the Paralysed and Epileptic. *British Medical Journal* 1 (2246): 117.

Guillemin, F.A., Rat, C., Mazieres, B., Pouchot, J., Fautrel, B., Euller-Ziegler, L., Fardellone P., et al. 2011. Prevalence of symptomatic hip and knee osteoarthritis: A two-phase population-based survey. *Osteoarthritis and Cartilage* 19 (11): 1314–1322.

Horne, G., McTernan, P., Visscher, T., and Peeters, A. 2014. BMC obesity: Expanding the BMC series into an important area of research. *BMC Obesity* 1 (1): 1.

Itoh, K., Okada, K., and Kawakita, K. 2004. A proposed experimental model of myofascial trigger points in human muscle after slow eccentric exercise. *Acupuncture in Medicine* 22 (1): 2–12.

Jemal, A., Bray, F., Center, M.M., Ferlay, J., Ward, E., and Forman, D. 2011. Global cancer statistics. *CA: A Cancer Journal for Clinicians* 61 (2): 69–90.

Kelly, M. 1945. The nature of fibrositis: I. The myalgic lesion and its secondary effects: A reflex theory. *Annals of the Rheumatic Diseases* 5 (1): 1.

Khorsan, R., Hawk, C., Lisi, A.J., and Kizhakkeveettil, A. 2009. Manipulative therapy for pregnancy and related conditions: A systematic review. *Obstetrical & Gynecological Survey* 64 (6): 416–427.

Korr, I.M. 1948. The emerging concept of the osteopathic lesion. *Journal of the American Osteopathic Association* 100 (7): 449–460.

Kwon, H., and Pessin, J.E. 2013. Adipokines mediate inflammation and insulin resistance. *Frontiers in Endocrinology* 4 (June): 71.

Licciardone, J.C., Buchanan, S., Hensel, K.L., King, H.H., Fulda, K.G., and Stoll, S.T. 2010. Osteopathic manipulative treatment of back pain and related symptoms during pregnancy: A randomized controlled trial. *Journal of Obstetrics* 202 (1): 1–43.

Lillios, S., and Young, J. 2012. The effects of core and lower extremity strengthening on pregnancy-related low back and pelvic girdle pain: A systematic review. *Journal of Women's Health Physical Therapy* 36 (3): 116–124.

Looker, A.C., National Center for Health Statistics (U.S.), et al. 2012. *Osteoporosis or low bone mass at the femur neck or lumbar spine in older adults, United States, 2005-2008.* U.S. Department of Health and Human Services, Centers for Disease Control and Prevention, National Center for Health Statistics. Accessed October 2012. http://www.cdc.gov/arthritis/

Lucas, K.R., Polus, B.I., and Rich, P.A. 2004. Latent myofascial trigger points: Their effects on muscle activation and movement efficiency. *Journal of Bodywork and Movement Therapies* 8 (3): 160–166.

Martin, C.L., Albers, J.W., Pop-Busui, R., et al. 2014. Neuropathy and related findings in the diabetes control and complications trial/epidemiology of diabetes interventions and complications study. *Diabetes Care* 37 (1): 31–38.

Mathers, C., Fat, D.M., and Boerma, J.T. 2008. *The global burden of disease: 2004 update.* Washington, DC: World Health Organization.

McPartland, J.M., and Simons, D.G. 2006. Myofascial trigger points: Translating molecular theory into manual therapy. *Journal of Manual & Manipulative Therapy* 14 (4): 232-239.

Mense, S. 2003. The pathogenesis of muscle pain. *Current Pain and Headache Reports* 7 (6): 419–425.

Murphy, L., and Helmick, C.G. 2012. The impact of osteoarthritis in the United States: A population-health perspective. *The American Journal of Nursing* 112 (3): S13–19.

Nguyen, U.D.T., Zhang, Y., Zhu, Y., Niu, J., Zhang, B., and Felson, D.T. 2011. Increasing prevalence of knee pain and symptomatic knee osteoarthritis: Survey and cohort data. *Annals of Internal Medicine* 155 (11): 725–732.

Nilsson-Wikmar, L., Holm, K., Öijerstedt, R., and Harms-Ringdahl, K. 2005. Effect of three different physical therapy treatments on pain and activity in pregnant women with pelvic girdle pain: A randomized clinical trial with 3, 6, and 12 months follow-up postpartum. *Spine* 30 (8): 850–856.

Oakley, C.B., Scher, A.I., Recober, A., and Peterlin, B.L. 2014. Headache and obesity in the pediatric population. *Current Pain and Headache Reports* 18 (5): 1–13.

Pennick, V., and Liddle, S.D. 2013. Interventions for preventing and treating pelvic and back pain in pregnancy. In *Cochrane Database of Systematic Reviews.* Cochrane Database of Systematic Reviews 2013, Issue 8. Art. No.: CD001139. doi:10.1002/14651858.CD001139.pub3.

Pivarnik, J.M., Perkins, C.D., and Moyerbrailean, T. 2003. Athletes and pregnancy. *Clinical Obstetrics & Gynecology* 46 (2): 403–414.

Radjieski, J.M., Lumley, M.A., and Cantieri, M.S. 1998. Effect of osteopathic manipulative treatment of length of stay for pancreatitis: A randomized pilot study. *Journal of the American Osteopathic Association* 98 (5): 264–272.

Ritchie, J.R. 2003. Orthopedic considerations during pregnancy. *Clinical Obstetrics & Gynecology* 46 (2): 456–466.

Salinas, C.M., and Webbe, F.M. 2012. Sports neuropsychology with diverse athlete populations: Contemporary findings and special considerations. *Journal of Clinical Sport Psychology* 6: 363-384.

Schett, G., Kleyer, A., Perricone, C., Sahinbegovic, E., Iagnocco, A., Zwerina, J., Lorenzini, R., et al. 2013. Diabetes is an independent predictor for severe osteoarthritis: Results from a longitudinal cohort study. *Diabetes Care* 36 (2): 403–409.

Schwartz, H. 1986. The use of counterstrain in an acutely ill in-hospital population. *The Journal of the American Osteopathic Association* 86 (7): 433–442.

Simons, D.G. 2004. Review of enigmatic MTrPs as a common cause of enigmatic musculoskeletal pain and dysfunction. *Journal of Electromyography and Kinesiology* 14 (1): 95–107.

Smith, H.S., Harris, R., and Clauw, D. 2011. Fibromyalgia: An afferent processing disorder leading to a complex pain generalized syndrome. *Pain Physician* 14 (2): E217–245.

Smythe, H.A., and Moldofsky, H. 1977. Two contributions to understanding of the "fibrositis" syndrome. *Bulletin on the Rheumatic Diseases* 28 (1): 928.

Stockman, R. 1920. *Rheumatism and Arthritis.* Edinburg: W. Green & Son.

Sytema, R., Dekker, R., Dijkstra, P.,U., Duis, H.,J., and Sluis, C.,K. 2010. Upper extremity sports injury: Risk factors in comparison to lower extremity injury in more than 25,000 cases. *Clinical Journal of Sport Medicine* 20 (4): 256–63.

Todd, J., Scally, A., Dodwell, D., Horgan, K., and Topping, A. 2008. A randomised controlled trial of two programmes of shoulder exercise following axillary node dissection for invasive breast cancer. *Physiotherapy* 94 (4): 265–273.

Toivanen, A.T., Heliövaara, M., Impivaara, O., Arokoski, J., Knekt, P., Lauren, H., and Kröger, H. 2010. Obesity, physically demanding work and traumatic knee injury are major risk factors for knee osteoarthritis: A population-based study with a follow-up of 22 years. *Rheumatology* 49 (2): 308–314.

Vincent, H.K., Heywood, K., Connelly, J., and Hurley, R.W. 2012. Obesity and weight loss in the treatment and prevention of osteoarthritis. *Physical Medicine and Rehabilitation* 4 (5): S59–67.

Von Stülpnagel, C., Reilich, P., Straube, A., Schäfer, J., Blaschek, A., Lee, S., Müller-Felber, W., Henschel, V., Mansmann, U., and Heinen, F. 2009. Myofascial trigger points in children with tension-type headache: A new diagnostic and therapeutic option. *Journal of Child Neurology* 24 (4): 406–409.

Wolfe, F., Simons, D.G., Fricton, J., Bennett, R.M., Goldenberg, D.L., Gerwin, R., Hathaway, D., McCain, G.A., Russell, I.J., and Sanders, H.O. 1992. The fibromyalgia and myofascial pain syndromes: A preliminary study of tender points and trigger points in persons with fibromyalgia, myofascial pain syndrome and no disease. *The Journal of Rheumatology* 19 (6): 944–951.

Wolfe, F., Smythe, H.A., Yunus, M.B., Bennett, R.M., Bombardier, C., Goldenberg, D.L., Tugwell, P., et al. 1990. The American College of Rheumatology 1990 criteria for the classification of fibromyalgia. *Arthritis & Rheumatism* 33 (2): 160–172.

World Health Organization. 2014. Obesity and overweight. Accessed August 1, 2014. www.who.int/mediacentre/factsheets/fs311/en.

Yunus, M.B. 2008. Central sensitivity syndromes: A new paradigm and group nosology for fibromyalgia and overlapping conditions, and the related issue of disease versus illness. *Seminars in Arthritis and Rheumatism* 37: 339–352.

Zidron, A., Escaño, I.G., Hendrix, A.N., McConnell, A.N., Ongito, J.O., Yogo, J., and Ice, G.H. 2005. Prevalence of somatic dysfunction among an elderly Kenyan population. *Journal of the American Osteopathic Association* 105 (1): 27–28.

Chapter 4

Bauer, T., Gaumetou, E., Klouche, S., Hardy, P., and Maffulli, N. 2014. Metatarsalgia and Morton's disease: Comparison of outcomes between open procedure and neurectomy versus percutaneous metatarsal osteotomies and ligament release with a minimum of 2 years of follow-up. *Journal of Foot and Ankle Surgery* 54 (3): 373–377.

Bolgla, L.A., and Malone, T.R. 2004. Plantar fasciitis and the windlass mechanism: A biomechanical link to clinical practice. *Journal of Athletic Training* 39 (1): 77.

Butterworth, P.A., Landorf, K.B., Gilleard, W., Urquhart, D.M., and Menz, H.B. 2014. The association between body composition and foot structure and function: A systematic review. *Obesity Reviews* 15 (4): 348–357.

Dowling, G.J., Murley, G.S., Munteanu, S.E., Franettovich Smith, M.M., Neal, B.S., Griffiths, I.B., Barton, C.J., and Collins, N.J. 2014. Dynamic foot function as a risk factor for lower limb overuse injury: A systematic review. *Journal of Foot and Ankle Research* 7 (53): 1–13. www.biomedcentral.com/content/pdf/s13047-014-0053-6.pdf.

Hill, C.L., Gill, T.K., Menz, H.B., Taylor, A.W., et al. 2008. Prevalence and correlates of foot pain in a population-based study: The North West Adelaide Health Study. *Journal of Foot and Ankle Research* 1 (2): 1–7.

Murphy, D.F., Connolly, D.A.J., and Beynnon, B.D. 2003. Risk factors for lower extremity injury: A review of the literature. *British Journal of Sports Medicine* 37 (1): 13–29.

Neal, B.S., Griffiths, I.B., Dowling, G.J., Murley, G.S., Munteanu, S.E., Franettovich Smith, M.M., Collins, N.J., and Barton, C.J. 2014. Foot posture as a risk factor for lower limb overuse injury: A systematic review and meta-analysis. *Journal of Foot and Ankle Research* 7: 55.

Schwenk, M., Jordan, E.D., Honarvararaghi, B., Mohler, J., Armstrong, D.G., and Najafi, B. 2013. Effectiveness of foot and ankle exercise programs on reducing the risk of falling in older adults: A systematic review and meta-analysis of randomized controlled trials. *The Journal of the Amercian Podiatric Association* 103 (6): 534-547.

Shibuya, N., Davis, M.L., and Jupiter, D.C. 2014. Epidemiology of foot and ankle fractures in the United States: An analysis of the national trauma data bank (2007 to 2011). *Journal of Foot and Ankle Surgery* 53 (5): 606–608.

Spink, M.J., Menz, H.B., Fotoohabadi, M.R., Wee, E., Landorf, K.B., Hill, K.D., Lord, S.R., et al. 2011. Effectiveness of a multifaceted podiatry intervention to prevent falls in community dwelling older people with disabling foot pain: Randomised controlled trial. *BMJ* 342. http://www.bmj.com/content/342/bmj.d3411.long.

Thomas, M.J., Roddy, E., Zhang, W., Menz, H.B., Hannan, M.T., and Peat, G.M. 2011. The population prevalence of foot and ankle pain in middle and old age: A systematic review. *Pain* 152 (12): 2870–2880.

Tong, J.W.K., and Kong, P.W. 2013. Association between foot type and lower extremity injuries: Systematic literature review with meta-analysis. *Journal of Orthopaedic & Sports Physical Therapy* 43 (10): 700–714.

Wong, C.K. 2012. Strain counterstrain: Current concepts and clinical evidence. *Manual Therapy* 17 (1): 2–8.

Wong, C.K., and Schauer-Alvarez, C. 2004. Effect of strain counterstrain on pain and strength in hip musculature. *Journal of Manual & Manipulative Therapy* 12 (4): 215–223.

Chapter 5

Bastien, M., Moffet, H., Bouyer, L.J., Perron, M., Hébert, L.J., and Leblond, J. 2015. Alteration in global motor strategy following lateral ankle sprain. *BMC Musculoskeletal Disorders* 15 (1): 436.

Cleland, J.A., Mintken, P., McDevitt, A., Bieniek, M., Carpenter, K., Kulp, K., and Whitman, J.M. 2013. Manual physical therapy and exercise versus supervised home exercise in the management of patients with inversion ankle sprain: A multicenter randomized clinical trial. *Journal of Orthopaedic & Sports Physical Therapy* 43 (7): 443–455.

Doherty, C., Delahunt, E., Caulfield, B., Hertel, J., Ryan, J., and Bleakley, C. 2015. The incidence and prevalence of ankle sprain injury: A systematic review and meta-analysis of prospective epidemiological studies. *Sports Medicine* 44 (1): 123–140.

Dowling, G.J., Murley, G.S., Munteanu, S.E., Franettovich Smith, M.M., Neal, B.S., Griffiths, I.B., Barton, C.J., and Collins, N.J. 2015. Dynamic foot function as a risk factor for lower limb overuse injury: A systematic review. *Journal of Foot and Ankle Research* 7 (53): 1–13.

Eisenhart, A.W., Gaeta, T.J., and Yens, D.P. 2003. Osteopathic manipulative treatment in the emergency department for patients with acute ankle injuries. *JAOA: Journal of the American Osteopathic Association* 103 (9): 417–421.

Franklyn-Miller, A., Wilson, C., Bilzon, J., and McCrory, P. 2011. Foot orthoses in the prevention of injury in initial military training: A randomized controlled trial. *The American Journal of Sports Medicine* 39 (1): 30–37.

Giandolini, M., Horvais, N., Farges, Y., Samozino, P., and Morin, J.-B. 2013. Impact reduction through long-term intervention in recreational runners: Midfoot strike pattern versus low-drop/low-heel height footwear. *European Journal of Applied Physiology* 113 (8): 2077–2090. doi:10.1007/s00421-013-2634-7.

Murphy, K., Curry, E.J., and Matzkin, E.G. 2013. Barefoot running: Does it prevent injuries? *Sports Medicine* 43 (11): 1131–1138. doi:10.1007/s40279-013-0093-2.

Nielsen, R.O., Buist, I., Sørensen, H., Lind, M., and Rasmussen, S. 2012. Training errors and running related injuries: A systematic review. *International Journal of Sports Physical Therapy* 7 (1): 58.

Newman, P., Witchalls, J., Waddington, G., and Adams, R. 2013. Risk factors associated with medial tibial stress syndrome in runners: A systematic review and meta-analysis. *Open Access Journal of Sports Medicine* 4: 229.

Peters, J.A., Zwerver, J., Diercks, R.L., Elferink-Gemser, M.T., and van den Akker-Scheek, I. 2015. Preventive interventions for tendinopathy: A systematic review. *Journal of Science and Medicine in Sport*, April. doi:10.1016/j.jsams.2015.03.008.

Smith, H.S., Harris, R., and Clauw, D. 2011. Fibromyalgia: An afferent processing disorder leading to a complex pain generalized syndrome. *Pain Physician* 14 (2): E217–245.

Swenson, D.M., Collins, C.L., Fields, S.K., and Comstock, R.D. 2013. Epidemiology of U.S. high school sports-related ligamentous ankle injuries, 2005/06-2010/11. *Clinical Journal of Sport Medicine: Official Journal of the Canadian Academy of Sport Medicine* 23 (3): 190–196. doi:10.1097/JSM.0b013e31827d21fe.

Valderrabano, V., Hintermann, B., Horisberger, M., and Shing Fung, T. 2006. Ligamentous posttraumatic ankle osteoarthritis. *The American Journal of Sports Medicine* 34 (4): 612–620.

Waterman, B.R., Owens, B.D., Davey, S., Zacchilli, M.A., and Belmont, P.J. 2010. The epidemiology of ankle sprains in the United States. *The Journal of Bone & Joint Surgery* 92 (13): 2279–2285.

Zadpoor, A.A., and Nikooyan, A.A. 2011. The relationship between lower-extremity stress fractures and the ground reaction force: A systematic review. *Clinical Biomechanics* 26 (1): 23–28.

Chapter 6

Bates, T., and Grunwaldt, E. 1958. Myofascial pain in childhood. *Journal of Pediatrics* 53 (2): 198–209.

Bauer, J., and Duke, L. 2011. Examining biomechanical and anthropometrical factors as contributors to iliotibial band friction syndrome. *Sport Science Review* 20 (1-2): 39–53.

Birmingham, T.B., Kramer, J., Lumsden, J., Obright, K.D., and Kramer, J.E. 2004. Effect of a positional release therapy technique on hamstring flexibility. *Physiotherapy Canada* 56 (3): 165–170.

Crowell, H.P., and Davis, I.S. 2011. Gait retraining to reduce lower extremity loading in runners. *Clinical Biomechanics* 26 (1): 78–83.

Danielson, P., Andersson, G., Alfredson, H., and Forsgren, S. 2008. Marked sympathetic component in the perivascular innervation of the dorsal paratendinous tissue of the patellar tendon in arthroscopically treated tendinosis patients. *Knee Surgery, Sports Traumatology, Arthroscopy* 16 (6): 621–626.

DiFiori, J.P., Benjamin, H.J.,. Brenner, J.S., Gregory, A., Jayanthi, N., Landry, G.L., and Luke, A. 2014. Overuse injuries and burnout in youth sports: A position statement from the American Medical Society for Sports Medicine. *British Journal of Sports Medicine* 48 (4): 287–288.

Felson, D.T., Niu, J., Gross, K.D., Englund, M., Sharma, L., Derek, T., Cooke, V., Guermazi, A., et al. 2013. Valgus malalignment is a risk factor for lateral knee osteoarthritis incidence and progression: Findings from the Multicenter Osteoarthritis Study and the Osteoarthritis Initiative. *Arthritis & Rheumatism* 65 (2): 355–362. doi:10.1002/art.37726.

Foss, K., Barber, D., Myer, G.D., Chen, S.S., and Hewett, T.E. 2012. Expected prevalence from the differential diagnosis of anterior knee pain in adolescent female athletes during preparticipation screening. *Journal of Athletic Training* 47 (5): 519–524. doi:10.4085/1062-6050-47.5.01.

Gage, B.E., McIlvain, N.M., Collins, C.L., Fields, S.K., and Comstock, R.D. 2012. Epidemiology of 6.6 million knee injuries presenting to United States emergency departments from 1999 through 2008. *Academic Emergency Medicine* 19 (4): 378–385. doi:10.1111/j.1553-2712.2012.01315.x.

Grimm, N.L., Shea, K.G., Leaver, R.W., Aoki, S.K., and Carey, J.L. 2012. Efficacy and degree of bias in knee injury prevention studies: A systematic review of RCTs. *Clinical Orthopaedics and Related Research* 471 (1): 308–316. doi:10.1007/s11999-012-2565-3.

Hägglund, M., Atroshi, I., Wagner, P., and Waldén, M. 2013. Superior compliance with a neuromuscular training programme is associated with fewer ACL injuries and fewer acute knee injuries in female adolescent football players: Secondary analysis of an RCT. *British Journal of Sports Medicine* 47 (15): 974–979.

Herbert, R.D., and Gabriel, M. 2002. Effects of stretching before and after exercising on muscle soreness and risk of injury: A systematic review. *BMJ* 325 (7362): 468.

Hewett, T.E., Di Stasi, S.L., and Myer, G.D. 2013. Current concepts for injury prevention in athletes after anterior cruciate ligament reconstruction. *American Journal of Sports Medicine* 41 (1): 216–224. doi:10.1177/0363546512459638.

Kaandeepan, M.M., Cheraladhan, E.S., Premkumar, M., and. Shah, S.K. 2011. Comparing the effectiveness of positional release therapy technique and passive stretching on hamstring muscle through sit to reach test in normal female subjects. *Indian Journal of Physiotherapy & Occupational Therapy* 5 (3): 58–61.

Kraus, T., Švehlík, M., Singer, G., Schalamon, J., Zwick, E., and Linhart, W. 2012. The epidemiology of knee injuries in children and adolescents. *Archives of Orthopaedic and Trauma Surgery* 132 (6): 773–779. doi:10.1007/s00402-012-1480-0.

Larsson, M.E.H, Käll, I., and Nilsson-Helander, K. 2012. Treatment of patellar tendinopathy: A systematic review of randomized controlled trials. *Knee Surgery, Sports Traumatology, Arthroscopy* 20 (8): 1632–1646.

Lavine, R. 2010. Iliotibial band friction syndrome. *Current Reviews in Musculoskeletal Medicine* 3 (1-4): 18–22.

Leetun, D.T., Ireland, M.L., Willson, J.D., Ballantyne, B.T., and McClay Davis, I. 2004. Core stability measures as risk factors for lower extremity injury in athletes. *Medicine & Science in Sports & Exercise* 36 (6): 926–934.

Michaelidis, M., and Koumantakis, G.A. 2014. Effects of knee injury primary prevention programs on anterior cruciate ligament injury rates in female athletes in different sports: A systematic review. *Physical Therapy in Sport* 15 (3): 200–210. doi:10.1016/j.ptsp.2013.12.002.

Murphy, D.F., Connolly, D.A.J., and Beynnon, B.D. 2003. Risk factors for lower extremity injury: A review of the literature. *British Journal of Sports Medicine* 37 (1): 13–29.

Neogi, T., and Zhang, Y. 2013. Epidemiology of osteoarthritis. *Rheumatic Disease Clinics of North America, Update on Osteoarthritis*, 39 (1): 1–19. doi:10.1016/j.rdc.2012.10.004.

Noyes, F.R., and Barber-Westin, S.D. 2014. Neuromuscular retraining intervention programs: Do they reduce noncontact anterior cruciate ligament injury rates in adolescent female athletes? *Arthroscopy: The Journal of Arthroscopic & Related Surgery* 30 (2): 245–255.

Rodriguez-Merchan, E.C. 2013. The treatment of patellar tendinopathy. *Journal of Orthopaedics and Traumatology* 14 (2): 77–81.

Sadoghi, P., von Keudell, A., and Vavken, P. 2012. Effectiveness of anterior cruciate ligament injury prevention training programs. *The Journal of Bone & Joint Surgery* 94 (9): 769–776.

Smith, H.C., Vacek, P., Johnson, R.J., Slauterbeck, J.R., Hashemi, J., Shultz, S., and Beynnon, B.D. 2012. Risk factors for anterior cruciate ligament injury a review of the literature—part 1: Neuromuscular and anatomic risk. *Sports Health: A Multidisciplinary Approach* 4 (1): 69–78.

Swenson, D.M.,. Collins, C.L., Best, T.M., Flanigan, D.C., Fields, S.K., and Comstock, R.D. 2013. Epidemiology of knee injuries among U.S. high school athletes, 2005/06–2010/11. *Medicine & Science in Sports & Exercise* 45 (3): 462–469. doi:10.1249/MSS.0b013e318277acca.

Van Gent R.N., Siem, D., and Middelkoop, M. 2007. Incidence and determinants of lower extremity running injuries in long distance runners: A systematic review. *British Journal of Sports Medicine* 41 (8): 469–480.

Chapter 7

Anderson, K., Strickland, S.M., Warren, R. 2001. Hip and groin injuries in athletes. *The American Journal of Sports Medicine* 29 (4): 521-533.

Cohen, S.P. 2005. Sacroiliac joint pain: A comprehensive review of anatomy, diagnosis, and treatment. *Anesthesia & Analgesia* 101 (5): 1440–1453.

Engebretsen, A.H., Myklebust, G., Holme, I., Engebretsen, L., and Bahr, R. 2010. Intrinsic risk factors for groin injuries among male soccer players: A prospective cohort study. *The American Journal of Sports Medicine* 38 (10): 2051–2057.

Gladwell, V., Head, S., Haggar, M., and Beneke, R. 2006. Does a program of Pilates improve chronic non-specific low back pain? *Journal of Sport Rehabilitation* 15 (4): 338.

Hopayian, K., Song, F., Riera, R., and Sambandan, S. 2010. The clinical features of the piriformis syndrome: A systematic review. *European Spine Journal* 19 (12): 2095–2109.

Khan, M., Adamich, J., Simunovic, N., Philippon, M.J., Bhandari, M., and Ayeni, O.R. 2013. Surgical management of internal snapping hip syndrome: A systematic review evaluating open and arthroscopic approaches. *Arthroscopy: The Journal of Arthroscopic & Related Surgery* 29 (5): 942–948.

Leetun, D.T., Ireland, M.L., Willson, J.D., Ballantyne, B.T., and Davis, I.M. 2004. Core stability measures as risk factors for lower extremity injury in athletes. *Medicine & Science in Sports & Exercise* 36 (6): 926–934.

Macedo, L.G., Maher, C.G., Latimer, J., and McAuley, J.H. 2009. Motor control exercise for persistent, nonspecific low back pain: A systematic review. *Physical Therapy* 89 (1): 9–25.

McGill, S. 2007. *Low back disorders: Evidence-based prevention and rehabilitation* (2nd ed.). Champaign, IL: Human Kinetics.

Morelli, V., and Weaver, V. 2005. Groin injuries and groin pain in athletes: Part 1. *Primary Care: Clinics in Office Practice* 32 (1): 163–183.

Peate, W.F., Bates, G., Lunda, K., Francis, S., and Bellamy, K. 2007. Core strength: A new model for injury prediction and prevention. *Journal of Occupational Medical Toxicology* 2 (3): 1–9.

Posadzki, P., Lizis, P., and Hagner-Derengowska, M. 2011. Pilates for low back pain: A systematic review. *Complementary Therapies in Clinical Practice* 17 (2): 85–89.

Rupert M.P., et al. 2009. Evaluation of sacroiliac joint interventions: A systematic appraisal of the literature. *Pain Physician* 12: 399–418.

Seidenberg, P., and Bowen, J.D. 2010. *The hip and pelvis in sports medicine and primary care.* New York: Springer.

Sharma, D., and Sen, S. 2014. Effects of muscle energy technique on pain and disability in subjects with SI joint dysfunction. *International Journal of Physiotherapy and Research* 2 (1): 305–311.

Speicher, T.E., Martin, R.D., and Desimone, R. 2006. Management of low back pain through the use of ADL education. *Athletic Therapy Today* 11 (6): 55–58.

Szadek, K.M., Van der Wurff, P., Van Tulder, M.W., Zuurmond, W.W., and Perez, R. 2009. Diagnostic validity of criteria for sacroiliac joint pain: A systematic review. *The Journal of Pain* 10 (4): 354–368.

Topol, G.A., Reeves, K.D., and Hassanein, K.M. 2005. Efficacy of dextrose prolotherapy in elite male kicking-sport athletes with chronic groin pain. *Archives of Physical Medicine and Rehabilitation* 86 (4): 697–702.

Valent, A., Frizziero, A., Bressan, S., Zanella, E., Giannotti, E., and Masiero, S. 2012. Insertional tendinopathy of the adductors and rectus abdominis in athletes: A review. *Muscles, Ligaments and Tendons Journal* 2 (2): 142.

Wong, C., and Schauer-Alvarez, C. 2004. Effect of strain counterstrain on pain and strength in hip musculature. *The Journal of Manual and Manipulative Therapy* 12 (4): 215-223.

Chapter 8

Andersson, G.B.J. 1999. Epidemiological features of chronic low-back pain. *The Lancet* 354 (9178): 581–588.

Baker, R.T., Nasypany, A., Seegmiller, J.G., and Baker, J.G. 2013. Treatment of acute torticollis using positional release therapy: Part 2. *International Journal of Athletic Therapy and Training* 18 (2): 38–43.

Belzberg, P.B., Hansson, T., Dorsi, M. 2010. Treatment for thoracic outlet syndrome. *Cochrane Database of Systematic Reviews* 1: 1-19.

Bartynski, W.S., Dejohn, L.M., Rothfus, W.E., and Gerszten, P.C. 2013. Progressive-onset versus injury-associated discogenic low back pain: Features of disc internal derangement in patients studied with provocation lumbar discography. *Interventional Neuroradiology* 19 (1): 110.

Bono, C.M. 2004. Low-back pain in athletes. *The Journal of Bone & Joint Surgery* 86 (2): 382–396.

Chirurgi, R., and Kahlon, S. 2012. Isolated torticollis may present as an atypical presentation of meningitis. *Case Reports in Emergency Medicine* Volume 2012, Article ID 193543, doi:10.1155/2012/193543.

Deane, L., Giele, H., and Johnson, K. 2012. Thoracic outlet syndrome. *British Medical Journal* 345: e7373.

Endean, A., Palmer, K.T., Coggon, D. 2011. Potential MRI findings to refine case definition for mechanical low back pain in epidemiology studies: A systematic review. *Spine* 15 (36): 160-169.

Furlan, A.D., Yazdi, F., Tsertsvadze, A., Gross, A., Tulder, M.V., Santaguida, L., Gagnier, J., et al. 2011. A systematic review and meta-analysis of efficacy, cost-effectiveness, and safety of selected complementary and alternative medicine for neck and low-back pain. *Evidence-Based Complementary and Alternative Medicine* Volume 2012, Article ID 953139: 1–61. doi:10.1155/2012/953139.

Hoy, D., Bain, C., Williams, G., March, L., Brooks, P., Blyth, F., Woolf, A., Vos, T., and Buchbinder, R. 2012. A systematic review of the global prevalence of low back pain. *Arthritis & Rheumatism* 64 (6): 2028–2037.

Hoy, D., Brooks, P., Blyth, F., and Buchbinder, R. 2010. The epidemiology of low back pain. *Best Practice & Research Clinical Rheumatology* 24 (6): 769–781.

Krismer, M., and Van Tulder, M. 2007. Low back pain (non-specific). *Best Practice & Research Clinical Rheumatology* 21 (1): 77–91.

Kuchera, M.L. 2008. Osteopathic manipulative medicine considerations in patients with chronic pain. *Journal of the American Osteopathic Association* 105 (Suppl. 4): S29–36.

Lal, S., Abbasi, A., and Jamro, S. 2011. Response of primary torticollis to physiotherapy. *Journal of Surgery Pakistan* (International) 16: 4.

Laulan, J., Fouquet, B., Rodaix, C., Jauffret, P., Roquelaure, Y., and Descatha, A. 2011. Thoracic outlet syndrome: Definition, aetiological factors, diagnosis, management and occupational impact. *Journal of Occupational Rehabilitation* 21 (3): 366–373.

Lewis, C., and Flynn, T.W. 2001. The use of strain-counterstrain in the treatment of patients with low back pain. *Journal of Manual & Manipulative Therapy* 9 (2): 92–98.

Lewis, C., Souvlis, T., and Sterling, M. 2011. Strain-counterstrain therapy combined with exercise is not more effective than exercise alone on pain and disability in people with acute low back pain: A randomised trial. *Journal of Physiotherapy* 57 (2): 91–98.

Livshits, G., Popham, M., Malkin, I., Sambrook, P.N., MacGregor, A.J., Spector, T., and Williams, F. 2011. Lumbar disc degeneration and genetic factors are the main risk factors for low back pain in women: The UK twin spine study. *Annals of the Rheumatic Diseases* 70 (10): 1740–1748.

Luo, X., Pietrobon, R., Sun, S.X., Liu, G., and Hey, L. 2004. Estimates and patterns of direct health care expenditures among individuals with back pain in the United States. *Spine* 29 (1): 79–86.

O'Brien, P.J., Ramasunder, S., and Cox, M.W. 2011. Venous thoracic outlet syndrome secondary to first rib osteochondroma in a pediatric patient. *Journal of Vascular Surgery* 53 (3): 811–813.

Patwardhan, S., Shyam, K., Sancheti, P., Arora, T., Nagda, and Naik, P. 2011. Adult presentation of congenital muscular torticollis a series of 12 patients treated with a bipolar release of sternocleidomastoid and z-lengthening. *Journal of Bone & Joint Surgery, British Volume* 93 (6): 828–832.

Per, H., Canpolat, M., Tümtürk, A., Gumuş, H., Gokoglu, A., Yikilmaz, A., Özmen, S., et al. 2014. Different etiologies of acquired torticollis in childhood. *Child's Nervous System* 30 (3): 431–440.

Povlsen, B., Belzberg, A., Hansson, T., and Dorsi, M. 2010. Treatment for thoracic outlet syndrome. *Cochrane Database of Systematic Reviews* 11. DOI: 10.1002/14651858. CD007218.pub3 .

Shankar, L., Abbasi, A.S., Jamro, S. 2011. Response of primary torticollis to physiotherapy. *Journal of Surgery Pakistan (International)* 16 (4): 153-156.

Shiri, R., Karppinen, J., Leino-Arjas, P., Solovieva, S., and Viikari-Juntura, E. 2010. The association between obesity and low back pain: A meta-analysis. *American Journal of Epidemiology* 171 (2): 135–154.

Todd, A.G. 2011. Cervical spine: Degenerative conditions. *Current Reviews in Musculoskeletal Medicine* 4 (4): 168–174.

Wong, C.K. 2012. Strain counterstrain: Current concepts and clinical evidence. *Manual Therapy* 17 (1): 2–8.

Yim, S.Y., Yoon, D., Park, M.C., Lee, I.J., Kim, J. H., Lee, M.A., Kwack, K.S., et al. 2013. Integrative analysis of congenital muscular torticollis: From gene expression to clinical significance. *BMC Medical Genomics* 6 (Suppl. 2): S10.

Chapter 9

Allen, L. 2013. Long head of biceps tendon. *UNM Orthopaedic Research Journal* 2: 21–23.

Andersen, J.H., Fallentin, N., Thomsen, J.F., and Mikkelsen, S. 2011. Risk factors for neck and upper extremity disorders among computers users and the effect of interventions: An overview of systematic reviews. *PLoS One* 6 (5): e19691.

Da Costa, B.R., and Vieira, E.R. 2010. Risk factors for work-related musculoskeletal disorders: A systematic review of recent longitudinal studies. *American Journal of Industrial Medicine* 53 (3): 285–323.

Das, K.P., Talukdar, D.C., Chowdhury, R.M., Islam, A., Datta, N.K., Shoma, F.K., and Islam, M.N. 2012. Patients' satisfaction of surgery for resistant cases of de Quervain's disease. *Journal of Dhaka Medical College* 20 (2): 146–152.

Ditsios, K., Agathangelidis, F., Boutsiadis, A., Karataglis, D., and Papadopoulos, P. 2012. Long head of the biceps pathology combined with rotator cuff tears. *Advances in Orthopedics* Volume 2012, Article ID 405472: 1-6. doi:10.1155/2012/405472.

Ebaugh, D., Spinelli, B., and Schmitz, K.H. 2011. Shoulder impairments and their association with symptomatic rotator cuff disease in breast cancer survivors. *Medical Hypotheses* 77 (4): 481–487.

Ellenbecker, T.S., and Cools, A. 2010. Rehabilitation of shoulder impingement syndrome and rotator cuff injuries: An evidence-based review. *British Journal of Sports Medicine* 44 (5): 319–327.

Fernandez-de-las-Penas, C., Gröbli, C., Ortega-Santiago, R., Fischer, C.S., Boesch, D., Froidevaux, P., Stocker, L., Weissmann, R., and González-Iglesias, J. 2012. Referred pain from myofascial trigger points in head, neck, shoulder, and arm muscles reproduces pain symptoms in blue-collar (manual) and white-collar (office) workers. *The Clinical Journal of Pain* 28 (6): 511–518.

Galasso, O., Gasparini, G., Benedetto, M., Familiari, F., and Castricini, R. 2012. Tenotomy versus tenodesis in the treatment of the long head of biceps brachii tendon lesions. *BMC Musculoskeletal Disorders* 13 (1): 205.

Gottschalk, A.W., Andrish, J.T. 2011. Epidemiology of sports injury in pediatric athletes. *Sports Medicine Arthroscopic Review* 19: 2-6.

Jacobson, E.C., Lockwood, M.D., Hoefner, V.C., Dickey, J.L., and Kuchera, W.L. 1989. Shoulder pain and repetition strain injury to the supraspinatus muscle: Etiology and manipulative treatment. *Journal of the American Osteopathic Association* 89 (8): 1037–1040.

Jain, N.B., Higgins, L.D., Losina, E., Collins, J., Blazar, P.E., and Katz, J.N. 2014. Epidemiology of musculoskeletal upper extremity ambulatory surgery in the United States. *BMC Musculoskeletal Disorders* 15 (1): 4.

Karthik, K., Carter-Esdale, C.W., Vijayanathan, S., and Kochhar, T. 2013. Extensor pollicis brevis tendon damage presenting as de Quervain's disease following kettlebell training. *BMC Sports Science, Medicine and Rehabilitation* 5 (1): 13.

Kietrys, D.M., Palombaro, K.M., Azzaretto, E., Hubler, R., Schaller, B., Schlussel, J.M., and Tucker, M. 2013. Effectiveness of dry needling for upper-quarter myofascial pain: A systematic review and meta-analysis. *Journal of Orthopaedic & Sports Physical Therapy* 43 (9): 620–634.

Koester, M.C., George, M.S., and Kuhn. J.E. 2005. Shoulder impingement syndrome. *The American Journal of Medicine* 118 (5): 452–455.

Krupp, R.J., Kevern, M.A., Gaines, M.D., Kotara, S., and Singleton, S.B. 2009. Long head of the biceps tendon pain: Differential diagnosis and treatment. *Journal of Orthopaedic & Sports Physical Therapy* 39 (2): 55–70.

Lucas, K.R., Polus, B.I., and Rich, P.A. 2004. Latent myofascial trigger points: Their effects on muscle activation and movement efficiency. *Journal of Bodywork and Movement Therapies* 8 (3): 160–166.

Umer, M., Qadir, I., Azam, M. 2012. Subacromial impingement syndrome. *Orthopedic Reviews* 4 (18): 79-82.

Ootes, D., Lambers, K.T., and Ring, D.C. 2012. The epidemiology of upper extremity injuries presenting to the emergency department in the United States. *Hand* 7 (1): 18–22.

Patel, K., Kashyap, R., Tadisina, K., and Gonzalez, M.H. 2013. De Quervain's Disease. *Eplasty* 13. Available at: http://www.eplasty.com/index.php?option=com_content&view=article&id=982&catid=49

Quan, D. 2013. Median nerve entrapment syndromes. *Upper Extremity Focal Neuropathies*: 7–9. Available at:

https://webportal.aanem.org/Resources/Files/Downloads/products/13CB.pdf#page=7

Rathbun, J.B., and Macnab, I. 1970. The microvascular pattern of the rotator cuff. *Journal of Bone & Joint Surgery* 52: 540–553.

Shanley, E., Rauh, M.J., Michener, L.A., Ellenbecker, T.S., Garrison, J.C., and Thigpen, C.A. 2011. Shoulder range of motion measures as risk factors for shoulder and elbow injuries in high school softball and baseball players. *The American Journal of Sports Medicine* 39 (9): 1997–2006.

Sytema, R., Dekker, R., Dijkstra, P.U., Duis, H., and Sluis, C. 2010. Upper extremity sports injury: Risk factors in comparison to lower extremity injury in more than 25,000 cases. *Clinical Journal of Sport Medicine* 20 (4): 256–263.

Wanivenhaus, F., Fox, A., Chaudhury, S., and Rodeo, S. 2012. Epidemiology of injuries and prevention strategies in competitive swimmers. *Sports Health: A Multidisciplinary Approach* 4 (3): 246–251.

Westrick, R.B., Miller, J.M., Carow, S.D., and Gerber, J.P. 2012. Exploration of the Y-Balance Test for assessment of upper quarter closed kinetic chain performance. *International Journal of Sports Physical Therapy* 7 (2): 139.

Chapter 10

Ahmad, Z.N., Siddiqui, N., Malik, S.S., Abdus-Samee, M., Tytherleigh-Strong, G., and Rushton, N. 2013. Lateral epicondylitis: A review of pathology and management. *Bone & Joint Journal* 95 (9): 1158–1164.

Andersen, J.H., Fallentin, N., Thomsen, J.F., and Mikkelsen, S. 2011. Risk factors for neck and upper extremity disorders among computers users and the effect of interventions: An overview of systematic reviews. *PLoS One* 6 (5): e19691.

Baker, R.T., Van Riper, M., Nasypany, A., and Seegmiller, J.G. 2014. Evaluation and treatment of apparent reactive tendinopathy of the biceps brachii. *IJATT* 19 (4): 14–21.

Bisset, L.M., Hing, W., and Vicenzino, B. 2011. The efficacy of mobilisations with movement treatment on musculoskeletal pain: A systematic review and meta-analysis. In *16th International Congress of the World Confederation for Physical Therapy*. www98.griffith.edu.au/dspace/handle/10072/43897.

Coombes, B.K., Bisset, L., and Vicenzino, B. 2010. Efficacy and safety of corticosteroid injections and other injections for management of tendinopathy: A systematic review of randomised controlled trials. *The Lancet* 376 (9754): 1751–1767.

Clar, C., Tsertsvadze, A., Hundt, G.L., Clarke, A., Sutcliffe, P., et al. 2014. Clinical effectiveness of manual therapy for the management of musculoskeletal and non-musculoskeletal conditions: A systematic review and update of *UK Evidence Report. Chiropractic & Manual Therapies* 22 (1): 12.

Creaney, L., Wallace, A., Curtis, M., and Connell, D. 2011. Growth factor-based therapies provide additional benefit beyond physical therapy in resistant elbow tendinopathy: A prospective, single-blind, randomised trial of autologous blood injections versus platelet-rich plasma injections. *British Journal of Sports Medicine* 45 (12): 966–971.

Da Costa, B.R., and Vieira, E.R. 2010. Risk factors for work-related musculoskeletal disorders: A systematic review of recent longitudinal studies. *American Journal of Industrial Medicine* 53 (3): 285–323.

Dean, B., Floyd, J., Franklin, S.L., and Carr, A.J. 2013. The peripheral neuronal phenotype is important in the pathogenesis of painful human tendinopathy: A systematic review. *Clinical Orthopaedics and Related Research* 471 (9): 3036–3046. doi:10.1007/s11999-013-3010-y.

De Vos, R.-J., Windt, J, and Weir, A. 2014. Strong evidence against platelet-rich plasma injections for chronic lateral epicondylar tendinopathy: A systematic review. *British Journal of Sports Medicine* 48 (12): 952–956.

Dommerholt, J., Bron, C., and Franssen, J. 2006. Myofascial trigger points: An evidence-informed review. *Journal of Manual & Manipulative Therapy* 14 (4): 203–221.

Drew, B.T., Smith, T.O., Littlewood, C., and Sturrock, B. 2012. Do structural changes (e.g., collagen/matrix) explain the response to therapeutic exercises in tendinopathy: A systematic review. *British Journal of Sports Medicine* 0: 1–8. doi:10.1136/bjsports-2012-091285

Hjelm, N., Werner, S., and Renstrom, P. 2012. Injury risk factors in junior tennis players: A prospective 2-year study. *Scandinavian Journal of Medicine & Science in Sports* 22 (1): 40–48.

Jewson, J.L., Lambert, G.W., Storr, M., and Gaida, J.E. 2015. The sympathetic nervous system and tendinopathy: A systematic review. *Sports Medicine* 45 (5): 727–743.

Lee, H.J., Kim, I., Hong, J.T., and Kim, M.S. 2014. Early surgical treatment of pronator teres syndrome. *Journal of Korean Neurosurgical Society* 55 (5): 296–299.

Meltzer, K.R., and Standley, P.R. 2007. Modeled repetitive motion strain and indirect osteopathic manipulative techniques in regulation of human fibroblast proliferation and interleukin secretion. *JAOA: Journal of the American Osteopathic Association* 107 (12): 527–536.

Olaussen, M., Holmedal, O., Lindbaek, M., Brage, S., and Solvang, H. 2013. Treating lateral epicondylitis with corticosteroid injections or non-electrotherapeutical physiotherapy: A systematic review. *BMJ Open* 3 (10): e003564. doi:10.1136/bmjopen-2013-003564.

Ootes, S., Lambers, K.T., and Ring, D.C. 2012. The epidemiology of upper extremity injuries presenting to the emergency department in the United States. *Hand* 7 (1): 18–22.

Orchard, J., and Kountouris, A. 2011. The management of tennis elbow. *BMJ* 342: d2687.

Quan, D. 2013. Median nerve entrapment syndromes. *Upper Extremity Focal Neuropathies*: 7-9. Available at: https://webportal.aanem.org/Resources/Files/Downloads/products/13CB.pdf#page=7.

Sanders, T.L., Kremers, H.M., Bryan, A.J., Ransom, J.E., Smith, J., and Morrey, B.F. 2015. The epidemiology and health care burden of tennis elbow: A population-based study. *The American Journal of Sports Medicine*, February, 0363546514568087. doi:10.1177/0363546514568087.

Scott, A., Docking, S., Vicenzino, B., Alfredson, H., Zwerver, J., Lundgreen. K., Finlay, O., et al. 2013. Sports and exercise-related tendinopathies: A review of selected topical issues by participants of the Second International Scientific Tendinopathy Symposium (ISTS), Vancouver 2012. *British Journal of Sports Medicine*, doi:10.1136/bjsports-2013-092329.

Shanley, E., Rauh, M.J., Michener, L.A., Ellenbecker, T.S., Garrison, J.C., and Thigpen, C.A. 2011. Shoulder range of motion measures as risk factors for shoulder and elbow injuries in high school softball and baseball players. *The American Journal of Sports Medicine* 39 (9): 1997–2006.

Shiri, R., and Viikari-Juntura, E. 2011. Lateral and medial epicondylitis: Role of occupational factors. *Best Practice & Research Clinical Rheumatology* 25 (1): 43–57.

Tyler, T.F., Nicholas, S.J., Schmitt, B.M., Mullaney, M., and Hogan, D.E. 2014. Clinical outcomes of the addition of eccentrics for rehabilitation of previously failed treatments of golfers elbow. *International Journal of Sports Physical Therapy* 9 (3): 365–370.

Ulrich, D., Piatkowski, A., and Pallua, N. 2011. Anterior interosseous nerve syndrome: A retrospective analysis of 14 patients. *Archives of Orthopaedic and Trauma Surgery* 131 (11): 1561–1565.

Wong, C.K., Moskovitz, N., and Fabillar, R. 2011. The effect of strain counterstrain (SCS) on forearm strength compared to sham positioning. *International Journal of Osteopathic Medicine* 14 (3): 86–95.

Chapter 11

Brown, J.S., Wheeler, P.C., Boyd, K.T., Barnes, M.R., and Allen, M.J. 2011. Chronic exertional compartment syndrome of the forearm: A case series of 12 patients treated with fasciotomy. *Journal of Hand Surgery* (European volume) 36 (5): 413–419.

Campbell, C.S. 1955. Gamekeeper's thumb. *Journal of Bone & Joint Surgery* (British volume) 37 (1): 148–149.

Collins, C.K. 2007. Physical therapy management of complex regional pain syndrome in a 14-year-old patient using strain counterstrain: A case report. *Journal of Manual & Manipulative Therapy* 15 (1): 25–41.

De Putter, C.E., Selles, R.W., Polinder, S., Panneman, M.J.M., Hovius, S.E.R., and van Beeck, E.F. 2012. Economic impact of hand and wrist injuries: Health-care costs and productivity costs in a population-based study. *The Journal of Bone & Joint Surgery* 94 (9): e56.

Fry, W.R., Wade, M.D., Smith, R.S., and Asensio-Gonzales, J.A. 2013. Extremity compartment syndrome and fasciotomy: A literature review. *European Journal of Trauma and Emergency Surgery* 39 (6): 561–567.

Gerwin, R.D, Dommerholt, J., and Shah, J.P. 2004. An expansion of Simons' integrated hypothesis of trigger point formation. *Current Pain and Headache Reports* 8 (6): 468–475.

Ghasemi-rad, M., Nosair, E., Vegh, A., Mohammadi, A., Akkad, A., Lesha, E., Mohammadi, M.H., et al. 2014. A handy review of carpal tunnel syndrome: From anatomy to diagnosis and treatment. *World Journal of Radiology* 6 (6): 284–300. doi:10.4329/wjr.v6.i6.284.

Koplay, M., Sivri, M., Kutahya, H., Erdogan, H., and Goncu, R.G. 2014. Gamekeeper's thumb: MR imaging findings. *Journal of Medical Diagnostics Methods* 2: 147.

Mahajan, M, and Rhemrev, S.J. 2013. Rupture of the ulnar collateral ligament of the thumb: A review. *International Journal of Emergency Medicine* 6 (1): 1–6.

Moseley, G. Lorimer, R.D., Herbert, T.P., Lucas, S., Van Hilten, J.J., and Marinus, J. 2014. Intense pain soon after wrist fracture strongly predicts who will develop complex regional pain syndrome: A prospective cohort study. *The Journal of Pain* 15 (1): 16–23.

Navalho, M., Resende, C., Rodrigues, A.M., Ramos, F., Gaspar, A., Pereira da Silva, J.A., Fonseca, J.E., Campos, J., and Canhão, H. 2012. Bilateral MR imaging of the hand and wrist in early and very early inflammatory arthritis: Tenosynovitis is associated with progression to rheumatoid arthritis. *Radiology* 264 (3): 823–833. doi:10.1148/radiol.12112513.

Ogawa, T., Tanaka, T., Yanai, T., Kumagai, H., and Ochiai, H. 2013. Analysis of soft tissue injuries associated with distal radius fractures. *BMC Sports Science, Medicine and Rehabilitation* 5 (1): 19.

Ootes, D., Lambers, K.T., and Ring, D.C. 2012. The epidemiology of upper extremity injuries presenting to the emergency department in the United States. *Hand* 7 (1): 18–22.

Patel, K., Kashyap, R., Tadisina, K., and Gonzalez, M.H. 2013. De Quervain's Disease. *Eplasty* 13. Available at: http://www.eplasty.com/index.php?option=com_content&view=article&id=982&catid=49

Patel, S., Potty, A., Taylor, E.J., and Sorene, E.D. 2010. Collateral ligament injuries of the metacarpophalangeal joint of the thumb: A treatment algorithm. *Strategies in Trauma and Limb Reconstruction* 5 (1): 1–10.

Schaefer, P.T., and Speier, J. 2012. Common medical problems of instrumental athletes. *Current Sports Medicine Reports* 11 (6): 316–322.

Sharan, D., and Ajeesh, P.S. 2012. Risk factors and clinical features of text message injuries. *Work: A Journal of Prevention, Assessment and Rehabilitation* 41: 1145–1148.

Siu, G., Jaffe, J.D., Rafique, M., and Weinik, M.K. 2012. Osteopathic manipulative medicine for carpal tunnel syndrome. *The Journal of the American Osteopathic Association* 112 (3): 127–139.

Speicher, T.E., and Draper, D.O. 2006. Top 10 positional-release therapy techniques to break the chain of pain—Part 1. *Athletic Therapy Today* 11 (5): 60–62.

Sytema, R., Dekker, R., Dijkstra, P.U., ten Duis, H.J., and van der Sluis, C.K. 2010. Upper extremity sports injury: Risk factors in comparison to lower extremity injury in more than 25,000 cases. *Clinical Journal of Sport Medicine* 20 (4): 256–263.

Villafañe, J.H., Cleland, J.A., and Fernandez-De-Las-Peñas, C. 2013. The effectiveness of a manual therapy and exercise protocol in patients with thumb carpometacarpal osteoarthritis: A randomized controlled trial. *Journal of Orthopaedic & Sports Physical Therapy* 43 (4): 204–213.

Werner, B.C., Hadeed, M.M., Lyons, M.L., Diduch, D.R., and Chhabra, A.B. 2014. Return to play and long-term clinical outcomes after suture anchor repair of thumb ulnar collateral ligament injuries in collegiate football athletes. *Orthopaedic Journal of Sports Medicine* 2 (2 Suppl.): 1-2.

Chapter 12

Abraham, V.C., Richmond, F.J.R., and Rose, P.K. 1975. Absence of monosynaptic reflex in dorsal neck muscle of the cat. *Brain Research* 92: 130–131.

Alsalaheen, B.A., Mucha, A., Morris, L.O., Witney, S.L., Furman, J.M., Camiolo-Reddy, C.E.,

Collins, M.W., Lovell, M.R., and Sparto, P.J. 2010. Vestibular rehabilitation for dizziness and balance disorders after concussion. *Journal of Neurologic Physical Therapy* 4: 87–93.

Baron, E.P., Cherian, N., and Tepper, S.J. 2011. Role of the greater occipital nerve block and trigger point injections for patients with dizziness and headache. *Neurologist* 17 (6): 312–317.

Becker, R.F. 1977. Cranial therapy revisited. *Osteopathic Annals* 5 (7): 13–40.

Bell, W.E. 1985. *Orofacial pain: Classification, diagnosis, management* (3rd ed.). Chicago: New Year Medical.

Biondi, D.M. 2005. Cervicogenic headache: Mechanism, evaluation and treatment strategies. *Journal of the American Osteopathic Association* 105 (Suppl. 2): 16S–22S.

Bogduk, N. 1998. Innervation and pain patterns of the cervical spine. In *Physical therapy of the cervical and thoracic spine*, ed. R. Grant. New York: Churchill Livingstone.

Bovin, G., Berg, R., and Dale, L.G. 1992. Cervicogenic headache: Anesthetic blockade of cervical nerves (C2-C5) and facet joints (C2-C3). *Pain* 49: 315–322.

Castenada, R. 1991. Occlusion. In *Temporomandibular disorders, diagnosis and treatment*, ed. A.S. Kaplan and L.A. Assael. Philadelphia: Saunders.

Chaitow, L. 1999. *Cranial manipulation therapy, theory and practice: Osseous and soft tissue approaches.* New York: Churchill Livingstone.

Cohen, M.J., and McArthur, D.L. 1981. Classification of migraine and tension headache from a survey of 10,000 headache diaries. *Headache* 21: 25–92.

D'Ambrogio, K.J., and Roth, G.B. 1997. *Positional release therapy: Assessment and treatment of musculoskeletal dysfunction.* St. Louis, MO: Mosby.

DeJarnette, M.B. 1975. *SacroOccipital Technique.* Rose Ertler Memorial DeJarnette Library, Chicago, IL.

DeJarnette, M.B. 1976. *SacroOccipital Technique.* Rose Ertler Memorial DeJarnette Library, Chicago, IL.

DeJarnette, M.B. 1977. *SacroOccipital Technique.* Rose Ertler Memorial DeJarnette Library, Chicago, IL.

DeJarnette, M.B. 1978. *SacroOccipital Technique.* Rose Ertler Memorial DeJarnette Library, Chicago, IL.

Dimitroulis. G. 1998. Temporomandibular disorders: A clinical update. *British Medical Journal* 317: 190–194.

Dreyfus, P., Michaelson, M., and Fletcher, A. 1994. Atlanto-occipital and lateral atlanto-axial joint pain patterns. *Spine* 19: 1125–1131.

Dutton, M. 2004. *Orthopedic examination, evaluation and intervention.* New York: McGraw-Hill.

Dworkin, S.F., et al. 1990. Epidemiology of signs and symptoms in temporomandibular disorders, clinical cases and controls. *Journal of the American Dental Association* 120: 273–281.

Ehni, G.E., and Benner, B. 1984. Occipital neuralgia and the C1 and C2 arthrosis syndrome. *Journal of Neurosurgery* 61: 961–965.

Fredrikson, T.A., Hovdal, H., and Sjaastad, O. 1987. Cervicogenic headache: Clinical manifestation. *Cephalalgia* 7: 147–160.

Friedman, M.H., and Nelson, R.J. Jr. 1996. Head and neck pain review: Traditional and new perspectives. *Journal of Orthopedic Sports Physical Therapy* 24 (4): 268–278.

Gelb, H.C., ed. 1977. *Clinical management of head, neck and temporomandibular pain: A multidisciplinary approach to diagnosis and treatment.* Philadelphia: Saunders.

Gladstone, J. 2009. From psychoneurosis to ICHD-2: An overview of the state of the art in post-traumatic headache. *Headache* 49 (7): 1097-1111.

Greenman, P.E. 2003. *Principles of manual medicine* (3rd ed.). Philadelphia: Lippincott Williams & Wilkins.

Greenwald, B.D., Kapoor, N., and Singh, A.D. 2012. Visual impairments in first year after traumatic brain injury. *Brain Injury* 26 (11): 1–22.

Griesbach, G.S., Houda, D.A., and Gomez-Pinella, F. 2009. Exercise induced improvements in cognitive performance after traumatic brain injury in rats is dependent on BDNF activation. *Brain Research* 1288: 105–115.

Headache Classification Committee of the International Headache Society. 1998. Classification and diagnostic criteria for headache disorders, cranial neuralgia and facial pain. *Cephalalgia* 7 (Suppl.): 1–551.

Herring, S.A., Canto, R.C., Guskiewicz, K., Putokiam, M., and Kibler, W.B. 2011. Concussion (mild traumatic brain injury) and the team physician: A consensus statement. 2011 update. *Medicine & Science in Sports & Exercise* 43 (12): 2412–2422.

Hunter, C.R., and Mayfield, F.H. 1949. Role of the upper cervical roots in the production of pain in the head. *American Journal of Surgery* 48: 743–751.

International Headache Society. 1988. Headache classification and diagnostic criteria for headache disorders, cranial neuralgias and facial pain. *Cephalalgia*, 8 (19–22): 71–72.

Janda, V. 1994. Muscles and motor control in cervicogenic disorders: Assessment and management. In *Physical therapy of the cervical and thoracic spine*, ed. R. Grant. New York: Churchill Livingstone.

Jones, L.H., Kusunose, R.S., and Goering, E.K. 1995. *Jones strain-counterstrain*. Boise, ID: Jones Strain-CounterStrain, Inc.

Kerr, F.W.L., and Olafsson, R.A. 1961. Trigeminal cervical volleys: Converging on single units in spinal grey at C1-C2. *Archives of Neurology* 5: 171–178.

Koren, T. 2006. The sphenoid pattern. *The American Chiropractor*: 26–30.

Kozlowski, K.F., Graham, J., Leddy, J.J., Divinney-Boymel, L., and Willer, B.S. 2013. Exercise intolerance in individuals with postconcussion syndrome. *Journal of Athletic Training* 48 (5): 627–635.

Kraus, S.L. 1994. *Temporomandibular disorders* (2nd ed.). New York: Churchill Livingstone.

McNeill, C. 1991. Temporomandibular disorders: Guidelines for diagnosis and management. *Journal of the California Dental Association* 19: 15–26.

Moore, K.I. 1985. *Clinically oriented anatomy* (2nd ed.). Baltimore: Williams & Wilkins.

Nicholson, G.G., and Gaston, J. 2001. Cervical headache. *Journal of Orthopedic Sports Physical Therapy* 31: 184–193.

Ochi, K., Ohashi, T., and Kinoshita, H. 2002. Acoustic tenser tympani response and vestibular evoked myogenic potentials. *Laryngoscope* 112: 2225–2229.

Reddy, C.C. 2011. Postconcussion syndrome: A psyiatrist's approach. *Physical Medicine and Rehabilitation* 3 (1052): S397.

Rocabado, M., and Iglarsh, Z.A. 1991. *Musculoskeletal approach to maxillofacial pain*. Philadelphia: Lippincott.

Salonen, L., and Hellden, L. 1990. Prevalence of signs and symptoms of dysfunction in masticatory system: An epidemiological study in an adult Swedish population. *Journal of Craniomandibular Disorders and Facial Oral Pain* 4: 241–250.

Selassie, A.W., Dulaney, A.W., Pickelsier, E.E., Voronca, D.C., Williams, N.R., and Edwards, J.C. 2013. Incidence of sports related traumatic brain injury and risk factors of severity: A population based study. *Annals of Epidemiology* 23 (12): 1–7.

Sharmann, S.A. 2001. *Diagnosis and treatment of movement impairment syndromes*. St Louis, MO: Mosby.

Simons, D.G., Travell, J.G., and Simons, L.S. 1999. *Travell and Simons' myofascial pain and dysfunction: Upper half of body*. Vol. 1. Baltimore: Lippincott Williams & Wilkins.

Stirimpakos, N. 2011. The assessment of the cervical spine, part 2: Strength and endurance/fatigue. *Journal of Bodywork and Movement Therapies*. 15 (4): 417–430.

Stohler, C.S. 1995. Clinical perspectives on masticatory and related muscle disorders. In *Temporomandibular disorders and related pain conditions: Progress in pain research and management*, ed. B.J. Sessle, P.S. Bryant, and R.A. Dionne. Seattle, WA: ISAP Press.

Sutherland, W.G. 1939. *The cranial bowl*. Mankato, MN: Free Press.

Treleaven, J. 2008. Sensorimotor disturbances in neck disorders affecting postural stability, head and eye movement control. *Manual Therapy* 13 (1): 2–11.

Upledger, J.E., and Vredevoogd, J.D. 1983. *Craniosacral therapy*. Seattle, WA: Eastland Press.

Warwick, R., and Williams, P.L. 1973. *Gray's anatomy, 35th British ed*. Philadelphia: W.B. Saunders Co.

Weightman, M.M., Bolgla, R., McCulloch, K.L., and Peterson, M.D. 2010. Physical therapy recommendations for service members with mild traumatic brain injury. *Journal of Head Trauma Rehabilitation* 25 (3): 206–218.

Willer, B., and Leddy, J.J. 2006. Management of concussion and postconcussion syndrome: Current treatment options. *Neurology* 8: 415–426.

Wilson, P.R. 1991. Chronic neck pain and cervicogenic headache. *Clinical Journal of Pain* 7 (1): 5–11.

INDEX

Timothy E. Speicher, PhD, ATC, LAT, CSCS, is president of the Positional Release Therapy Institute. He is considered a leading expert in positional release therapy (PRT). Speicher discovered and developed the fasciculatory response method (FRM), which has revolutionized the way PRT is applied, practiced, and taught. He established the Positional Release Therapy Institute to provide education on the FRM and PRT through the institute's courses while allowing for its application to a patient population at the institute in Ogden, Utah.

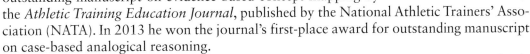

Speicher frequently speaks on PRT to professional organizations and at conferences, and his research has been published in academic journals. In 2014 he received the first-place award for outstanding manuscript on evidence-based concept mapping by the *Athletic Training Education Journal*, published by the National Athletic Trainers' Association (NATA). In 2013 he won the journal's first-place award for outstanding manuscript on case-based analogical reasoning.

Speicher, who has held several faculty and research appointments at various academic institutions, is a member of the NATA and was on the board of directors of NATA Research & Education Foundation. Currently, Speicher holds two faculty appointments: affiliate faculty for the University of Idaho, where he teaches neuroscience for the master's degree in athletic training program, and assistant professor at Rocky Mountain University of Health Professions, where he provides instruction in evidence-based medicine for the doctorate in health science.

About the Contributor

Regis Turocy, DHCE, MPT, PRT-c, received a bachelor of science degree from West Virginia University, a certificate in physical therapy from the University of Pittsburgh, a master of science degree in orthopedic physical therapy from the University of Pittsburgh, a master of arts in health care ethics from Duquesne University, and a doctorate in health care ethics from Duquesne University. Dr. Turocy has extensive experience in orthopedic physical therapy and alternative care approaches to physical therapy. He has taught orthopedic manual therapy, electrotherapeutic modalities, health care ethics, and complementary approaches to health care. Dr. Turocy has provided numerous educational presentations at the local, district, regional, state, and national levels, emphasizing the clinical use of positional release, neural tension, and muscle energy techniques. He is engaged in clinical practice through the treatment of patients at Catholic Charities Free Health Care Clinic in Pittsburgh.

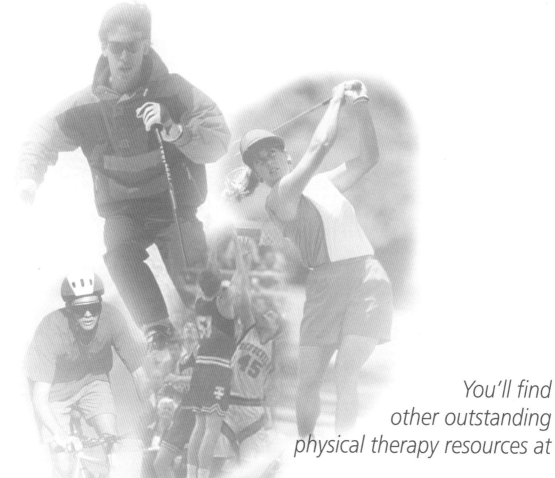